Medicine at Michigan

Medicine at Michigan

A History of the University of Michigan Medical School at the Bicentennial

Dea H. Boster and Joel D. Howell

University of Michigan Press
Ann Arbor

Published in the United States of America by
the University of Michigan Press

Manufactured in the United States of America

♾ Printed on acid-free paper

2020 2019 2018 2017 4 3 2 1

A CIP catalog record for this book is available from the British Library.

ISBN 978-0-472-13061-0 (hardcover : alk. paper)
ISBN 978-0-472-12342-1 (e-book)

Contents

Foreword

This year, we are celebrating the two-hundred-year anniversary of the founding of the University of Michigan in 1817. The university has achieved countless achievements and milestones since its beginnings, one of those being the creation of the University of Michigan Medical School, today a top-ranked institution in the United States. Upon opening its doors in 1850, the Department of Medicine and Surgery became the university's first professional school. The first class of students paid five dollars per year for a two-year education. Since those early days, the University of Michigan Medical School has graduated almost fifteen thousand students and trained even more residents and fellows, and it is now recognized as one of America's great medical schools.

In this book, Dea Boster and Joel Howell recount the rich history of the medical school. This includes some of the major distinctions that reflect the leadership and innovation we have contributed to medical practice in the nation. Michigan was the first university to own and operate its own university hospital, which was created to serve the needs of the medical students and the university. We were also an early major medical school to admit women, graduating our first female physician, Amanda Sanford, in 1871. The next year, W. Henry Fitzbutler, the son of a slave, became the first recognized African American graduate of the program. And we were one of the few early schools to incorporate science and the idea of changing knowledge as core elements of education.

Boster and Howell cover such notable historical episodes, but they also delve into hard times and less flattering episodes, many of which led to changes that today define the school. Drawing on extensive archival research as well as on published primary and secondary sources, this is the first book to frame the history of the medical school in a broad social context. The main focus of this book is on the core medical education of students at Michigan that has existed since its founding. Boster and Howell consider the question of why this major institution came into existence in the small, Midwestern town of Ann Arbor, and why it has stayed here. They examine the close relationships of the medical school with the university, the local community, and the broader society at large. As we look toward the future, this book reminds us that the school has always been changing and will continue to change in ways that none of us can predict. We draw inspiration from looking at the medical school's milestones and achievements despite past challenges.

As dean of the University of Michigan Medical School, I am extremely proud to be leading this educational institution into the future to better serve all of our students and trainees.

I hope you will enjoy learning about the path we took to get here.

Marschall S. Runge, M.D., Ph.D.
Dean, University of Michigan Medical School
Executive Vice President for Medical Affairs,
University of Michigan
CEO, Michigan Medicine

Acknowledgments

The authors are grateful for the support of many talented individuals who have contributed to this work. In particular, Terrence J. McDonald, Malgosia Myc, and the rest of the staff at the University of Michigan's Bentley Historical Library have provided invaluable assistance for archival visits, requests, and queries over several years. The administrators and staff members at the University of Michigan Medical School have been enthusiastic about the project from its inception, and we thank them for their contributions and support. We thank James Woolliscroft, then dean of the medical school, for suggesting that we write this book to be part of the bicentennial celebration. The work has also benefited from conversations and input from a variety of our colleagues—including Bruce Fye, Susan Lawrence, Kenneth Ludmerer, Martin Pernick, Alexandra Stern, and John Harley Warner—and many others who expressed their excitement and interest in our work. We also thank the editorial staff at the University of Michigan Press, particularly Scott Ham and Danielle Coty, for their guidance and patience, and the anonymous peer reviewers whose thoughtful feedback helped direct the book to its fruition.

Introduction

Michigan's Medical School

In 2017 the University of Michigan celebrated its bicentennial. The celebration offered an opportunity to reflect on the history of the institution, to consider what has happened in the centuries since its founding, and to think about how history can help us contemplate what lies ahead. This book offers a brief history of one part of the university, the medical school. From its beginning as a department with one building and five faculty members, the medical school has become home to thousands of faculty members and dozens of buildings. But despite the huge difference in scale (and much else), some constants remain. Just as they did in 1850, entering medical students come to Ann Arbor hoping to become exceptional physicians. Since 1850 some consistent questions have confronted the school, such as which students to admit, what those students should study, where they should study, and what ought to be the relationship of the medical school with the larger university. But this history does not limit itself to the medical school or even to the university. When University of Michigan president Harlan Hatcher marked the university's sesquicentennial in 1967, he noted, "The student of social history soon discovers that social institutions both influence and are influenced by the society of which they are a part. . . . [C]ertainly this is true of the Medical School of the University of Michigan."[1] Fifty years later, Hatcher's words remind us of the importance of community connections in an institution's history. The university and its medical school have always had a deep and complex relationship with the town of Ann Arbor and the people of Michigan, one that has shaped the development of this remarkable institution and its educational mission since it was founded.

In writing this history, we have been aided by medical historian Kenneth Ludmerer's synthetic analysis of the history of medical education. He has shown that many medical schools founded in the nineteenth-century United States were proprietary and wholly didactic, but a number of changes—the rise of university systems, the influence of European laboratory and scientific practices, new state and federal regulatory structures, and the philanthropy of wealthy industrialists—began to transform medical education and practice by the onset of the twentieth century.[2] Much of this description applies to the University of Michigan. Many historians have written histories of specific medical schools, each with its own conceptual model of how to approach such a task.[3] We have attempted to learn from these earlier works and to take an approach that reflects not only larger national trends but also the specific circumstances surrounding the experience at Michigan. We have tried to remain aware of the choices, disputes, and failures that informed medical decision making and the development of knowledge and practice in the hospital, laboratory, and classroom to understand how medicine and medical education changed within specific social and cultural contexts. Local communities in particular are vital for understanding health and illness, patient experiences and expectations for treatment and expertise, professional identities and reputations, political support for institutional advancement, and the growth of the medical field.[4]

The local community has played a particularly important role in the history of the University of Michigan Medical School, given its location in a small Midwestern town. Ann Arbor offered important, tangible support to the early school, and many of Michigan's medical faculty have had significant ties with the local community: as private practitioners who cared for Ann Arbor residents, as public health advocates (both locally and nationally), as politicians, and as entrepreneurs. The medical school has always been part of a state university, which introduces a set of dynamics somewhat different from those that existed for other, private schools. All of these relationships have affected the decisions made at Ann Arbor's medical school—regarding professional identities, student admissions, curricula, budgeting, hiring and firing, clinical instruction, and hospital facilities and renovations—and those decisions have not always followed what might seem like a "logical" progression. They have been influenced by a variety of specific political, social, and cultural factors, all of which are part of the historical fabric.

The University of Michigan Medical School provides fertile ground for such a contextual history. Reuben Peterson, an early-twentieth-century faculty member in obstetrics and gynecology, as well as an amateur historian, remarked perceptively that the Michigan medical school, a new department of a new state university in a "new" part of the country, did not "flow on gently from year to year"; instead, it had to set precedents for administrative, pedagogical, and clinical policies in a young, Midwestern state.[5] The precedents resulted from a specific historical context, and many had national significance: Michigan was one of the first major U.S. medical schools to adopt a four-year curriculum, was the first to own and operate its own university hospital, and became a pioneer for both laboratory instruction and clinical clerkships. It is often considered to be the first major university medical school in the United States to regularly admit women and one of the first to recognize the value of and support clinical research. Its instructors were among the earliest American medical professors to become full-time university faculty members.[6] Sinclair Lewis's *Arrowsmith*, one of the first American novels that focused on cultures of science, was inspired by alumnus Paul de Kruif's experiences at the school and in Ann Arbor.[7] While many graduates of the school have gone on to distinguished careers, the school has also experienced its share of public controversies, such as its association with the controversial Jack Kevorkian, who graduated from the program and completed two years of a pathology residency at Michigan.[8]

The school has a rich history of interdisciplinary collaborations with other branches of the university, as well as community outreach and education initiatives for both health-care providers and patients. It has relied on Michigan citizens to present themselves as research subjects or teaching patients. Historians and physicians have lauded Michigan's notable achievements in education and research, as well as its "long tradition of service to all of the state's residents."[9] In a 2000 article in the *Journal of the American Medical Association* commemorating the school's sesquicentennial anniversary, faculty physician and medical historian Howard Markel described Michigan as "an example worthy of imitation" and highlighted the school's transition from "frontier medical outpost" to a frontrunner of modern medical education and research. Horace Davenport, a Michigan faculty member and chair of the physiology department for many years, published the most comprehensive history of the medical school to date (in addition to his other books on medical school professor George Dock and specific departments within the school) and identified the institution as "not just any medical school."[10]

Because the University of Michigan Medical School is a complex and long-lived institution, any attempt to write a history must necessarily be limited in scope. We have not attempted to balance our coverage of individual departments. It would be impossible to devote equal weight to all the departments that have existed or currently exist, particularly since they have not all played steady roles in the changing medical school. Readers wishing to read more about a specific topic or department will find guidance in the "Note on Sources" section below.

In writing this history we emphasize the medical school's position as a national forerunner of modern medical education (in both clinical instruction and academic medicine) but at the same time maintain a focus on the complex relationships between the school and its social and physical location. Ann Arbor, for many years, seemed an unlikely place to build a modern medical institution, and ongoing concerns about Michigan's reputation as a leader of medical education played a significant role in the development of the school's curriculum, physical plant, patient base, and student populations. Appreciating this connection allows us to ask more questions about the people who came to the school as faculty members, students, and patients: Where did they come from, and why did they come to Ann Arbor? What social interactions and controversies in Michigan have helped shape the policies, practices, and missions of the school? Rather than chronicling the school's milestones from an exclusively academic or professional perspective, this book seeks to investigate the medical school's position (both physical and social) within a larger community.[11]

Michigan's evolution from a small, rural medical school to a large, modern medical complex did not follow a straight, upward trajectory. The social, political, and cultural landscapes of Michigan both supported and challenged the school in significant ways. Conflicts with the state's medical sectarian organizations (particularly homeopaths), concerns about the ability to train doctors in a small town rather than an urban center like Detroit, proximity (physical and administrative) to other departments within the university, and "selling" the germ theory of disease to Michigan's practitioners and public were among the major issues that influenced the medical school's growth and progress during its earliest decades. However, even after such conflicts had ebbed and Michigan had earned its national reputation as a top-ranking medical school, the institution still had to contend with a number of pressures: economic support for research and construction, changing politics and populations in the state of Michigan, and expectations of faculty, students, patients, and supporting communities. The conflict between private practice and academic interests, different opinions about premedical requirements and the medical curriculum, patient fees at the University Hospital, debates over affiliations with other hospitals, and controversies over academic subject matter were all issues that arose numerous times over the past 150 years. We hope that this broad glimpse into the history of the University of Michigan Medical School will contribute to a deeper understanding of the social and cultural forces that have shaped, and continue to shape, medical education and the profession in Michigan and the United States.

Note on Terminology

In this book we discuss the development of the University of Michigan Medical School from its 1837 inception as the Department of Medicine and Surgery until the twenty-first century. We need to make our terminology clear. In the interests of clarity, and because our intended audience is not only professional historians but also medical school students, faculty, staff, alumni, and the general public, we have made a slight change in the terms used to describe the school. In 1837, the medical branch was officially designated the Department of Medicine and Surgery at the University of Michigan and was often referred to as the "Medical Department" well into the twentieth century. At the same time, it was occasionally referred to as the "medical school." Moreover, some units, such as surgery, pediatrics, and obstetrics and gynecology, were also referred to as "departments" (as were departments no longer in existence, such as the Department of the Theory and Practice of Medicine). The variable usage of terminology attracted criticism from national organizations such as the Carnegie Foundation for the Advancement of Teaching. Thus, in 1915 the Board of Regents attempted to remedy what they termed "the ugly and troublesome inconsistency and confusion" associated with existing terminology and recommended that the school simply be called the "Medical School."[12] We follow their lead. Rather than using a variety of terms to describe the administrative unit over the course of the book, for the sake of clarity, except when part of a direct quotation, we usually refer to the institution as "the medical school."

Note on Sources

The collections of the University of Michigan's Bentley Historical Library have been indispensable for this project. Not only does the library maintain official medical school and hospital administrative records, but it also houses the papers of many individual professors, deans, and university regents. Faculty meeting minutes, correspondence, annual reports, promotional materials, speech drafts, and a variety of other types of evidence have provided useful glimpses from different perspectives of the medical school's development. The library's collection of books and journals—a collection initiated by the prescient nineteenth-century decision of Victor Vaughan to subscribe to every major medical journal—has also been extremely valuable. In addition, the medical school kept files on individual students and their organizations, including journals, correspondence with faculty members, and publications, which enabled us to analyze and give historical context to medical student experiences at Michigan from the mid-nineteenth century until the present. A number of digitized sources—Board of Regents proceedings and the university's *University of Michigan: An Encyclopedic Survey, Bicentennial Edition*—have also been very helpful. Visual sources (maps, photographs, and building plans) provide a useful record for changes in the physical growth of the school and University Hospital and developments in its spatial relation to the rest of the university and the town of Ann Arbor.

We also examined a variety of sources from outside the university, particularly articles and editorials published in local newspapers (most of which have been archived by the Ann Arbor District Library). Public opinion about the medical school and its faculty and general ideas about health and disease illuminate significant connections between the medical school and the "lay" community that are not always clear in the institutional archive. From the late nineteenth century to the early twenty-first, local newspaper reporting took a strong interest in the medical school's curriculum, particularly cadaver use in gross anatomy instruction, major events and traditions like graduations and Match Day ceremonies, leadership changes, and (of course) scandals.

We have benefited from several published departmental histories. In addition, the university has taken the initiative to update its entries for the *Encyclopedic Survey* as part of the university's 2017 bicentennial celebration. The Bentley Historical Library administers this Faculty History Project, and those digitized survey updates that departments have completed (currently unpublished but soon to be added to the *Survey*'s website) have been useful for our research into the school's more recent history. We decided not to include oral histories of former or current medical school faculty members, mainly for pragmatic reasons. The school's faculty and staff have grown so large that it would be impractical to schedule and record a representative number of interviews, and interests of privacy would complicate our records and citations.[13] In that interest, we have also chosen to eliminate the names of students and patients of the University Hospital and its clinics, unless those names were included in published sources. We seek to use this primary evidence to illuminate significant historical trends and themes and, we hope, inspire future scholars to investigate elements of the medical school's fascinating story.

ONE

Beginnings

The Development of the Medical School

The University of Michigan was first conceived of as the "Catholepistemiad," or "University of Michigania," in 1817, before the state of Michigan even existed. The Catholepistemiad was more than what we now think of as a university. It was intended to offer a coordinated system of education spread throughout the Territory of Michigan, based on thirteen *didaxiim*, or professorships, of which one was to be in the medical sciences. A building for this new institution was begun in Detroit. In 1821 it was renamed the University of Michigan, and education continued in this building (mostly at a primary-school level) only for another six years.

When Michigan became a state in 1837, one of the first things the new legislature did was to pass an act establishing the University of Michigan. The legislature specified that the university was to consist of at least three departments, one of which was to be a "Department of Medicine." By including medicine as one of three elements of this new university—the other two were the liberal arts college and the law school—lawmakers made medical education a clear priority. Given the many other needs of a new, rural, western state, that decision to prioritize medical education for the very young state was remarkable, if not prescient. A state university, the University of Michigan was unusual for its time in lacking any religious affiliation.[1] Its governance structure also allowed for important elements of academic freedom. Since 1837 the university has reported not to the state legislature but to a Board of Regents, which has been an elected body since 1850. That did not, however, completely prevent the legislature from dictating what would be taught, even only a few decades later.

Also in 1837 the university was moved from Detroit to Ann Arbor, about forty-five miles to the west and the seat of Washtenaw County. The fact that the university moved to, and remained in, Ann Arbor has played an important role in the history of the institution. As we discuss, the location not only offered a hospitable environment but also provided very tangible support at key moments. Founded in 1824, Ann Arbor had become a small town of around two thousand residents, one with considerable civic pride and planning. The city street names paid tribute to members of its cofounder John Allen's family (particularly his daughters, Ann and Catherine) as well as patriotic heroes of the young United States (Washington, Jefferson, Madison, and Monroe). Within the town's first decade, several churches, mills, factories, and banks had opened, and quite a few German immigrant families had settled there. Local newspapers, like the *Ann Arbor Argus*, had begun printing by the 1830s, and other periodicals were established by mid-century; in 1847, the town's first telegraph line was extended from Detroit. Yet Ann Arbor was close enough to the frontier that Native Americans visited the town and patronized its businesses during the first half of the nineteenth century. The University of Michigan quickly became the focal point of the Ann Arbor community, and its presence was to be one of the most significant factors in the town's physical and economic growth. The first seven students arrived at the university in 1841.[2]

However, despite petitions from local physicians about the need for such an institution, it took almost another decade for the medical school to be realized. Construction difficulties certainly contributed to the delay. Although the facility was supposed to open in 1849, the original three-story medical building was not completed until the autumn of 1850. The sandstone Greek Revival structure—"by far the handsomest on campus"—included a dramatic portico at the entrance, bordered by brick columns with cast-iron capitals. As physiology professor and historian Horace Davenport describes it, the first medical school was located on a dirt road on the eastern side of the forty-acre university pasture, in a building with "lecture rooms required by the curriculum, offices for the five professors, a small chemical laboratory, . . . a room under a dome on the roof dedicated to anatomical dissections," and no clinical facilities.[3]

But before describing this fledgling medical school, it is worthwhile to consider the state of general medical education in the United States in the middle of the nineteenth century. The medical profession at that time was not as prestigious, structured, or lucrative as it would later become. Many "doctors," particularly in rural areas, could not support themselves and their families through medical practice alone and so earned their subsistence through farming, pharmacy, or another form of business.[4] Physicians also had a widespread reputation for various forms of debauchery, in particular excessive drinking; as Michigan physician J. H. Beech noted somewhat bitterly in 1858, any "Bacchanalian ring has long been considered incomplete, unless Dr. SOMEBODY was there; and it would be well for us to lose such unenviable notoriety."[5] Given such opinions, physicians at that time were conscious of the need to present an image of "propriety and respectability" to assert their professional authority, however precarious.[6]

One reason for the lack of respect for the profession was that medical education in the United States was sparse and unregulated. By 1850, there were forty-two medical schools in the nation, and many of those had been operating for only a few years. A number of the newer schools were founded in rural, "western" regions and operated on small budgets, most of which were derived from students' tuition. The reliance on tuition at such proprietary schools created a pronounced disincentive for those schools to adopt strict (or any) standards. For example, at Castleton Medical School in Vermont—where Abram Sager, the first dean at Michigan's medical school, received his training—students who paid for their diplomas never failed their examinations. The curriculum (to the extent that there was one) varied widely from school to school, unconstrained by state requirements for licensure. Unsurprisingly, many schools churned out large numbers of "physicians" with minimal education and dubious skills.[7]

But there was another equally legitimate (and perhaps even more popular) path to becoming a physician. Instead of attending a formal medical school, many mid-nineteenth-century practitioners, especially in rural areas, received their training through apprenticeships with practicing physicians. It was typical for an aspiring physician to work with a more experienced preceptor for several years, often living in the preceptor's household and providing assistance in the quotidian care of patients. The quality of such training varied widely, being a function of the expertise of the supervising physician and his interest in teaching. The education also depended on the diseases that were prevalent. A student could learn a great deal about the care of a common disease, but if a disease happened not to occur in the supervisor's practice during the preceptorship, the student would learn little about it. Before the medical school at the University of Michigan was founded, the state's more adventurous apprentices supplemented their practical instruction by traveling to schools in the East for didactic lectures, or even for an M.D. degree. Others stayed closer to home and received anatomy instruction in informal student groups that met in physicians' offices or basements. Some, for instance, witnessed dissections upon local indigent or unclaimed cadavers, including corpses exhumed from Detroit's potter's field (a cemetery for the destitute to be buried at public expense) and at least one veteran of the Mexican War.[8] Members of the medical profession certainly were aware of the problems surrounding medical education and had taken steps to reform and improve the training of doctors. The American Medical Association (AMA), founded in 1847, spearheaded curricular reform as well as attempts to standardize licensing and medical ethics.

From its inception the AMA recognized that, as historian John Harley Warner has noted, "the physician's proper interactions with patients and fellow practitioners, as much as his mastery of medical knowledge, were critical to the regular profession's effectiveness and authority."[9] Such an objective was significant in the mid-nineteenth century, when the medical profession in the United States was characterized by dubious reputations, intense hostility and competition among practitioners, and "sectarian" divisions and antagonisms between groups of people with very different ideas about the healing mission. It was in this fluid setting that the original students and faculty members of the University of Michigan's Department of Medicine and Surgery gathered.

The Early Medical Faculty

Detroit physician, several-time Detroit mayor, and future AMA president Zina B. Pitcher played a key role in establishing the medical school.[10] A member of the Board of Regents, he chaired the committee that reported to the board on the need for a medical school and helped to select the original faculty. On January 19, 1848, the Department of Medicine and Surgery began with five faculty members: Dean Abram Sager (diseases of women and children), Silas H. Douglas[11] (chemistry), Samuel Denton (medicine and pathology), Moses Gunn (surgery and anatomy), and Jonathan Adams Allen, Jr. (physiology). Together, they taught a curriculum made up of two six-month terms, leaving students free to pursue other activities during the other half of the year. Over the next several decades, as the medical school grew and changed, these initial chairs would be expanded, renamed, combined, and recombined in a number of configurations.[12]

The close relationship with the university has always been a central element of the medical school's identity. From its inception, the medical school

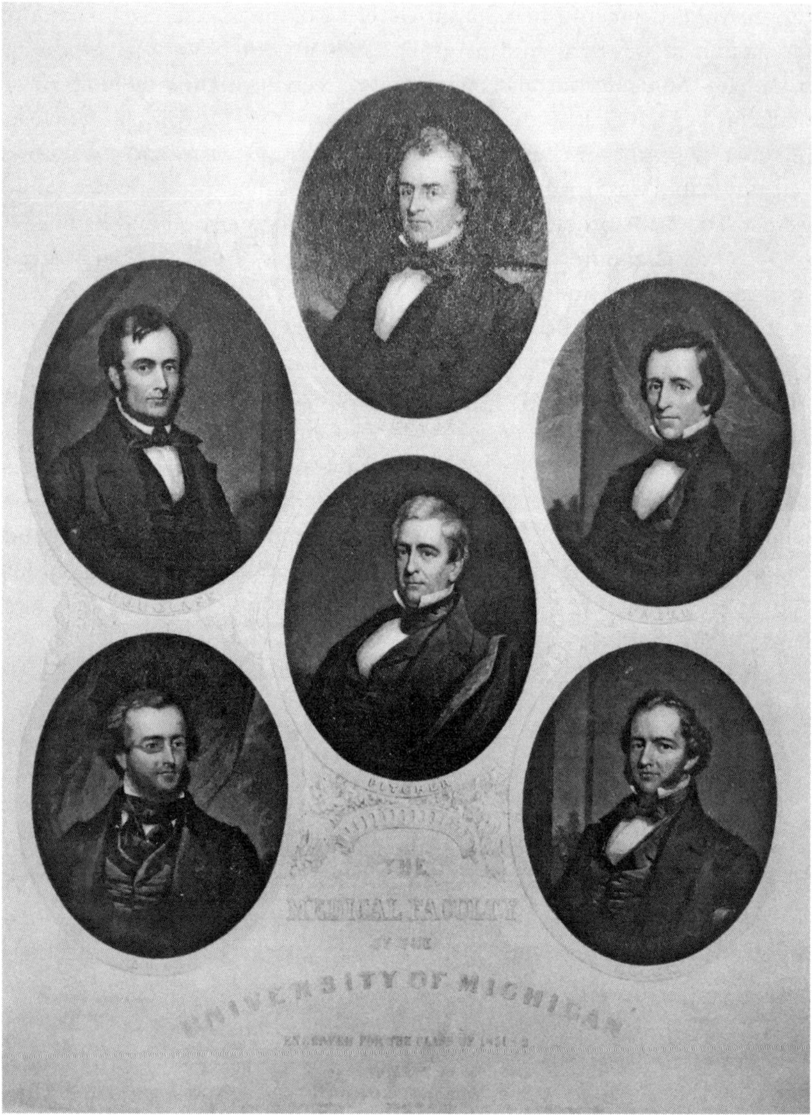

Medical faculty, 1851–1852 (clockwise, from bottom left): Moses Gunn, Silas H. Douglas, Samuel Denton, Abram Sager, Jonathan Adams Allen, Jr., and Regent Zina B. Pitcher (center). Engraved by J. Sartain. Bentley Historical Library, University of Michigan, Ann Arbor.

was considered to be an integral component of the larger university. Its faculty members were considered University of Michigan professors, which was unique among American medical schools at the time, even those affiliated with older universities such as Harvard or Columbia. Annual faculty salaries of $1,000 were paid by the state of Michigan, and Pitcher was proud that the medical school was "the only medical school in the country endowed by the government and regulated by state authority."[13]

However, hiring and keeping good medical professors was a challenge. Maintaining private medical practice was an integral part of the experience of faculty members in medical schools throughout the country. Gunn argued that "professorships . . . require for their incumbents practical men, men engaged in daily practice of their profession."[14] The biggest problem, one that presaged many future debates, was that Ann Arbor was a small town with limited clinical opportunities, and for many faculty, private practice income in Ann Arbor was not enough to supplement university pay. Gunn believed that "Ann Arbor is unable to furnish practice for all practical men which it is necessary to combine in a faculty of a medical college."[15] He moved from Ann Arbor to Detroit in 1853 to expand his surgical practice and work as coeditor for the *Peninsular and Independent Medical Journal* (formerly the *Medical Independent*). For most of the next fourteen years Gunn commuted to Ann Arbor twice weekly via the Michigan Central Railroad to teach at the university and even served one year as the dean. Students were not overly pleased with the arrangement, complaining that he hurried through class because "the rail cars were coming."[16] L. Corydon Ford (who arrived from Geneva Medical College in New York to take over as anatomy professor in 1854) was the only faculty member who did not maintain an active private practice and for quite some time "was the closest to being a full-time staff member."[17] Professor and surgeon Theodore McGraw remembered the Ann Arbor of the 1870s as "a small village, and the University teachers could not add much to their meagre salaries by outside practice."[18]

Another solution to small-town living was to hold a simultaneous professorship somewhere else, even outside the state. Alonzo Palmer, hired to teach medicine at Michigan in 1852, later held a chair at the Berkshire Medical College in Pittsfield, Massachusetts, and both he and Ford lectured there during the summer. Detroit physician Henry Lyster, who was hired to teach surgery in 1868, stayed at the university for only one year because the regents wanted him to relocate to Ann Arbor. In 1872, the medical faculty considered the matter of allowing a member to hold "a double relation to the University and the Detroit Medical College" and ultimately voted "that it is not for the interest of the Medical Department of the University that such relation such [*sic*] exist between the Department and any other school"; somewhat tellingly, Professor Ford was the only member who voted against the resolution, and Professors Palmer and McGraw abstained from the vote.[19] After the medical school lengthened its annual term from six to nine months in 1877, out-of-city residence and simultaneous faculty appointments—even with institutions close to Ann Arbor—became even more problematic and controversial.[20]

Although small, Ann Arbor was filled with people who took an active interest in school affairs, decisions, and expansions and supported the university and its students.[21] For instance, town residents supplied about $10,000 in funds "by subscription" to expand the medical school's facilities in the early 1860s, which was more than the building had originally cost to construct fewer than two decades earlier.[22] Many early faculty members and other professionals took pride in the "rural city" of Ann Arbor and its "hospitable citizens."[23] Palmer lauded the town as "one of the most healthy localities anywhere to be found."[24] But the placid, small-town nature of Ann Arbor during the first years of the medical school stood in increasingly stark contrast to nearby Detroit, which expanded steadily and dramatically. The completion of the Erie Canal in 1826, together with the application of steam power to boats, provided an easy route for Midwestern agricultural produce to travel from Detroit to the East Coast. A rail line reached west to Lake Michigan and then to Chicago, linking two promising Great Lakes cities. Detroit's population grew from forty thousand to seventy thousand residents in the 1850s alone.[25]

Detroit's booming success in such close proximity undoubtedly accentuated the fear that despite Ann Arbor's pastoral beauty, locating a major state university—not to mention a medical school—in the rural town could be disadvantageous. Observers opined that as long as the university's medical school remained in Ann Arbor, it could "never become anything more than a respectable country school."[26] Unsurprisingly, it did not take long for medical faculty members, particularly those who already lived and worked in Detroit, to propose moving the school from Ann Arbor to Detroit. The earliest recorded mention of such a plan appears to be in the minutes of a faculty meeting from December 29, 1856, less than a decade since the school had opened its doors, during which Samuel Denton argued "that the removal of the medical college of the University to the city of Detroit would promote the true interests of the University, and especially those of its Medical Department."[27] Three months later, the faculty voted against the move.

Although the school remained in Ann Arbor, faculty decided to use the resources of the growing city nearby and recommended "a course of Clinical Instruction in Detroit to commence on the 15th day of June & continue till the first day of October, to which all students who shall have attended one full course of Lectures in the University of Michigan and shall have passed an examination approved by the Faculty shall be admitted."[28] During that time, professors were expected to lead small groups of students on "deliberate walks through the wards" to give "thorough instruction at the bed-side of the sick" for several hours each day of the week except Sundays. These visits were to take place at the U.S. Marine Hospital (supported by a tax on sailors and open only to seamen, who were treated without charge) or St. Mary's Hospital. Pitcher lauded the summer clinical course as an important innovation in American medical instruction, in keeping with modern European practices.[29] However, despite Pitcher's recommendations to make the clinical course in Detroit a degree requirement and to establish an endowed clinical professorship, relatively few students could be induced to take advantage of the opportunity, and the course was discontinued after just two years. Although Pitcher supported the urban clinical program, he (along with the other regents) did not approve of relocating the entire medical school.[30]

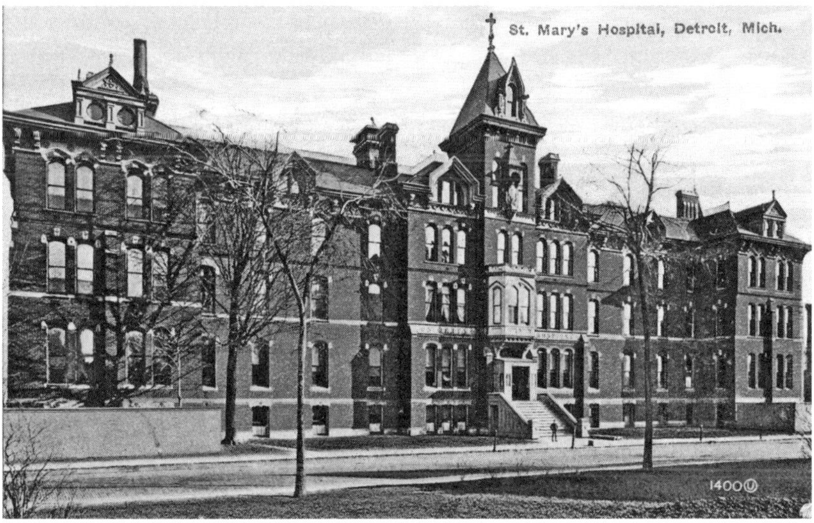

St. Mary's Hospital (House of Invalids), founded in Detroit in 1845. The structure shown here was the hospital's third building, constructed in 1879. Detroit Historical Society.

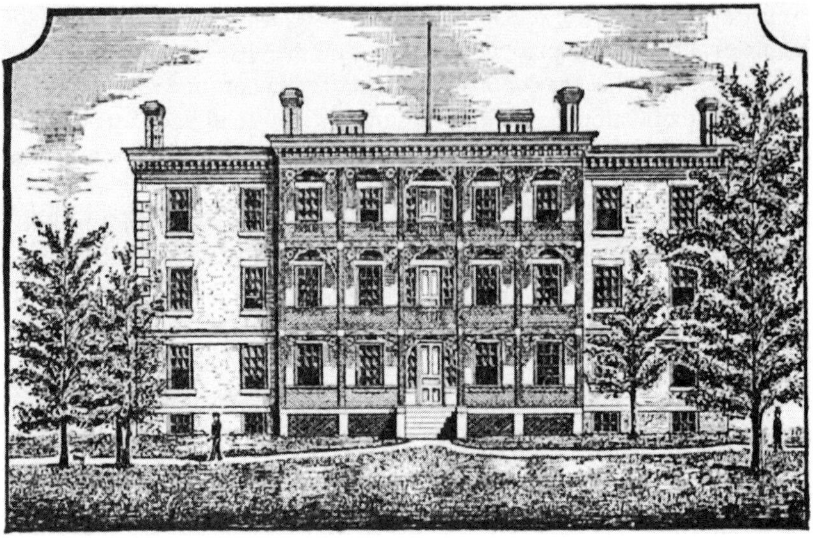

U.S. Marine Hospital, built in Detroit, 1857. Silas Farmer, *History of Detroit and Wayne County and Early Michigan*, vol. 1, 3rd ed. (Detroit: Silas Farmer, 1890), 923.

Although the regents certainly opposed moving the university's medical school to Detroit, some early faculty members continued to support the idea, most notably Moses Gunn. He claimed that medical schools located outside major cities were "an anachronism."[31] Moving beyond the obvious self-interest inherent in arguing for the move (as Gunn had already "voted with his feet" and decamped to live in Detroit), he maintained in an 1858 article in the *Peninsular and Independent Medical Journal* that "the Department should be transferred from its present location to one where greater advantages could be enjoyed, a higher standard of education be attained, and, consequently, a greater amount of glory be shed upon the University, and a greater degree of benefit be experienced by the people of Michigan." Citing other calls for compulsory clinical education, and contrasting the American situation with European schools that had been offering clinical education for many years, Gunn claimed that competition had prevented most American medical schools outside major cities from instituting such a demanding requirement. As "the only prosperous country medical school in the United States," the University of Michigan's school was uniquely poised to establish such a significant reform, which Gunn described as a "sacred duty."[32] In his view,

> the question, then . . . is: Can the Medical Department attain this high ground in its present locality? There can be but one answer: *Never.* . . . But let the transfer to Detroit be made, where a rich College Medical and Surgical Clinic can be enjoyed, Hospitals be opened to candidates for the Doctor's degree, *one year's attendance upon which shall be a* CONDITION *of graduation*, and the University of Michigan may realize in its Medical Department a character *second to none in the country.*[33]

Gunn's use of language in his stirring article is telling of his perspective on the school's rural identity. His description of the University of Michigan's medical school as a "country medical school" clearly differentiated it from institutions in cities like New York and Philadelphia, where "Hospital-teaching," though imperfect, was attracting many more students and providing a more complete education. He also cited a professor at Chicago's Rush Medical College, another school in a growing urban location, who argued for the necessity of "'access to the wards of a well regulated hospital.' . . . This indicates the disposition of our neighbors; and shall the *endowed* University of Michigan . . . be backward in taking equally high ground?"[34] Toward the end of the article, Gunn adopted an even more alarmist tone, suggesting the emergent need to provide broader clinical exposure to graduating students. Appealing directly to the university's Board of Regents, Gunn made this earnest plea:

> Are you furnishing to the State men fully qualified, *safely* to assume the charge of human life, when invaded by disease and threatened by death? or must these your graduates derive their *first* experience from patients *who look to them alone* for aid? Have they been enabled to *observe* the phenomena of disease and the effects of remedies, under your guidance and direction, until they are familiar with both? or do you turn them out upon the world, armed with *theories* alone? What answer could we make with these interrogatories? Alas! what answer![35]

The regents were unmoved. Several months after Gunn's article appeared, they again voted to keep the medical school in Ann Arbor. They addressed the consideration of a move to Detroit "or elsewhere" in part by stipulating that all professors would be required to live near the university during the term of the course. Unsurprisingly, the regents also severely censured Gunn for publicizing his opinions, and he ultimately left the school in 1867.[36]

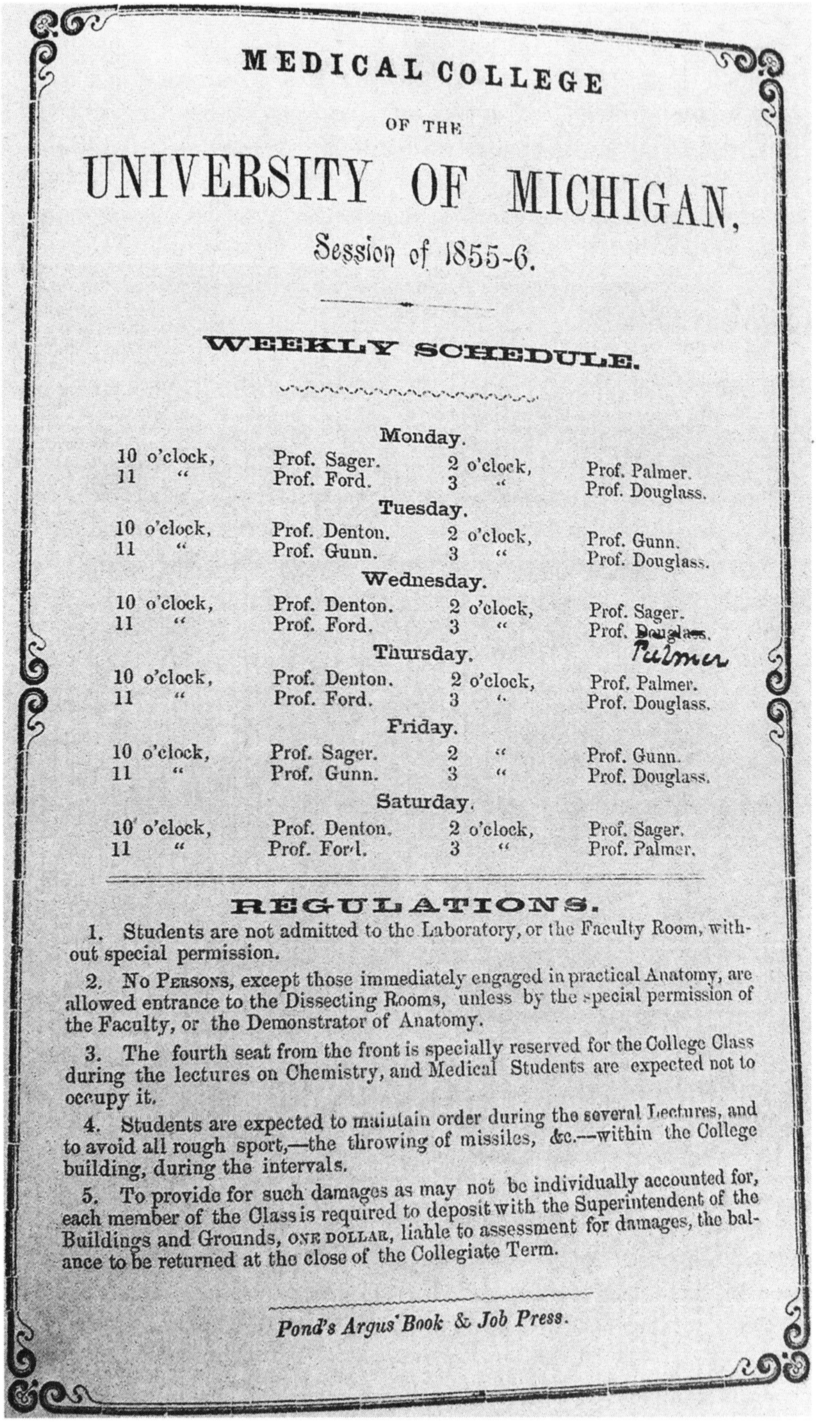

MEDICAL COLLEGE

OF THE

UNIVERSITY OF MICHIGAN,

Session of 1855-6.

WEEKLY SCHEDULE.

Monday.			
10 o'clock,	Prof. Sager.	2 o'clock,	Prof. Palmer.
11 "	Prof. Ford.	3 "	Prof. Douglass.
Tuesday.			
10 o'clock,	Prof. Denton.	2 o'clock,	Prof. Gunn.
11 "	Prof. Gunn.	3 "	Prof. Douglass.
Wednesday.			
10 o'clock,	Prof. Denton.	2 o'clock,	Prof. Sager.
11 "	Prof. Ford.	3 "	Prof. ~~Douglass~~. Palmer
Thursday.			
10 o'clock,	Prof. Denton.	2 o'clock,	Prof. Palmer.
11 "	Prof. Ford.	3 "	Prof. Douglass.
Friday.			
10 o'clock,	Prof. Sager.	2 "	Prof. Gunn.
11 "	Prof. Gunn.	3 "	Prof. Douglass.
Saturday.			
10 o'clock,	Prof. Denton.	2 o'clock,	Prof. Sager.
11 "	Prof. Ford.	3 "	Prof. Palmer.

REGULATIONS.

1. Students are not admitted to the Laboratory, or the Faculty Room, without special permission.

2. No Persons, except those immediately engaged in practical Anatomy, are allowed entrance to the Dissecting Rooms, unless by the special permission of the Faculty, or the Demonstrator of Anatomy.

3. The fourth seat from the front is specially reserved for the College Class during the lectures on Chemistry, and Medical Students are expected not to occupy it.

4. Students are expected to maintain order during the several Lectures, and to avoid all rough sport,—the throwing of missiles, &c.—within the College building, during the intervals.

5. To provide for such damages as may not be individually accounted for, each member of the Class is required to deposit with the Superintendent of the Buildings and Grounds, ONE DOLLAR, liable to assessment for damages, the balance to be returned at the close of the Collegiate Term.

Pond's Argus' Book & Job Press.

Weekly schedule of the Medical College, 1855–1856. Medical School (University of Michigan) Records, 1850–2010, Bentley Historical Library, University of Michigan, Ann Arbor.

The Curriculum

The initial medical curriculum consisted of instruction in "anatomy, physiology, pathology, practical medicine and surgery which include the directions for arresting morbid action, removing its products and repairing the injuries arising from accident, materia medica, obstetrics, chemistry, [and] medical jurisprodence [*sic*]."[37] Students attended a total of two six-month terms, with annual commencements scheduled in late March. Their fees were considerably lower than those of many other medical schools in the United States at the time.[38] For the first few decades professors simply repeated the same material for both classes of students, making the medical school's first- and second-year lectures virtually identical. Faculty did this because they believed that students would find the repeated lecture "much more interesting . . . and profitable than the first."[39] They also felt that the amount of required material could be covered in only one year. The desire to have to prepare only one lecture also may have played a role.

Before 1878, prospective graduates were also required to submit a written thesis, based on published material rather than on original research. Some students included examples from their personal experience. Topics ranged widely, from common diseases and conditions (such as tetanus and pregnancy) to the use of new medical technology (such as physical diagnosis and electricity) to drugs and substances (such as tobacco and lead).[40] In addition to encouraging students to learn about a topic in some depth, the thesis requirement was intended to make students both capable and "morally bound" to present their findings to others, suggesting (though not yet clearly stating) that graduates were expected to participate in the advancement (or at least the spread) of knowledge. Professors traditionally read the best submissions aloud as part of the commencement. In 1853, for example, two medical theses—G. W. Carter's "Touch" and D. L. Heath's "Modus Operandi of Medicines"—were presented as shining examples of student work.[41]

The school maintained a limited library and a "museum" of materia medica, initially consisting of a collection of Parisian chemicals purchased from the struggling University of Louisiana.[42] It began acquiring equipment for an "anatomy museum" during its first full year of operation, purchasing tables, charts, display cases, and other items "necessary for the lodgement and preservation of specimens in healthy and morbid anatomy."[43] Ford created many of his own teaching models, made anatomical charts, and prepared specimens for the collection to address the dearth of available laboratory materials for students.[44] Medical faculty meetings in early decades were concerned primarily with schedules, expense reports, library and anatomical museum acquisitions, and student behavioral problems (including low test scores and nonattendance), rather than educational reforms.[45]

One critical area of instruction for University of Michigan medical students was gross anatomy. Despite some concerns that the dissection experience could be dangerous or morally corrupting, the use of cadavers for anatomical instruction and surgical experimentation was a crucial element of medical identity and advancement. As historian Michael Sappol has observed, "socially and professionally [dissection] was . . . designed to transform the student, to inure him to the body and to death."[46] The practical need to acquire bodies, however, posed a challenge in the mid-nineteenth century. In many parts of the country, there were no legal means to procure bodies for medical education, institutional or otherwise. Gunn supposedly performed the first anatomical dissection in Ann Arbor (and possibly the entire state of Michigan) using a cadaver he brought to Ann Arbor in 1846 from New York's Geneva Medical College. Gunn dissected that body over a four-week period for a small, informal audience.[47] The Michigan state legislature attempted to legalize anatomical dissections that same year; its revised 1846 statutes included a provision that the bodies of criminals who died while serving a prison sentence of at least six months would be offered to state and local medical societies. That provision, however, was overturned five years later, prompting Zina Pitcher to complain, "the midnight assassin and the inquiring medical student are liable to become inhabitants of the same cell in the Michigan State Prison."[48]

The professor of anatomy was aided by a hired demonstrator, whose job included obtaining and preparing specimens for instruction by any means available and necessary. The first person to hold that position was Robert Clark Kedzie, an 1851 Michigan graduate who began working in the anatomical laboratory as a senior medical student. He noted in his memoir that many people were in awe of the university's dissecting room: "The question 'where do you get your subjects,' had a strange fascination for many people. The reply, 'we *raise* 'em,' did not seem to satisfy the inquiring mind."[49] Nor did townspeople see this as a humorous topic. Grave robbing horrified Michigan locals. Evidence of the practice—such as desecrated graves in nearby cemeteries—could lead to bitter hostilities and even mob violence aimed at the medical school. On one occasion townspeople discovered a recently emptied gravesite, with a broken coffin and torn burial shroud serving as proof of what had transpired. A mob gathered with the intent of burning

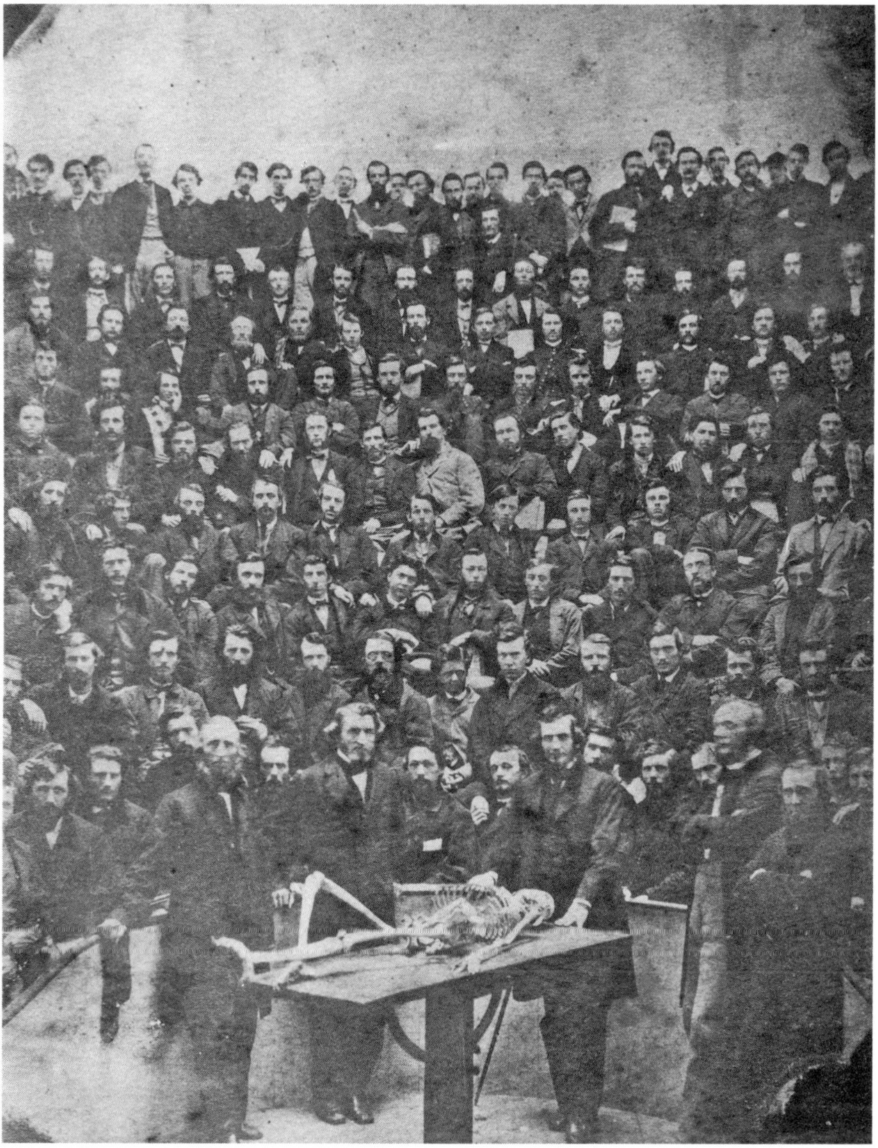

Students in amphitheater and medical faculty at front (standing, left to right): Abram Sager, Alonzo Palmer, Corydon Ford, Moses Gunn, and Silas Douglas, March 1865. Medical School (University of Michigan) Records, 1850–2010, Bentley Historical Library, University of Michigan, Ann Arbor. Ford was disabled from infantile paralysis as a child and used a gold-capped cane supposedly made of timber from Oliver Hazard Perry's ship (presumably the flagship *USS Lawrence*) and inscribed in bronze with, "We have met the enemy and they are ours," spoken by Perry at the Battle of Lake Erie. A cane is visible behind the examining table, on Ford's right. See Donald F. Huelke, "The History of the Department of Anatomy, the University of Michigan: Part I, 1850 to 1894," *University of Michigan Medical Bulletin* 27 (1961): 10–12.

the medical building and "scattering the young crop of sawbones that would not let the dead sleep in the graves." Medical students infiltrated the mob and mounted a guard (said to have been armed) to protect the building until tempers cooled.[50]

The jobs of the demonstrator and anatomical laboratory assistants became even more challenging when, in the 1860s, the faculty resolved "that students be required to dissect at least one half of a subject."[51] Earlier in the decade, the medical school required only between fifteen and twenty-five cadavers for student use each year, but the steady growth of class sizes greatly increased the need for bodies. Although "the demonstrator seldom robbed graves himself, . . . he bought cadavers from those who did."[52] Another demonstrator, Edmund Andrews, who also had been a member of the medical school's first class, found himself "authorized & required by the great State of Michigan to buy, steal, or in any other manner pro-cure subjects for dissection, and to give instructions thereon, with a provision in the statutes that if I did this duty faithfully, I should serve out a term in the States Prison." According to Andrews's description of his plan and corroborating accounts, the school would purchase bodies taken from only almshouse cemeteries or potter's fields, since "nobody would spend money" over the loss of "friendless paupers." None of these bodies was exhumed from Ann Arbor. Sometimes agents in cities like Detroit, Buffalo, Toledo, and Chicago sent bodies "by express" for a considerable fee; the Buffalo agent charged twenty-five dollars per cadaver.[53] However, in reality there was virtually no oversight of these suppliers, and Michigan faculty members simply could not verify the sources of their anatomical specimens.

According to legend, when Gunn left Ann Arbor for Chicago's Rush Medical College in 1867 he continued (and amplified) his earlier habit of taking bodies from one place to another, stealing the Michigan medical school's entire supply of about forty cadavers. Donald Huelke claims that Gunn "is supposed to have bound and gagged the janitor of the Medical Building and locked him in a room to prevent him from sounding the alarm. . . . Gunn claimed that [the regents] would not proceed against him for this would reveal the method by which anatomical material was procured."[54] Even after the state of Michigan amended its "Anatomical Law" in the 1870s, there were still reports of extralegal body-snatching. In 1876, one student wrote to his mother that two other medical students had shipped the bodies of two gunmen from Jesse James's gang in paint barrels from Northfield, Minnesota, to Ann Arbor for the anatomical laboratory.[55] In an 1880 statement to the

Board of Regents, anatomy professor William J. Herdman acknowledged public outrage about grave robbing but assumed a reactionary tone to seek empathy and respect "instead of that wholesale abuse and criticism which it has become the fashion to heap upon me." Herdman claimed to "have labored early and late and have tested every honorable method that has been suggested" to satisfy the medical school's annual required supply of cadavers, which he estimated to be between ninety and one hundred. However, "the peculiar location and facilities of our University" were problematic for procuring bodies, and Herdman agitated for the state of Michigan to allow for more of its dead to be used, legally, for educational purposes, rather than forcing the Ann Arbor school to rely upon the "clandestine business" of grave-robbing.[56]

Some other fields of study, notably surgery and obstetrics, faced their own pedagogical challenges. For example, instruction in surgery was originally limited to passive observation of operations conducted in lecture halls. After the mid-1860s, surgical demonstration became possible in an operating amphitheater in the medical building addition. Instruction was also challenged by a lack of available patients, which was a problem for many medical institutions, but especially so for those in rural areas. When Gunn appealed to local physicians to send surgery patients to the medical school for educational purposes, he would "remind the profession that operations are made before the medical class free of charge."[57] The conditions frustrated many early surgery lecturers and professors and certainly contributed to fairly rapid turnover in that field's department chair position. Canadian physician Donald Maclean, who had held positions in Edinburgh and Ontario, was appointed lecturer of surgery at Michigan in 1872 and assumed the chair the following year. A superb clinician, Maclean would hold that position for nearly two decades, which up to that point was the department's longest tenure for the surgery professorship.[58]

Obstetrics had an even more significant problem, and not just because Michigan was a rural medical school. It was not uncommon in the mid-nineteenth century for American medical students to have no access to obstetrics and gynecology patients. Clinical obstetrics was virtually nonexistent for decades at the University of Michigan. The few women who consented to serve as demonstration patients were not very useful for students, since the decorum of the time dictated that gynecological exams take place under a sheet; the male doctor's "gaze" was perceived to be more threatening to a woman's modesty than his touch.[59] Furthermore, the question of using parturient female patients for instruction presented instructors with a dilemma. The prevalent assumption was that only morally dubious, unmarried mothers would avail themselves of the free services of a teaching hospital, and such women might be hazardous to impressionable, young, mostly male students. Even after the creation of a functioning university hospital, most Ann Arbor women—particularly those who would have been considered "respectable" enough to be brought before the class—gave birth at home or (less frequently) in private clinics, rather than subjecting themselves to the lack of privacy and potential contamination of a hospital ward. During this period most deliveries in the United States took place at home, with only the occasional involvement of physicians. Thus, for the first forty years of its existence the medical school did not require its graduates to witness labor and childbirth, let alone participate in a delivery.[60]

Educational patterns change slowly, and the apprenticeship model of medical education did not immediately go away with the creation of a functional medical school. Similarly to those people who for much of the nineteenth century trained to be physicians only through an apprenticeship, Michigan medical students were also required to supplement their didactic instruction with a three-year preceptorship "with some respectable practitioner of medicine."[61] Although the preceptorship was explicitly mandated by the university Board of Regents in 1850, in reality the rule was often interpreted to include the two full lecture terms in the school. Nonetheless, the early faculty and regents promoted the importance of medical apprenticeships, particularly with physicians in private practice. Before 1857, the medical school's annual announcement stated that "the hasty walk through the wards of a hospital . . . furnishes but a sorry substitute for the close and accurate study of cases." The withdrawal of this statement from the school's publications indicates a growing awareness of the significance of formal clinical instruction in medical education, as well as the recognition that private physicians could not be effectively regulated as preceptors.[62] But the apprenticeship tradition continued to be noted for at least another twenty years. Between 1877 and 1890, the medical school's list of acceptable preceptors decreased, and Michigan professors were listed more often in that role, just to fulfill the requirement for their students. When the four-year curriculum was adopted in 1890, the formal preceptorship was dropped altogether.[63]

The content of the medical curriculum was also starting to change, perhaps most notably by including laboratory science. For this revolution,

Michigan's medical school was an early American convert. University presidents like James B. Angell were strong supporters of scientific medicine and encouraged an emphasis on basic sciences, particularly chemistry and physiology.[64] The university's first chemical laboratory, "the first building in an American university to be devoted entirely to chemistry," was built adjacent to the medical school in 1856, under the auspices of Professor Silas Douglas.[65] In an attempt to apply basic scientific methods to understandings of disease, all University of Michigan medical students were required to complete a practical laboratory course in chemistry, which was rare in U.S. schools before the 1870s. Later in the century, the medical school also implemented a required experimental physiology course (designed in part to rival a new course at Harvard), and physiology chair Henry Cheever, hired in 1872, became one of the first full-time faculty members to focus exclusively on teaching and research.[66]

The medical school did not only look inward, toward the laboratory bench and the microscope. It looked outward as well, toward the health needs of the larger community. Jonathan Adams Allen, Jr., the school's physiology professor until 1854, was a vocal advocate for the collection of accurate and useful mortality statistics (birth and death registries) and epidemiological data for endemic and epidemic diseases in Michigan.[67] He reputedly had a sarcastic sense of humor, and when seeking accurate data on epidemics, he dismissed isolated reports as "comparatively valueless," saying that "what Dr. So-and-so saw, or thought he saw; what wonder-working charms he carried in his dilapidated saddle bags . . . are hardly worth the paper on which he communicates them." What was needed, he argued, was accurate counting of births, deaths, and the causes of deaths.[68] Years later, the university would host a bacteriological ("hygienic") laboratory, which assisted medicolegal authorities with chemical analysis and autopsies for years before state facilities in Lansing were opened. Through systematic attention to the issue of health for the larger population, the medical school operated as a de facto school of public health, although at that time the boundaries between medicine and public health were so blurred as to be almost nonexistent.[69]

In the midst of these changes came the U.S. Civil War, which historian Margaret Humphreys has described as "the greatest health disaster that this country has ever experienced."[70] The war certainly played a major role in catalyzing fundamental transformations in American medicine. The unprecedented casualty rate of the conflict—from both disease and battlefield trauma—created a pressing need for more effective medical training and treatment, as well as better systems of emergency evacuation, triage, and convalescence. Hospital architecture also underwent an important change. Wartime hospitals in the United States began to feature more modern design elements, based in part on the recommendations of British nurse Florence Nightingale. These hospitals were characterized by spacious, open wards and high windows for better light and fresh air. They minimized the number of closed walls and corridors that inhibited cross-ventilation.[71] The medical school tried, unsuccessfully, to have the federal government build a military hospital on campus during the Civil War in 1863 and 1864.[72]

A new generation of doctors, nurses, sanitary commissioners, social workers, and emergency medics who worked with military forces and the government during the Civil War developed revolutionary ideas for reforming American medical practice and started implementing those ideas in medical schools and other institutions even before the war ended. Many Michigan faculty members and students enlisted to serve the Union Army, where they could come in contact with these new ideas. Moses Gunn, for example, was absent from the university during the Civil War while he served as a surgeon in the 5th Michigan Regiment of the Army of the Potomac, and Donald Maclean worked in Union hospitals in St. Louis, Missouri, and Louisville, Kentucky. Of the class of 1861, thirty of forty-four students enlisted in the army. For example, Richard Swanson Vickery served in Company F, 2nd Michigan Infantry, for the duration of the war and then returned to the Michigan medical school, writing his thesis titled "The Duties of the Surgeon in Action."[73]

After the war ended in 1865, enrollments soared at the University of Michigan in general and its medical school in particular. In 1867, the medical school had a total of 525 students enrolled, the highest number before 1900.[74] The annual curriculum expanded from its original ungraded six-month term to a nine-month term in 1877, one of only three U.S. medical schools to have nine-month terms (along with Harvard and the University of Pennsylvania). Medical school officials worried that enrollment might drop precipitously with this change, as there certainly were places where students could obtain a degree and spend less time in school. But being a public university that drew significant support from the state, and hence being less dependent on tuition, Michigan was in a position to take the risk. Enrollment did not fall significantly; nor did it decline much in 1879, when the total program length was expanded from two to three years. As the University of Michigan president's report from 1879 noted, "if it has heretofore been true that in no department of education was improvement more sadly needed than in medical education, it may now be said that in no department of education is improvement more rapidly going on at the present time."[75]

The Students

From its earliest years, the medical school had relatively high standards for admission. Successful applicants were required to have a high school education, knowledge of Greek and Latin, "evidence of good moral character," and, preferably, apprenticeship experience with a "respectable" physician. None of the original class had graduated from college. Starting in 1875 the school decided to tighten standards by requiring students to pass an entrance examination. Most applicants passed, but some, who displayed "profound" ignorance, did not. The exam tested general knowledge; the ability to read, write, and spell; and basic numeric skills. The president's report noted that students felt to be unqualified for Michigan were nonetheless able to be admitted to other schools. While no other medical schools had such a requirement in place at that time, the Michigan report indicated that Harvard, Dartmouth, and Bowdoin soon planned to initiate entrance exams.[76]

Members of the freshmen class were between the ages of eighteen and thirty-one, but most were at least twenty-three years old at the time of matriculation.[77] In common with many other nineteenth-century medical school students, they shared a reputation for immaturity and rowdy behavior. The school's printed weekly schedule for the 1855–1856 year includes the statement that all students were "expected to maintain order during the several Lectures, and to avoid all rough sport—the throwing of missiles, &c.—within the College building, during the intervals."[78] Years later, in 1878, the faculty discussed the expulsion of several medical students who were involved in a "riotous attack" on a Second Street house on Halloween night.[79]

The students also lived in a world replete with infectious diseases. In 1873, for example, a smallpox outbreak afflicted the medical school; classes continued, but four medical students died. While there is no clear evidence that this was the motivation, the Michigan Board of Health started promoting vaccinations that year, and the incidence of the disease fell sharply.[80]

Most of the school's students during its earliest decades came from the state of Michigan. With the exception of Canadian matriculants (who in 1864 composed 13 percent of the medical school student body), there were relatively few international students.[81]

UNIVERSITY OF MICHIGAN.

DEPARTMENT OF MEDICINE AND SURGERY.

Examination of Candidates for Admission, 6th October, 1875.

1. Write your name *in full.*

2. When were you born? [Give day, month and year.]

3. Where were you born? [Give town, county and State.]

4. What is your present residence? [Give town, county and State.]

5. What educational advantages have you had? [Name the schools you have attended, and, approximately, the time spent in each.]

6. What studies have you pursued, and, in a general way, to what extent have you pursued them?

7. In what other occupation have you been engaged than that of student, and how long were you thus employed?

8. When did you commence the study of medicine? [Give month and year.]

9. How many months of actual medical study have you had up to this date?

10. Have you attended a course of lectures at any school or college? If so, state at what one and when?

11. With what preceptor (or preceptors) have you studied? [Give names and present residence as fully as possible?

---

1. What is a peninsula? Give an example from our own country.

2. What are the principal rivers of North America?

3. Name the States of the Union which lie on the left bank of the Mississippi river giving them in order from North to South.

4. What are the principal countries in Europe?

5. Name the five great lakes of North America? Where and through what river do they empty?

6. What body of water lies between Europe and Africa, and what straits connect it with the Atlantic Ocean?

Medical school entrance examination, 1875. Folder FImu/C41: Medical School Miscellaneous and General, University of Michigan Photographs Vertical File, Bentley Historical Library, University of Michigan, Ann Arbor.

It is not clear when the University of Michigan admitted its first African American students, since demographic data were not kept systematically, and lighter-skinned students may have simply "passed" as white. One memoir suggests the presence of a "student of color" in a chemistry class early in the Civil War—somewhere around 1860 or 1861. But we do not know the name of that student, or in which school he was enrolled.[82] Recent historical studies have revealed the medical school experiences of a young, dark-skinned (presumably mixed-race) student named Alpheus W. Tucker, who attempted to enroll in 1863. He was initially able to enter the class of 343 men, only to be greeted with jeers and shouts of "Take him out!" After about a week, he was asked to leave, and his name was unceremoniously erased from the student ledger. While Tucker may have left the school quietly, he made his feelings clear in a letter to the *Detroit Advertiser and Tribune,* noting that, although a "native of the State, a supporter of the University through my taxes," he was denied attendance because, "from an accident of birth I am a shade or two darker than my fellow students." He blamed an unnamed faculty member for supporting the people who drove him out, writing that "a negro-hating faculty will soon make negro-hating students." Tucker went on to complete his degree at the Iowa College of Physicians and Surgeons and eventually established a practice in Washington, D.C. Around the same time as Tucker, another person of color, John Rapier, Jr., enrolled in the medical school as a Jamaican (though he had been born in Alabama) and, perhaps because he was considered a foreigner and had a relatively light complexion, was not forced to leave. Although Rapier maintained his seat at Michigan, he decided to leave Ann Arbor. Like Tucker, he completed his medical degree at Iowa, and he obtained a commission in the U.S. Army.[83]

William Henry Fitzbutler, of Louisville, Kentucky, is generally said to be the first black graduate of Michigan's medical school, in 1872. However, there is no indication that the medical school enrolled very many students of color in its early classes. Some African American students may have withdrawn before completing the program because of the sorts of discrimination and harassment that Tucker had experienced.[84]

The admission of women to the University of Michigan was considered as early as 1851, but it was not until 1870 that the regents provided for the admission of any person, including a woman, who "possesses the requisite literary and moral qualifications."[85] When the medical school did begin to enroll women in 1870, it became the first major American medical school to become coeducational. Although Elizabeth Blackwell, the first woman to get a medical degree in the United States, had graduated from the small

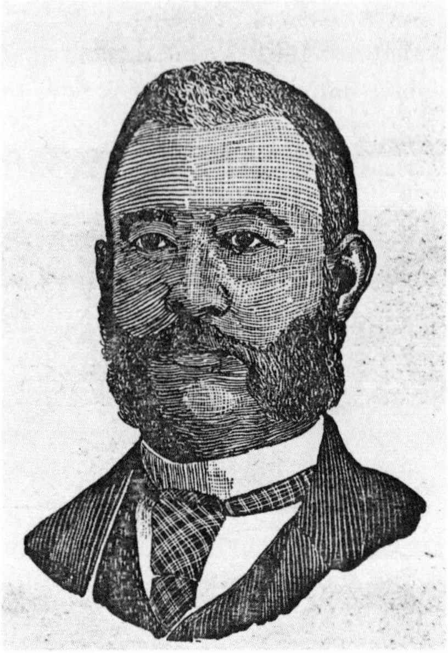

William Henry Fitzbutler, 1872 medical school graduate. BMC Media Services Records, Bentley Historical Library, University of Michigan, Ann Arbor.

Geneva Medical College in 1849, that college was not seen then as a major institution and ceased to exist as an independent school a few decades later. The first woman to earn her medical degree at Michigan, Amanda Sanford, was also the first woman to graduate from the university as a whole. She graduated in 1871 with honors and fulfilled her thesis requirement by writing a paper titled "Puerperal Eclampsia," about a dreaded complication of pregnancy.[86]

Over the next decade, the number of female medical students at Michigan increased steadily and dramatically. Michigan was for many years one of very few schools in the United States that provided women with the opportunity to obtain high-quality medical training. Many female applicants to the medical school had better foundations and qualifications for admission than their male counterparts. The entering group of women obtained slightly higher grades than did the men, including grades from professors who had previously voiced opposition to the admission of women. At the 1872 commencement, six women (from Michigan, New York, and Connecticut) were listed as graduates. That number doubled the following year; by 1881, women comprised about 20 percent of the medical school's matriculating class.[87]

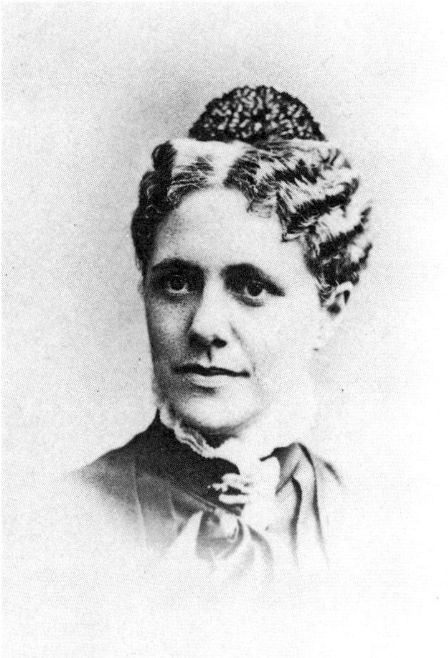

Amanda Sanford (Hickey), 1871 medical school graduate. Amanda Sanford Hickey Photograph Collection, Bentley Historical Library, University of Michigan, Ann Arbor.

Despite President Angell's support for women's coeducation at the University of Michigan,[88] the first female students in the medical school faced intense hostility. Early in 1870, months before the first women were admitted to the program, the medical faculty sent a statement to the Board of Regents claiming that "the medical co-education of the sexes is at best an experiment of doubtful utility, and one not calculated to increase the dignity of man, nor the modesty of women." This statement echoed broader concerns about opening the profession to female practitioners. Many feared that the indelicacies of medical education (particularly anatomical dissection) would "unsex" women.[89] Furthermore, the faculty argued that it was dangerous for women (who, in their view, were "during a large fraction of each month . . . quasi-invalid") to study medicine and work as physicians. They also maintained that "as child-bearing would be an insuperable obstacle in the way of a female physician, the danger would be that foeticide and infanticide, already alarmingly frequent, would become still more so."[90]

Initially, the medical school recommended separate classes for women, a policy that required adjusting the entire lecture schedule and effectively doubled the faculty teaching load. This, the faculty maintained, was the most expedient way "of restraining improprieties of deportment, and checking insubordination, in large classes of mixed students assembled in a common

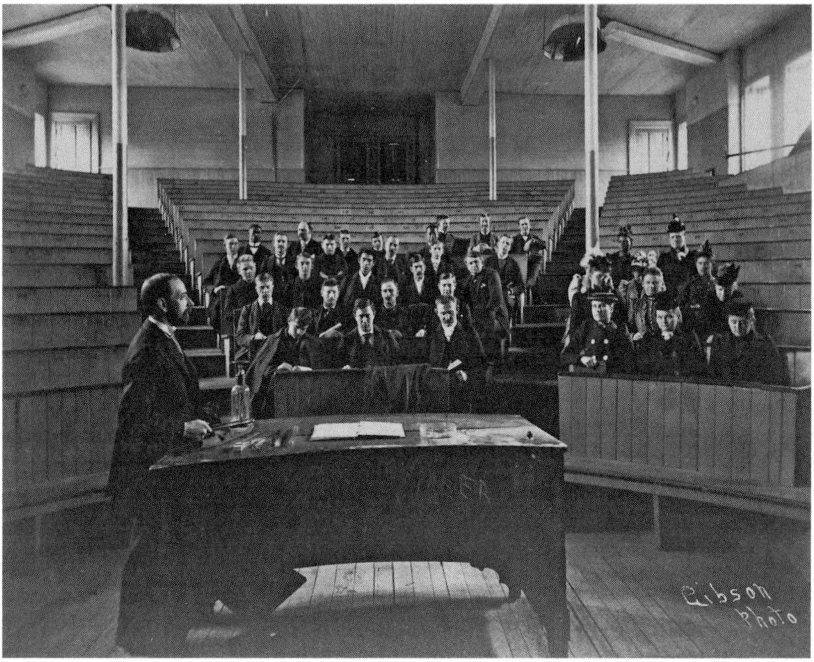

Physics lecture in the medical school showing segregation of female students, ca. 1893. Medical School (University of Michigan) Records, 1850–2010, Bentley Historical Library, University of Michigan, Ann Arbor.

lecture room," especially given the propensity of medical students for uncivil behavior.[91] The regents approved the plan—and a $500 salary increase per instructor to compensate for the extra lectures—with only one board member voicing dissent.[92] This plan, however, proved difficult to sustain, and by 1872 some faculty members asked not to repeat their lectures for male and female classes. When Silas Douglas made the request for his chemistry classes, for example, the board approved but required him to "arrange his lectures . . . so as to avoid introducing the students of both sexes into a common lecture room"; apparently, Douglas had the women sit in an adjacent preparation room, where the male class members could not see them. By the spring of 1874, the regents reversed the policy and required the medical faculty to combine their lectures for men and women without extra compensation, a system that has continued to the present day.[93]

Even after women were allowed to sit in the same lectures as men, early female medical students at Michigan faced discrimination and harassment.

Although lectures were ostensibly coeducational, individual faculty members often separated the women in their classes, demarcating their places with curtains or a red line on the floor. Women who dared to cross that line would be driven back by male medical students chanting, "Red line, red line." An exception to the integration of teaching was the gross anatomy laboratory, supposedly to deter abuse and denigration from male students, particularly in the dissection room. Sappol has argued that nineteenth-century anatomy instruction was established as a particularly masculine "rite of passage" for aspiring physicians and often involved "high-spirited" rituals and pranks to demonstrate courage in the face of dead bodies.[94] Gross anatomy laboratories remained segregated until the early 1900s, with female students initially relegated to an attic space in the original medical building.[95]

The medical faculty in the early 1870s noted several behavioral "improprieties" in coeducational classes, and records indicate that male students pestering their female counterparts was fairly common. For example, in January 1873, Douglas charged a male student with "disorderly and insulting deportment to the class of lady medical students on their entrance into the Lecture room." While the student admitted to the charge, and the faculty ultimately resolved that he should be suspended, he "affirmed that his deportment was not worse than that of many others."[96] When Sanford received her degree in 1871, she reportedly was "hooted and showered with abusive notes from young men students" at the ceremony. Women were also not afforded the honor (or dignity) of being treated as full members of the class. For the 1872 commencement, the six female medical graduates were listed alphabetically in the program after all of the male graduate names, and none of them was included in the class photo.[97] Thus, despite clear support for coeducation at the University of Michigan, the admission of women to the medical school incited discomfort and hostility among the (all-male) faculty and male students alike for a number of years. Even so, women did well, and the experience at Michigan was closely watched and led to inquiries from other universities around the United States and in Europe about how to successfully integrate women into a previously all-male medical school.

Homeopathy at the University of Michigan: The "War of the Pathies"

During the nineteenth century, American society grappled with the question of which was to be the dominant system of medical knowledge.[98] Various ways of understanding the human body in health and disease competed in the medical marketplace. Some medical systems based their understanding on the use of plant materials; others saw great efficacy in the healing powers of water. In many parts of the nation, the popularity of "irregular" medical "sects" was perceived as threatening competition for the orthodox profession—that is, "regular" physicians who believed in the system of practice that led to the M.D. degree, sometimes referred to as "allopathic" physicians. This tension certainly contributed to the founding of the AMA, which sought to limit the influence of and opportunities for alternative practitioners.[99] As early as the mid-1830s, Michigan's territorial government allowed irregular medical societies to grant licenses.[100]

Reasons for the popularity of irregular medical practice are not hard to discern. Regular medicine in the early nineteenth century often advocated drastic and painful (if not fatal) treatments such as aggressive bloodletting and the use of purgatives. Irregular practitioners often used less toxic therapies and relied more on nature's healing powers. So it is not surprising that there was professional, political, and public support in Michigan for sectarian medical practices. For many of the state's inhabitants, the often less drastic alternative remedies simply seemed more effective and attractive. The alternative medical sects of the nineteenth century also used conventions of professionalization similar to those of the regular physicians—educational standards, licensure, publications, and professional societies—and despite heated campaigns on the part of regular practitioners to marginalize or exclude sectarians, they had a deeply reflexive and mutually constructive relationship. The failures of one medical philosophy or treatment could be used to highlight the successes of another and encouraged all medical schools of thought to develop higher standards of practice and instruction.

Of the various options, homeopathic medicine was a particularly attractive one. Founded decades earlier by the German physician Samuel Hahnemann, homeopathy is based on the principle of *similia similibus curantur*, or "like cures like." As medical historian Jacalyn Duffin describes it, "the best remedy will be the one which, taken in large doses, produces symptoms similar to the disease to be cured; treatment then consists of giving that remedy in small 'homeopathic doses.'"[101] Such ideas and practices ran deep in Michigan. The state's first homeopathic medical society coincided with the formation of the AMA, and its *Michigan Journal of Homeopathy* (first issued in 1848) was the first medical periodical in the state. I. N. Eldridge, a homeopathic physician from New York who opened an Ann Arbor practice in 1847, proudly recalled that homeopathic remedies were more effective than "old school treatment" during an 1850 epidemic of "bloody flux" and noted that when the wife of one of his biggest orthodox critics, South Lyons physician E. F. Olds, became ill, Olds hired Eldridge to treat her with homeopathic remedies.[102] Such crossover of techniques ought not be too surprising. As one anonymous Michigan observer noted, reacting to an inflammatory 1854 article about medical eclecticism in the *Detroit Daily Tribune*, "Every honest physician must be, and is, an Eclectic physician, as far as his knowledge extends; that is, he selects from all the measures and remedies known to him."[103] The author reflected the widespread diversity of medical belief and practice in the mid-nineteenth-century United States. While today we may divide sectarians into dualities of orthodox and unorthodox, or regular and irregular groups, such distinctions often overlook important similarities and relationships in underlying practice.

Given the state legislature's early attention to medical education, it is not surprising that in the late 1840s, homeopaths began petitioning the university and the legislature to establish a homeopathic medical school, or at least a chair of homeopathic medicine in the proposed Department of Medicine and Surgery.[104] These suggestions did not find a positive response from the physicians who founded the university's medical school. They were regular, or orthodox, physicians, and most saw little reason to support the formal institutionalization of sectarian medicine such as homeopathy within the university. In 1858, respected local physician J. H. Beech confidently told the graduates of the University of Michigan's medical school that sectarian medicine was nonsense, "concentrated *nothingness* waxed in phantom light," and assured them that "*Regular Medicine* has nothing to fear from such parasites," as he deemed irregular practitioners.[105] Despite strongly believing that homeopathic ideas were baseless, many university administrators and medical faculty considered homeopathy to be a significant threat to the established institution, and with good reason. During the first year that the university's medical school was open, the Board of Regents received a number of requests to install a chair of homeopathic medicine, or even to dissolve the regular medical school and replace it with a homeopathic one. In 1851, after a protest led by Detroit homeopathic physician John Ellis, the state repealed an older law that had required all Michigan physicians and surgeons to obtain practice licenses from state or county medical societies. Regular physicians and administrators feared this trend toward less regulated medicine in Michigan, claiming that once "all barriers against the indiscriminate admission of persons to practice medicine were removed . . . the medical law of our revised statutes is of no value to the physician and of no safeguard to the people."[106] Zina Pitcher and other professionals clearly envisioned the new medical school as a resolutely orthodox institution, which would defiantly (and often illegally) resist the integration of alternative medical faculty and instruction for decades.

The homeopathy question went to the highest levels of the university. Regents went to great lengths to protect the "regular" interests of the school and its new medical department from the influences of homeopathy. In the spring of 1852, when the Board of Regents was considering who should be president of the new university, a rumor that nominee Henry Philip Tappan had once sought medical advice from a homeopathic practitioner persuaded Regent Pitcher that Tappan ought not to be allowed to become president. Trying to gather more information about Tappan's sympathies toward homeopathy, Pitcher wrote to the physician—a Dr. Vanderburgh from New York—using an assumed name. Pitcher then used that information to sway the board to consider two other candidates. However, they both declined the offer, and Tappan ultimately did become the university's first president that August.[107] Homeopathic medicine continued to be an issue for potential university leaders. Reuben Peterson, in his history of the University Hospital, suggests that one of the main reasons James B. Angell at first declined the university presidency was because of "the Homeopathic question." Angell eventually accepted in 1871 after the regents assured him that a homeopathic medical school would not be located in Ann Arbor—an assurance they were unable to keep.[108]

Despite strong opposition from university administrators and regular medical professors, the state's homeopaths remained confident and persistent. The *Michigan Homeopathic Journal* argued that the "truth" of homeopathy frightened regular medical instructors at orthodox schools and that homeopaths "alone can cure without making sick, or cure with any degree of certainty; and sooner or later they 'will be borne by grateful people, to all chairs at the college building of the Medical Department of the State University at Ann Arbor.'"[109] In 1855, the Michigan legislature mandated the appointment of at least one professor of homeopathy in the university's medical school. Tappan, who was by then the university's president, supported the state legislature's mandate (indicating that Pitcher may have been accurate in his initial concerns), but the Board of Regents refused to enforce it.[110] Implementation of the law was further slowed by internal dissent within the homeopathic community. Some of the state's homeopathic professionals disagreed with the law, arguing that their interests would be better served with a separate department, perhaps located in Detroit. The founding of the unaffiliated Michigan Homeopathic Medical College at Lansing in 1871 also distracted homeopathy's advocates.[111]

The Board of Regents and medical school faculty remained firm in their opposition to homeopathy. They successfully defied the state law for more than twelve years, claiming that "these two principles of medicine cannot be taught in the same institution."[112] In the late 1860s Silas Douglas (then dean) explained that a professor of homeopathy would be a severe impediment to the educational process. It would "destroy all good discipline in the medical class," invite insults from students, violate AMA codes, and damage the reputation of the medical school in general. According to Douglas, "we, the Faculty and graduates, would be outcasts from the profession, and our diplomas would not be worth the parchment upon which they are printed."[113] Some professors even may have considered defecting from the university to open an independent school.

But there were limits as to how long the medical school could hold out against the state legislature. After a Michigan Supreme Court case brought by S. B. Thayer, chair of the state's Homeopathic Medical Society, the Board of Regents—also facing increased competition from medical schools in Detroit and Lansing, and a threatened loss of revenue—finally relented, to some extent.[114] While adamantly refusing to incorporate homeopathy into the regular structure of the university's medical school, the board did vote to create a separate Homeopathic Medical College on the Ann Arbor campus. The college opened in 1875 with Samuel Arthur Jones as its first dean. Jones was a homeopathic physician who moved from New York, where he had been a member of the first New York State Board of Medical Examiners. His position on that official board indicates the extent to which homeopathic medicine had entered the medical mainstream. The Ann Arbor homeopathic school had two professors—one for materia medica and therapeutics, the other for theory and practice. Homeopathic students received the rest of their basic education in the regular medical school. They took the same entrance examinations, paid the same fees as the rest of the students, and were subject to the same curriculum and graduation standards.[115]

This action certainly did not resolve the conflict between regular and irregular medicine. The mandated integration of medical courses was a key factor in Abram Sager's decision to resign as dean in 1875. Several faculty members in the regular department openly denounced homeopathy in their science lectures, even in the presence of homeopathic students.[116] Having legislators mandate the content of academic instruction also did not sit well with the faculty or dean. Following Sager's departure Acting Dean Edward

Dunster noted to the AMA that relationships between the two schools remained tense and that popular pressures and the desire for revenue had led the state legislature "to practically invade the constitutional function of the Regents . . . and to dictate to them."[117] Furthermore, Dunster found it insulting that the state medical society had appointed its "Committee of Nine" to consider barring any Michigan medical school graduate (regular or homeopathic) from membership; this "attack," as Dunster described it, was "not prompted by a desire to remove homeopathy from the University, but by a desire to crush the regular medical department in order to further certain private interests."[118]

But other orthodox faculty members argued in favor of the integration. For example, ophthalmology chair George E. Frothingham, who received his medical education at Michigan and was later memorialized for his "powers as a controversialist," believed that the best approach was to subject homeopathic ideas to discussion and critical scrutiny. He claimed that, "as knowledge had ever been the most effective antidote to superstition and false theories, the plan proposed would prove a most effectual blow to homeopathy." When the Michigan State Medical Society denounced his position in the mid-1870s, Frothingham angrily resigned from the organization.[119] Some students in the regular medical school complained about asymmetry in access to education. Although the homeopathic students had full access to the regular medical curriculum and facilities, the regular students were not exposed to homeopathic practice. In 1875, students sent a petition to the Board of Regents requesting access to homeopathic patients so they could "have opportunity to observe any advantages resulting from this system and detect any errors that may be concealed by the present system of the management of their cases." It is not clear whether they made this request because they felt that there was value in homeopathic medicine or they wanted a chance to expose failures in the practice; in either case, the petition (and its 115 accompanying signatures) indicates a widespread awareness of inequalities in the integrated medical school.[120]

The coexistence of the two schools was never harmonious, and the propriety of teaching homeopathy at the University of Michigan remained controversial. In a letter to the editor of the *Detroit Free Press*, one observer remarked on the threat of "medical quackery" in the state and noted that "no thoughtful and unprejudiced person will deny that it is of vital importance that the general public should be able to discriminate between the qualified, regularly educated physician and the ignorant quack; and yet, according to the present law of this State, it is impossible to do so, and there is nothing whatever to prevent any tinker, cobbler, loafer, or common impostor, from dubbing himself 'Doctor.'"[121] Another Michigan newspaper noted in 1879 that a "war of the pathies" was under way.[122] The University of Michigan would remain a significant battlefield in that conflict for decades to come.

Establishing a University Hospital

When the medical school first opened its doors, it had no clinical facilities, and the town of Ann Arbor had no community hospital. Clinical facilities may not at first have seemed essential, as all students presumably already would have had clinical experience as part of an apprenticeship before arriving at medical school. But some early medical faculty members, such as Jonathan Adams Allen, Jr., urged the establishment of a state hospital under the auspices of the university's medical school. In Allen's view, the Michigan public (whom he described as apathetic and ignorant of medical training) could simultaneously improve medical education and serve the common welfare by being patients for clinical instruction.[123] The need for some type of clinical instruction in medical school was slowly becoming discussed by the profession; Pitcher tried (and failed) to establish a regular clinical rotation in Detroit hospitals during the 1850s. In 1867, the AMA held a convention (attended by Michigan professor Alonzo Palmer) on curricular reform. Attendees supported extending medical programs to three years, with the final year devoted to clinical training in a hospital setting.

Although regular and effective clinical training was common in Germany and France in the mid-nineteenth century, it had been adopted by only a few medical schools in the United States (the University of Virginia, Yale, and Harvard among them). Michigan faculty certainly appreciated the value of clinical instruction and sought to provide students with some exposure to patients. During a single day in 1865, for example, Moses Gunn demonstrated procedures for treating gunshot wounds, strabismus, and a swollen trachea due to an enlarged thyroid.[124] Some Michigan medical students had taken advantage of the school's clinical training opportunities in Detroit hospitals in the mid-1850s or spent their semester breaks interning with doctors and hospitals in other cities. But student access to hospitals was always contingent on the goodwill of the hospital and the physicians who cared for patients there. Students could easily find their access severely constrained, or cut off altogether. Only owning and operating a hospital could allow the medical school and its students to have controlled, regular access to the clinical setting.

However, the decision to endorse a university hospital was not made without some reasoned opposition. In March 1860 the Board of Regents heard from medical school faculty opposed to teaching clinical medicine. Arguing by analogy, faculty members pointed out that the university trained people in the skills necessary to build railroads but did not itself run a railroad. The university had a law school but did not run a court, as "the court is not the theater of the University."[125] Similarly, the university had no business running a hospital, or a course that involved patient care, even if the instructors were university employees. But another factor making the case in favor of running a hospital was clinical demand—patients wanted to be seen at the University of Michigan. In 1868, the faculty reportedly received more than three hundred people seeking consultation or care as "teaching" patients, treated in anatomical lecture rooms. After weighing the competing rationales, the regents decided to establish a university hospital.

This decision made the University of Michigan the first university in the United States to own and operate its own hospital in connection with its medical school. It served as a national model for medical schools all over the country, many of which elected to establish their own university hospitals over the following decades. In Ann Arbor, once again the local environment shaped the course of the medical school. As later faculty member and hospital director Reuben Peterson remarked, "It was fortunate there was no Ann Arbor City Hospital. This compelled the University to establish and control its own hospital from the start. In other words, local conditions compelled the adoption of the right system."[126] But the responsibilities went both ways. The primary intent in creating the hospital was to create space to serve the educational needs of the university. Hence, patients were to be admitted only "upon the condition of willingness to contribute, directly or indirectly, to the main object of the institution, in such manner as the hospital staff shall direct."[127]

The original University Hospital was located on North University Avenue. It was a two-story stucco building (previously a campus residence for professors), with a total of four rooms off of central hallways with space for twenty patient beds.[128] It could offer services throughout the entire year, although the academic term was much shorter. The building's initial conversion cost $582.18. In September 1869, Abram Sager and Alonzo Palmer were named heads of a committee to plan and oversee the hospital's organization, and John Carrington was employed as hospital steward. Carrington and his

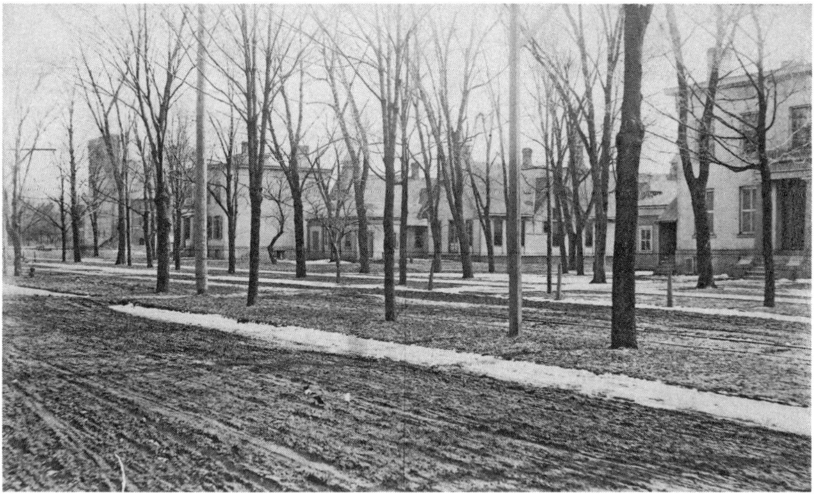

Professors' residences on North University Avenue, built in 1840 and later converted into hospital buildings—such as the first University Hospital in 1869. University of Michigan Photographs Vertical File, Bentley Historical Library, University of Michigan, Ann Arbor.

family were allowed to "use so much of the basement of the east dwelling house on the north side of the University grounds as may be necessary for . . . convenience and comfort" and also received a fuel and light allowance. The steward initially earned seventy-five cents per week for every admitted patient and was required to "keep the fires, & wash & otherwise cleanse the rooms & make the beds as often as in the opinion of the Hospital staff a proper hygiene may require."[129] What constituted "proper" hygiene, however, was not clearly defined in Carrington's duties, and early sanitary procedures in Michigan's hospital were woefully inadequate by modern standards, particularly for surgical patients.

For the first decade of the University Hospital's existence, faculty members performed most surgical procedures not in the hospital, but in the lecture halls of the medical building. This posed hygienic problems for several reasons. Not only were patients carried across campus to and from lecture halls on the upper floors, but operations were done in the same space where anatomical demonstrations on cadavers had taken place only a few hours before. An 1871 article in the *Michigan University Medical Journal* described Sager's performance of a Caesarian section on a "rachitic dwarf" (one of the earliest of such procedures documented in the state) in these conditions and noted that the patient died of peritonitis following the operation.[130] Michigan's physicians expressed concern about the dearth of useful postoperative facilities and the fact that patients recovering from surgical procedures had no choice but to receive care from poorly trained nurses and family members. Recalling his term as a lecturer in surgery at the University of Michigan during the 1871–1872 academic year, Detroit physician Theodore A. McGraw noted that "the clinics were small and very unsatisfactory. I had as surgeon, enough material for a weekly clinic, but had no proper place to treat patients after operation."[131] Thus, even though aseptic and antiseptic sanitary measures would not be standardized in U.S. or European regular medical practice for several more decades (and the germ theory of disease was still a decade away), early Michigan faculty members worried about the risks of major surgical procedures and their limiting effect on patient availability.

After just a few years, it became apparent that a new hospital building was necessary. But who should pay for it? The regents had hoped that the hospital would support itself, but many Ann Arbor residents (especially women) balked at paying a fee—even a small one for maintenance, food, and medicines—to "go before the class" and receive care as demonstration patients in the current facilities.[132] McGraw, recalling the struggle to obtain money from the state, avowed that Michigan was only "pretending to teach medicine" by refusing to grant funds to maintain an adequate hospital. When McGraw approached state legislators to discuss the issue, "the stereotyped reply was, why should the people be taxed to educate doctors? To the laity, the Medical Department of the University, with its two or three hundred students, was considered a great success. Why not let it alone?"[133] However, in 1875, the state legislature finally agreed to appropriate $8,000 for a new University Hospital. Once again, the mutually supportive relationship between the medical school and the town came into play. Ann Arbor again contributed half as much, another $4,000.

The new Pavilion Hospital was composed of two new frame structures (each 114 feet by 30 feet). It was built onto the existing hospital building and opened in 1876. The new facility's design was inspired by the most modern, "healthy" hospital concept of the mid-nineteenth century. Florence Nightingale described a pavilion hospital as "a separate detached hospital, which has . . . as little connexion in its ventilation with any other part of the hospital" for optimal light and fresh-air circulation.[134] Michigan's new pavilion expanded the hospital's patient capacity to sixty beds and allowed for more clinical focus on fields like ophthalmology.

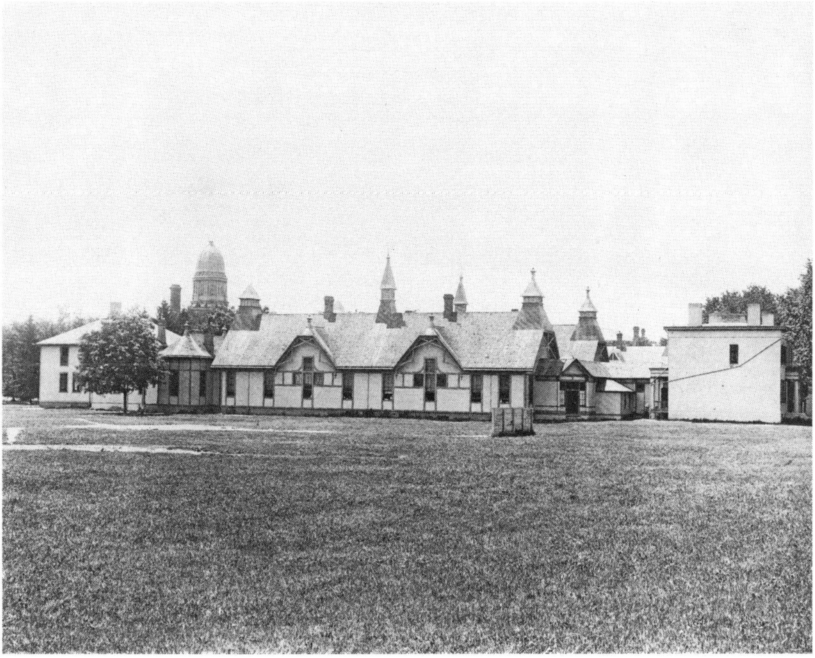

University Hospital, 1887. The original hospital is seen on the right, with the 1876 Pavilion Hospital addition built on the rear of the original structure. The surgical amphitheater addition is visible on the left. University of Michigan Photographs Vertical File, Bentley Historical Library, University of Michigan, Ann Arbor.

Despite its benefits, the Pavilion Hospital still posed challenges for patients and physicians. It was never intended to be permanent. Its basic frame construction was designed to allow it to be burned down when it became "hopelessly saturated with germs of disease" after a few years. It lacked a basement and adequate ventilation and also did not originally include an operating theater. In 1879, the university created a separate Homeopathic Hospital (including a surgical amphitheater) on the north side of campus, which housed that department until 1891.[135] This was the first time the medical school's "regular" hospital was equipped with its own dedicated space for surgical procedures.[136]

Training in obstetrics continued to pose a problem because the number of gynecological patients remained very low (only three cases were seen in 1877). Even fewer parturient women presented themselves as demonstration patients in the Pavilion Hospital. In 1879 Dunster, as obstetrics professor, issued a purchase request for the school's first obstetrical "manikin," a model to be used for clinical instruction, arguing that "from our position, we are unable to have clinics."[137] Manikins were widely used to teach deliveries, with some faculty claiming that such instruction was adequate to prepare a student to deliver babies. Even after the University Hospital expansion, Michigan faculty continued to grapple with conventions of modesty and gender expectations in the treatment of pregnant women. Sager presciently noted in his 1869 report to the regents that "the necessity of discriminating between patients who may or may not . . . with propriety be brought before the class will be obvious from a moments [*sic*] consideration."[138]

In the 1880s, the state passed legislation to provide for the free care of public University Hospital patients. They could receive treatment (and provide clinical instruction) free of charge. The medical faculty specifically indicated that the hospital was never meant to serve as a "public charity" but also should not restrict its services only "to those who were competent to meet the necessary charge." Instead, as Sager claimed, "the main object of a Hospital here is, and should ever be, to utilize for practiced instruction all the clinical material that may present itself for medical and surgical treatment."[139] The understanding was that all University Hospital patients, regardless of their financial means or social class, could be used for demonstration, study, or both. For a time in the early 1870s, the regents' committee on the medical school strongly recommended creating a large, modern state hospital (following the model set by Massachusetts), which would be attached to the medical school and provide service for the rich and poor alike. As one advocate stated, "not only are our alms-houses the repositories of many persons who are thus incarcerated to languish, suffer on and die without that aid to which the suffering poor are justly entitled, but many persons of wealth and refinement labor from diseases which if treated at all by the private practitioner, are treated but poorly, and with indifferent and unsatisfactory results." Sending these patients to the University of Michigan, described as "the best place 'in the West' for pursuing the 'higher clinical field of thought,'" therefore would be beneficial to all.[140]

Many of Michigan's medical professionals, however, believed that large clinics were not ideal for clinical instruction and refused to send paying patients to a teaching hospital. Conversely, the university worried that charging hospital fees would dissuade potential patients from availing themselves of the facility and seemed reluctant to request state funds for hospital construction. To be sure, Michigan's first University Hospital did not actually suffer a dearth of "teaching material"—in fact, additional beds had to be secured after its first full year of operation—but the Board of Regents remained concerned about striking a balance between operating a "free" teaching hospital and allowing that hospital to be self-supporting—a tension that remained well into the twentieth century.[141]

Conclusion

By the 1870s, the University of Michigan Medical School had experienced significant growth and found itself poised at the forefront of major reforms in medical education in the United States. At the start of that decade, requirements for admission remained relatively low, and each year's six-month academic term mostly consisted of didactic lectures and anatomical dissection. As historian Kenneth Ludmerer observes, "Students would graduate without having attended a delivery, without having witnessed an operation, and often without having examined a patient."[142] The recruitment of faculty members devoted to more innovative medical science and laboratory instruction, the creation (and subsequent expansion) of the University Hospital, and the change to a nine-month academic term in 1877 heralded a significant shift for Michigan's medical students and provided them with groundbreaking opportunities for laboratory and clinical education that were uncommon in the late nineteenth century.[143] However, the university would continue to contend with limitations and controversies that had been present at the medical school's inception. In particular, the school's location would remain a major concern for state legislators, the Board of Regents, and medical professors for years to come. What Ann Arbor's size, demographics, and geographic location would signify for faculty recruitment, hospital facilities, and patient availability, and the propriety of housing a homeopathic institute at the University of Michigan, would cause heated debates and scandals to erupt around the "country" medical school that was, by the end of the century, considered one of the best in the United States.

TWO

Finding an Identity

Leading Major Changes in American Medicine

Scientific theory started to change radically beginning around the mid-1870s, and medical practice followed not long thereafter. Foundational work in microbiology and bacteriology by scientists like the Frenchman Louis Pasteur and the German Robert Koch found an enthusiastic audience in both academic and popular circles. "Koch's postulates" for establishing the bacteriological causes of disease opened the floodgates to a near mania for identifying and cultivating the microscopic origins of infectious diseases, starting with tuberculosis and gonorrhea and rapidly moving on to anthrax, rabies, cholera, diphtheria, and typhoid fever. From all over the world people went to Europe to learn about new tools and techniques from the masters. In 1888 Michigan professors Victor Vaughan and Frederick Novy made the transatlantic trip. They attended Koch's Hygienic Institute at the University of Berlin and then visited Pasteur's laboratory in Paris, along the way acquiring not only ideas but also laboratory equipment to take back to Ann Arbor.[1]

Bacteriology advocates on both sides of the Atlantic built on the nascent movements of sanitary science and public health to publicize their innovative discoveries and to implement them in medical education, a transition made physically manifest by the laboratory tools and techniques used to study microorganisms.[2] As historian Kenneth Ludmerer concludes, "No development carried more force than the germ theory of disease and the emergence of modern bacteriology. . . . [The germ theory] prepared the way for the acceptance of a laboratory-based medical education more than any other single scientific event."[3] That acceptance, however, did not come without debate as late-nineteenth-century changes in medical thinking led to tensions about the relationships between theory and practice. Ludmerer describes the years between 1871 and 1893 as a period of both innovation and conflict at "pivotal" medical schools (including Michigan), characterized by "continuing skepticism about the utility of scientific knowledge in clinical practice."[4]

Other changes (and conflicts) of the time involved the increase of clinical exposure in the medical curriculum. Following the AMA's 1867 recommendations, medical schools in the United States began to discuss ways to incorporate patient care into education, but by the end of the 1870s, only five of them had adopted required clinical rotations for all graduates as part of a graded, three-year curriculum: Rush Medical College in Chicago, Harvard, the University of Pennsylvania, Syracuse, and the University of Michigan.[5] Institutions worried that educational reforms—laboratory instruction and research, clinical experience in a three-year program, or both—would necessitate higher admission standards, which could lead to devastating drops in enrollment. But new facilities meant added expenses and increasing operating costs, so schools that ultimately adopted these reforms had to establish and maintain limits on class size.[6]

At the University of Michigan administrators and faculty members were quick to embrace the heightened expectations of scientific medical training and to implement the improvements necessary to put the university at the forefront of progressive education. University president James B. Angell pushed for more stringent entry requirements for medical students in the mid-1870s, arguing that "efforts at inspired medical teaching" would be wasted on unprepared students.[7] Ophthalmology chair George E. Frothingham (an alumnus of Michigan's program) argued against "the so-called classical education, that is, a profound knowledge of the dead languages," as suitable preliminary education for medical students and instead called for more modern, scientific requirements.[8] According to Vaughan, "'the University of Michigan Medical School was from the start a scientific in contradistinction to a practical or clinical institution.'"[9] Such enthusiasm in Ann Arbor, however, was not without disagreement. Speaking from the platform of the Michigan Medical Society, a number of local doctors (some of whom were faculty members) worried that too much emphasis on scientific theory and research would lead to a decline in the quality of treatment and that practitioners should focus less on the microscopic origins of disease and more on other factors, including air quality, climate, and location. Whatever the content of the instruction was to be, the issue of social context was particularly close to Vaughan's heart. Well aware of the sometimes questionable reputation of the medical profession, he wanted instead to emphasize the

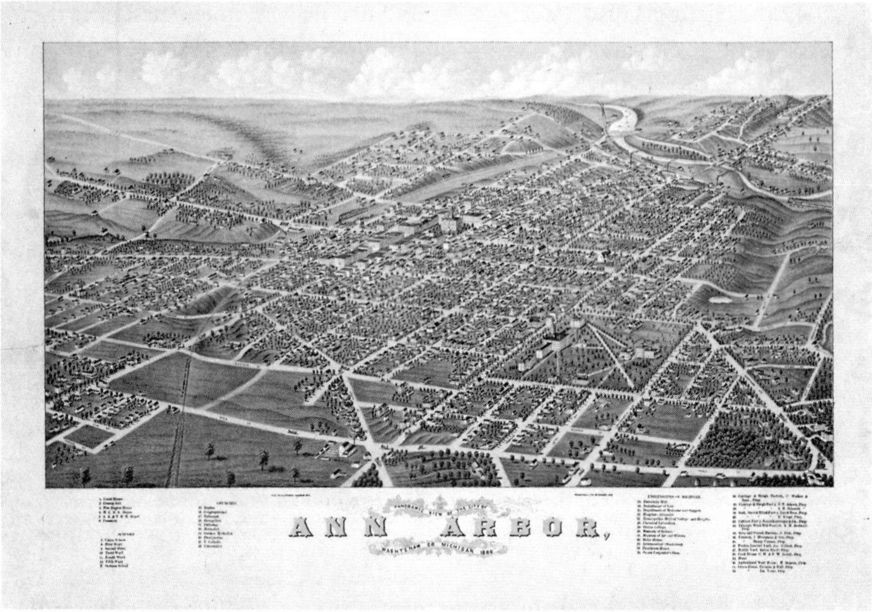

Bird's-eye view of Ann Arbor, Washtenaw County, Michigan, 1880. A. Ruger. Bentley Historical Library, University of Michigan, Ann Arbor.

importance of gentlemanly "cultivation" among the medical school faculty. In other words, he wanted to create a thriving, collegial productive community of scholars in the small town.[10] The school at times found itself torn between the impulse to provide new, more scientific instruction and research capabilities and the responsibility to provide doctors who would care for Michigan residents.[11]

Ann Arbor Moves into the Twentieth Century

After the Civil War, new railroad lines connected Ann Arbor with surrounding communities. From 1837 the Michigan Central Railroad (running east to west) had linked the town to industries in Detroit, but from 1878 the Ann Arbor Railroad ran north to south. By the end of the next decade, the town had constructed an impressive new stone railroad depot in Romanesque style (now a seafood restaurant) and built nearby freight facilities to enable the increase in railroad traffic. In 1890, the first streetcars began operating, with an interurban line between Ann Arbor and neighboring Ypsilanti opening the following year and an electric car line to Detroit in operation by 1898. Telephone exchanges in Ann Arbor began to appear in the late 1880s, and the first "modern" garbage removal and incineration program was introduced in 1905.[12]

Through all of these changes the university and its medical school remained defining features of the town. In 1891, an article in the *Ann Arbor Register* titled "Michigan's Pride" stated, "at one time the [University of Michigan's] college of medicine and surgery enjoyed the distinction of being the largest in the United States. It still is firmly established in public estimation as one of the best."[13] Certainly, Ann Arbor residents lauded their medical school and the services it provided, particularly during local outbreaks of diseases such as smallpox, typhoid fever, and malaria.[14] But in many other ways, it was the university as a whole that was the heart of Ann Arbor's society and commerce and contributed to the town's growth and modernization.

The University of Michigan experienced its most significant growth during the late nineteenth and early twentieth centuries; by the 1880s it rivaled Harvard University in size. According to one historian, "Word spread widely that at Michigan there was a spirit of democracy and tolerance in the student body that was inviting. . . . Ann Arbor was hospitable."[15] Residents exhibited considerable civic pride in their status as a "university town" and offered funding for a number of university facilities, including those associated with the medical school and a 4,300-seat auditorium. The Ann Arbor Civic Association's motto, adopted in 1913, lauded the town as a "City of Knowledge and Homes."[16]

Ann Arbor, however, was clearly not a big city, and its small size was especially apparent given the town's proximity to Detroit. From 1900 to 1910, the population of Ann Arbor grew from 14,509 to 14,817, but that of Detroit grew from 285,704 to 465,706.[17] In fact, historian Jonathan Marwil argues that the university population created "something of a mirage" as regards the size of Ann Arbor and that the university's presence and reputation masked the fact that the town's resident population growth and industrial development were slow compared with other Michigan cities.[18] The expansion of public transportation networks linking Ann Arbor to other markets and industries led local businesses to worry about competing with their more urban counterparts. The *Ann Arbor Democrat* noted that "merchants were worrying about 'a certain class of people' who preferred taking their trade to Detroit, 'imagining that in no smaller city than Detroit can they satisfy their wants.'"[19] Thus, even as Ann Arbor and its university grew and prospered,

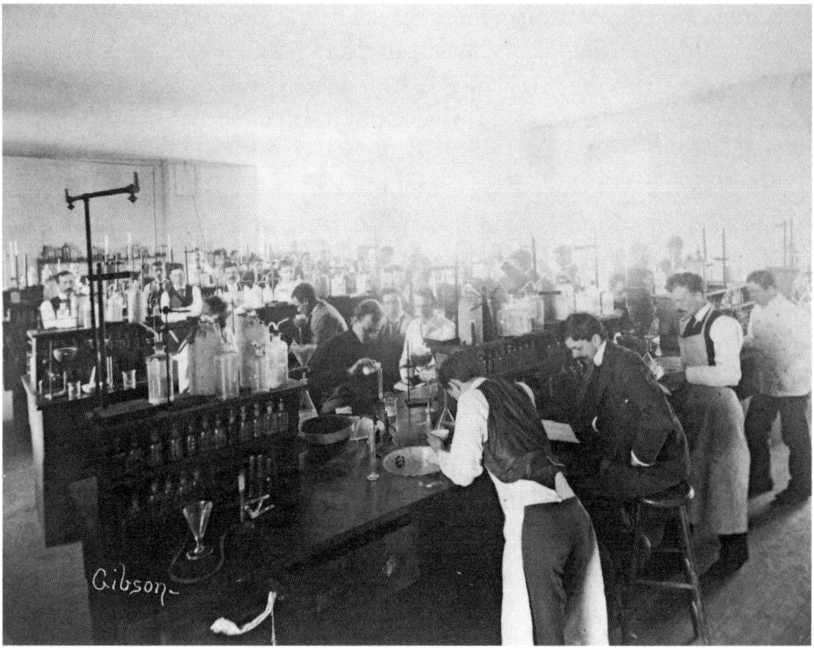

Physiological chemistry laboratory, ca. 1893. Medical School (University of Michigan) Records, 1850–2010, Bentley Historical Library, University of Michigan, Ann Arbor.

there was a constant, self-conscious comparison with their nearby urban neighbor. That contrast exerted a tremendous influence on a variety of institutions and developments in the modernizing town and university, not least on the quickly growing medical school.

New Directions at the Medical School

The medical school was one of a handful of medical schools in the United States to implement several revolutionary changes to its basic curriculum and requirements during the late nineteenth century. After 1879, the three-year program became mandatory—making Michigan one of the first medical schools in the nation to institute such a reform—with a regent-approved committee of "local physicians in practice" to report on its success.[20] Scientific laboratory work was an integral element in the expansion. Unlike the original curriculum, in which students sat through the same class twice, the

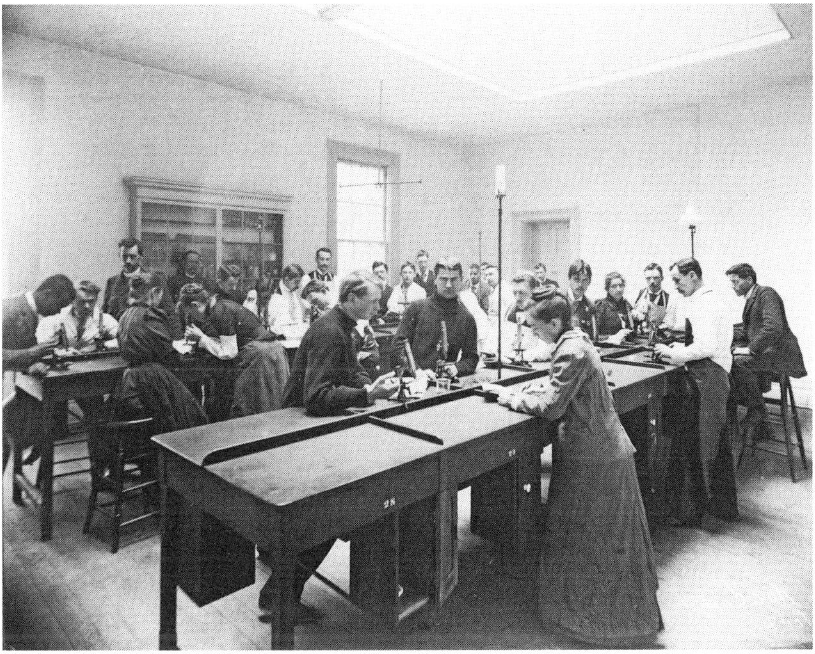

Physiological chemistry microscopic work, ca. 1893. Medical School (University of Michigan) Records, 1850–2010, Bentley Historical Library, University of Michigan, Ann Arbor.

school now offered different classes each year. Students were required to take both organic chemistry and "chemical laboratory" coursework in each of the first two years, and bacteriology and "practical hygiene" were offered in the senior (third) year.[21] However, to some members of the faculty, even three years did not seem sufficient to teach the rapidly expanding world of medical knowledge along with clinical instruction. In the fall of 1887, Professor Victor Vaughan sent a resolution to the Board of Regents that "the Science and Art of Medicine in its present and prospective expansion, with the many specialties into which it tends to be divided, requires a much longer period of study and of College and Hospital instruction than is provided for in the ordinary Medical Schools of this Country." Vaughan suggested that a fourth year, "devoted chiefly to Clinical Specialties," would be necessary.[22] In 1890, the Michigan medical school's curriculum was extended to become one of the nation's first four-year programs. It included a combination of lecture and laboratory courses in all semesters of the first three years (with an

647

UNIVERSITY OF MICHIGAN,

DEPARTMENT OF MEDICINE AND SURGERY.

ORDER OF EXERCISES, SECOND SEMESTER, 1889-90.

SENIORS.

	Mon.	Tues.	Wed.	Thur.	Fri.
Theory and Practice	5-R	11:30 1:30C	----	----	11:30 1:30C
Obstetrics and Gynæcology	11:30	10:30 2:30C	5-R	11:30	2:30C
Diseases of Children	----	----	11:30	----	----
Surgery	10:30 2:30C	----	10:30	2:30C	10:30 5-R
Hygiene	----	----	----	10:30	----
Pathology	9:30	----	----	9:30	----
Ophthalmology, Otology and Diseases of Upper Air Passages	1:30C	----	9:30	1:30C 5-R	----
Minor Surgery and Bandaging	----	5	----	----	----
Diseases of the Nervous System	----	9:30	2:30C	----	9:30
Practical Pathology and Bacteriology	2	2	2	2	2
Practical Hygiene	2-5	2-5	2-5	2-5	2-5

JUNIORS.

	Mon.	Tues.	Wed.	Thur.	Fri.
Theory and Practice	----	11:30	----	----	11:30
Physiology	11:30	----	11:30	11:30	----
Surgery	10:30	----	10:30	----	10:30
Surgical Anatomy, Operative Surgery,	----	10:30	----	10:30	----
Organic Chemistry	----	9:30	9:30R	9:30	----
General Therapeutics and Materia Medica,	9:30	----	----	----	9:30
Practical Anatomy	2-5	2-5	2-5	2-5	2-5
Chemical Laboratory	2-5	2-5	2-5	2-5	2-5
Practical Physiology	----	----	----	2-5	2-5

FRESHMEN.

	Mon.	Tues.	Wed.	Thur.	Fri.
Hygiene	11:30	----	11:30	11:30	----
Physiology	----	11:30	----	----	11:30
Descriptive Anatomy	10:30	----	10:30	----	10:30
Materia Medica and Therapeutics,	9:30	10:30	----	10:30	9:30
Organic Chemistry	----	9:30	9:30R	9:30	----
Practical Histology	2-5	2-5	2-5	----	----
Chemical Laboratory	2-5	2-5	2-5	2-5	2-5

C—Clinic R—Recitation. [OVER] *Courier Print.*

Weekly schedule of classes, 1889–1890. Miscellaneous, 1894–1903, Box 135, Medical School (University of Michigan) Records, 1850–2010, Bentley Historical Library, University of Michigan, Ann Arbor.

expanded, three-month laboratory course in bacteriology) and a senior year containing "theory and practice" credits for surgery, ophthalmology, gross pathology, gynecology, dermatology, and diseases of the nervous system, as well as "medical jurisprudence" in the second semester.[23]

The growing emphasis on bacteriology at the medical school dovetailed with a focus on laboratory science in other departments of the university. Beginning in 1877, the Physiological Laboratory established instruction in microscopy and histology, and in 1881 the faculty called for the creation of a chair in experimental physiology. The following year, the physiologist Henry Sewall from Johns Hopkins took on that position, and during his short tenure at Michigan, he inaugurated a new approach to medical instruction that revolutionized the school's curriculum not just in physiology but in a number of its other subjects.[24] Students were expected to play a more active role in their own education. This was true even in subjects that had long been part of the curriculum. For example, beginning in 1889 the anatomical laboratory course required students to dissect and prepare their own materials, which was a considerable investment for the school's resources and students' schedules.[25]

During this transition, the medical school also began its shift to follow a German-inspired "modern" standard of medical education, which imitated what many notable faculty members had experienced in their own studies abroad. This created the medical school's first significant cohort of "academic physicians"—that is, faculty members who devoted their primary attentions to research rather than private practice. In 1891 John Jacob Abel, for example, became the first professor of experimental pharmacology in the United States (with vivisection demonstrations as part of his lectures) and one of the first prominent medical school instructors to abandon private practice opportunities in favor of a full-time research career.[26] He was soon followed by other professors who shared his devotion to research. Looking back on his experiences as chair of the school's internal medicine department, Professor Albion Walter Hewlett applauded the phenomenon of expecting physicians to search for new knowledge, noting that Michigan's emphasis on research and its necessary facilities had been, and would continue to be, a driving force in the institution's development.[27] Certainly, such an expectation for instructors was not always financially advantageous—in the 1890s, Vaughan jokingly admitted that Michigan's "unsurpassed" medical professors constituted "a full time faculty on less than half time pay"[28]—but it elevated the medical school in Ann Arbor to a new, higher standard of faculty accomplishment. This trend helped the University of Michigan to have one of the first and most notable scientific medical schools in the country.

Praise for the medical school sometimes arrived from quarters that may seem unexpected from a modern perspective. Arguably the leading industrial group in the United States at the turn of the twentieth century was the railroad industry (also a leader in sending patients to seek medical care after industrial accidents). Managerial and organizational innovations from railroads were eagerly imitated by many other industries, including health care.[29] It is therefore noteworthy that in 1896 the railroad publication *Ann Arbor Headlight* proudly stated that "the [medical] Faculty has constantly endeavored to give the courses of instruction in the most scientific manner . . . at a time when such instruction was not given elsewhere in this country except in the most superficial manner."[30] Clearly, Michigan's approach to medical instruction and practice was celebrated in a number of circles, professional and public alike.

Laboratory work often involved looking at small objects under a microscope. But the new scientific ideas also led people to look outward and apply bacteriological insights to matters involving the health of the larger community. Academic physicians and medical educators were often in the vanguard of public health and sanitary movements during the Progressive era, being "as important to that movement as they were to the development of medical education."[31] The field we now know as "public health" had not yet differentiated from that of medicine, and it was not unusual for medical school leaders, most notably Victor Vaughan, to play a major role in studying and advocating for community health.

Victor C. Vaughan and Other Scientists

In many ways, Vaughan was the exemplar of Michigan's move toward scientific medical instruction, the rise of the academic physician, and the role of the medical school in community health.[32] But his early years in Ann Arbor did not presage the important part that he ultimately played in the institution's development. After receiving his Ph.D. in chemistry (one of the first two doctorates conferred by the University of Michigan), Vaughan was denied promotion to full-time faculty status because of charges of "atheism."[33] However, he continued teaching at the institution's Chemical Laboratory as a temporary assistant while attending the medical school and eventually received a permanent appointment. After earning his medical degree in 1878,

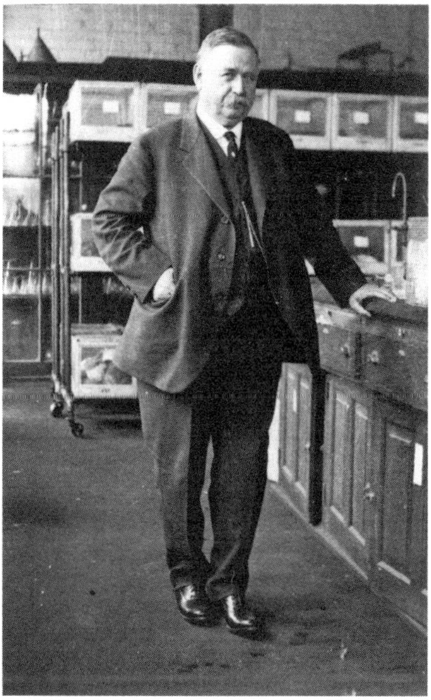

Victor C. Vaughan, ca. 1915. Victor C. Vaughan Papers, Bentley Historical Library, University of Michigan, Ann Arbor.

he began teaching and practicing medicine at the university and in the larger community. Within just a few years, Vaughan's involvement in local sanitary and public health interventions catapulted him to national attention. He eventually became one of the most influential deans in the country, as well as in the medical school's history. Never one to shy away from a national spotlight, Vaughan was a major and a division surgeon during the Spanish-American War, and he coauthored an influential report on the spread of typhoid fever in military camps during that conflict. He then worked with the U.S. Army and the U.S. Surgeon General's Office, for which he was in charge of communicable diseases and was active in helping control the influenza pandemic in the late 1910s. He advocated for the creation of the Hygienic Laboratory, the first in the United States to provide systematic practical instruction in bacteriology.[34] Vaughan served as dean from 1891 to 1921 and played a key role in establishing the relatively new field of preventive medicine.[35]

One of Vaughan's early investigations was of an apparently cheese-based toxin. This episode exemplifies how what we would now call a local public health investigation could link with laboratory science and have national implications. In August 1883, more than a dozen people in Oxford, Michigan (north of Detroit), experienced the near-simultaneous onset of sudden, violent nausea, dryness and constriction in the throat, and diarrhea.[36] Searching for the chemical origins of the outbreak, Vaughan found "sick" cheese in a dairy in Lenawee County, Michigan. Laboratory analysis identified a crystalline alkaloid that Vaughan named "tyrotoxicon" (combining the Greek words for "cheese" and "poison") and classified as a "ptomaine," or "chemical poison [that] might be generated by the growth of bacteria."[37] Such a "cadaveric alkaloid" had already been identified in meats, but Vaughan was the first American scientist to claim that ptomaines also could be found in dairy products. Vaughan first tested its toxicity by feeding the crystals to puppies and kittens. He then tested the substance on human subjects (his students, as well as himself). The test material reproduced the characteristic symptoms of throat dryness, nausea, vomiting, and diarrhea, demonstrating that it was the cause of the illness.[38]

Despite the fact that no clearly fatal cases were reported,[39] the disease evoked considerable fear, not least because tyrotoxicon seemed impossible to identify without laboratory analysis. According to the *Ann Arbor Courier*, "sick" cheese was virtually indistinguishable from good cheese, and "there is no certain means aside from a chemical examination, by which a poisonous cheese can be distinguished from a wholesome one."[40] Vaughan was able to assuage these fears in part by demonstrating that grocers and the general public could use a simple litmus test to determine whether cheese might be "suspicious": a piece of blue litmus paper (available at many drugstores, the newspaper expressly stated) pressed against a freshly cut cheese surface would redden "instantly and intensely" if tyrotoxicon was present.[41] Although Vaughan had heightened public alarm about the poisoning outbreak, he was able to also provide a simple solution to ease those fears. His methods derived from, and enhanced the power of, the new techniques of laboratory science.

These findings brought Vaughan national attention and acclaim. Tyrotoxicon (as well as other ptomaines) became a popular trend in early bacteriological research.[42] More importantly, Vaughan's investigations established him as an expert in the rapidly growing fields of bacteriology and public health. He argued that tyrotoxicon was linked with other widespread diseases such as cholera infantum and typhoid. Vaughan published his findings in both professional journals and popular magazines, including *Popular Science Monthly*, and his achievements became the source of considerable local pride. An 1893 column in the *Ann Arbor Argus* took issue with the claim that Vaughan was "better known in England than America, and more appreciated in New York than in Michigan," stating proudly that "the east is beginning to find out that low-necked clams, long-tailed coats and the gold standard never yet discovered tyrotoxicon in cheese."[43]

In 1885, Vaughan received the American Public Health Association's Lomb Prize for his essay on domestic hygiene in the working classes. His success put him in a position to influence the Michigan legislature and the university's Board of Regents to fund the school's Hygienic Laboratory in 1887. Originally located in the West Physics Building, the laboratory was the first university facility (and only the second worldwide) designed to serve the state by being able to analyze water, food, and other substances that could affect health in the United States. Before 1907 the laboratory was the state public health board's sole facility and was instrumental in identifying the bacteria responsible for typhoid fever epidemics and other outbreaks of disease.[44]

For some of its more zealous supporters, the germ theory seemed to promise an end to all human maladies. The ability to identify the causative bacterial agents for food poisoning and typhoid fever contributed significantly to bacteriology's dominance as "scientific orthodoxy" in medical training, research, and practice by the turn of the twentieth century.[45] However,

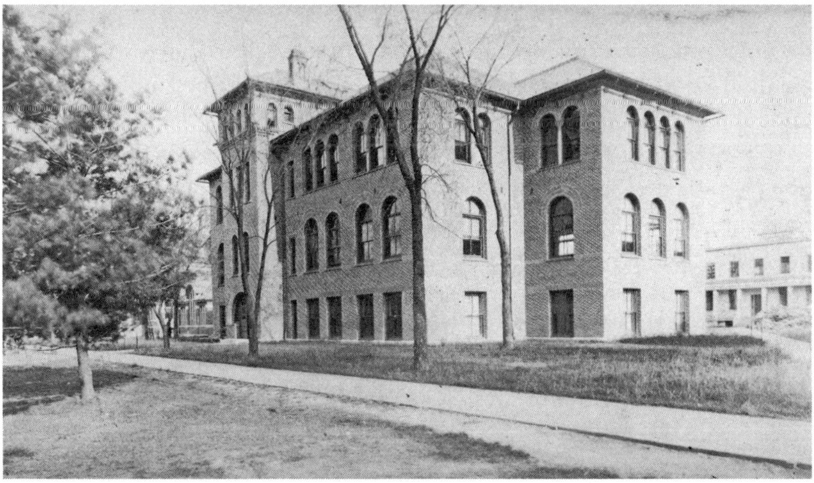

West Physics Building, ca. 1900 (completed in 1888). The Hygienic Laboratory was located on its upper floors until 1903. University of Michigan Photographs Vertical File, Bentley Historical Library, University of Michigan, Ann Arbor.

skeptics hesitated to accept Vaughan's conclusions. Some Michigan physicians disavowed the microbiological explanations for cheese poisoning, while others claimed that chemical preservatives used in dairies and groceries (and often recommended by sanitary reformers) were to blame.[46] Moreover, Vaughan himself later determined that tyrotoxicon, and ptomaines more generally, were not the sole cause of dairy food toxicity. Some samples of "sick" products showed no signs of the crystalline substance. The disease gradually abated, and by the early 1900s there were hardly any reports of tyrotoxicon poisoning. Whether that was due to improved sanitation in food preparation and storage or because tyrotoxicon never actually existed is difficult to determine. In 1909, Vaughan admitted that "practically nothing is known regarding the precise chemical nature of these bacterial poisons."[47] Vaughan's 1926 memoir hardly mentions his tyrotoxicon investigations at all.[48] Nonetheless, his involvement with and discoveries during Michigan's "sick" cheese and other dairy poisoning outbreaks unquestionably brought him and the University of Michigan to national attention and became a significant source of local pride. Notoriety and public acceptance of scientific, laboratory-based medicine, along with demonstrations of its practical utility, enhanced the growing focus on chemistry and bacteriology at the medical school. Bacteriology had become a standard requirement of the curriculum as early as 1885. In 1891, it was divided into two separate courses, bacteriology and hygiene (the latter of which Vaughan continued to teach until he retired in 1921).

Other notable scientists taught and conducted research in the rapidly expanding worlds of laboratory science. Frederick Novy trained under Vaughan at Michigan, joined Vaughan on his European tour in 1888, and became assistant director of the Hygienic Laboratory before he received his M.D. in 1891.[49] After that, he joined the Michigan faculty as assistant professor of hygiene and physiological chemistry. Novy wrote a seminal text, *Directions for Laboratory Work in Bacteriology*; developed revolutionary methods for cultivating anaerobic bacteria; was the first scientist to obtain cultures of *Trypanosoma brucei* in blood infected with tsetse fly disease; and was commissioned to investigate the 1900 San Francisco bubonic plague outbreak. Henry Sewall also gave lectures on bacteriology and conducted his own research on ptomaines. His pioneering work on antivenom serum therapy for rattlesnake bites in 1887 showed that the toxin's effects on experimental animals (pigeons) could be ameliorated by repeated exposure.[50] The medical school also worked with the pharmaceutical industry, teaming up with Detroit firm Parke, Davis and Co. to produce diphtheria antitoxin in the

1890s to be used to inoculate horses in Detroit. Their blood would be used to develop a serum for treatment in humans, an early, dramatic example of a life-saving laboratory medicine. In 1902 George Dock conducted a major study on malaria. He personally gathered data on Ann Arbor mosquitoes by tromping through the surrounding countryside to find mosquito larvae, extending the research field outside the world of the scientific laboratory, both figuratively and literally.[51] All of these interventions were potentially beneficial to the local Michigan community. Vaughan (among others) certainly was aware that the school's research and involvement in public health could lead to significant financial aid for the institution, and he has been called one of several "exceptional fund-raisers" in the history of American medical science.[52]

However, not all faculty members at the University of Michigan supported such activity. As early as 1883, John Jacob Abel complained that then-professor Vaughan was ignoring his university work (or delegating it to his assistants) to focus on so many other duties and "local political ambitions."[53] Others questioned the growing focus on bacteriological investigations and raised fundamental questions about "germ theories" of disease more generally. In 1888, pathology chair Heneage Gibbes began offering coursework in practical bacteriology in the anatomical laboratory. Earlier in his career Gibbes had been a member of the British Cholera Commission, which was sent to India to investigate Koch's claim that he had identified the organism responsible for cholera. Gibbes was skeptical of assertions that the bacillus was in fact the cause of the disease. He argued instead that cholera and tubercle bacilli "were merely adventitious organisms" rather than causative agents—that is, that although they might well be present in people with the disease, those organisms were not actually the cause, but a result of the disease. In 1894, Gibbes even stated that he had "accidentally inoculated himself with active tuberculosis bacilli yet did not contract the disease."[54] Gibbes was certainly not alone in his skepticism among Michigan practitioners; a number of other physicians were convinced that diseases (particularly epidemics) were related more to urbanization and poor sanitation than to germs and questioned the ethics of microbiological research. However, those views were facing increasing disfavor in many circles. Even Robert Koch had heard of Gibbes; Vaughan recollected that during a visit to Berlin, "Koch spoke bitterly of Gibbes . . . [and] condemned the University for having a professor . . . who did not accept the 'germ theory' as fact."[55] Back in Ann Arbor, the Board of Regents voted in 1895 to "unseat" Gibbes and installed George Dock as chair of both medicine and pathology. Gibbes's subsequent career is yet another reminder of how long it takes disease theories to change. Although he had been dismissed from the University of Michigan for doubting the new scientific theory, Gibbes continued teaching at the Michigan Medical College in Detroit and became the health officer of the city of Detroit, a position for which his views opposing the germ theory seem not to have disqualified him.[56]

Curricular Innovations of the Progressive Era

The emphasis on research and scientific medicine influenced not only the intellectual milieu but also the physical structure of the medical school. Older buildings were renovated and new ones were built. In addition to the new Hygienic Laboratory and the University Hospital on Catherine Street in 1891 (discussed later in this chapter), a two-story anatomy building was erected in 1887, and the West Medical Building was completed in 1903 for $200,000, more than fivefold the cost of all previous medical school structures combined. This new facility, on West University Street, housed most preclinical departments and was intended to support scientific research using laboratory animals. The building was designed around an open court, with a carriageway for the delivery of anatomical and vivisection specimens, mainly dogs.[57]

The tremendous amount of medical knowledge being generated and published (at Michigan and elsewhere) opened the possibility of a new approach to maintaining a medical library. When Michigan's medical school opened, there seemed to be little reason to subscribe to medical journals. The first graduates of the school had been encouraged to learn medicine from the ancient Greeks, whose understanding of the body was said to be the equal of any person of the time.[58] Only thirty years later this sort of worship of ancient ideas was no longer possible. Instead, it was understood that knowledge was constantly changing and that the medical school needed to keep abreast of those changes. Vaughan persuaded each professor in the school to allocate his annual book allowance (which Davenport claims was a staggering $200, or approximately $5,000 in 2017 dollars) to the medical library, reflecting in his memoir that "a medical school without a good research library is like an automobile without gasoline; it will not go."[59] By 1905 the school's library contained 13,455 volumes and held subscriptions to 266 journals (including eighty-nine complete sets). Vaughan realized that while science was progressing in the United States, most of the major new ideas in medicine continued to come from the more established medical institutions abroad. As a result, Michigan was one of the nation's first medical schools to prioritize subscriptions to international medical journals.[60] More knowledge meant that physicians had more to keep up with once they left school. To respond to that need, in 1892 the medical school also approved a postgraduate education program, allowing physicians to enter six-week summer courses in a number of subjects, including hygiene and bacteriology. The changes in medical science illuminated a need for ongoing professional development, and the University of Michigan continued offering that particular summer program until the 1920s.[61]

The late nineteenth and early twentieth centuries also saw the growth of medical specialization, a trend that was reflected in the establishment of new or expanded medical school departments at Michigan.[62] Syphilis was a common disease. It was ubiquitous especially in the teaching of medical students: one oft-quoted aphorism was "The physician who knows syphilis knows medicine." Because of the striking cutaneous manifestations of the disease, "dermatology and syphilology" were seen as a nearly inextricable pairing. Courses on the subject started in 1890, and when a specialized department was established in 1912, Michigan became one of the few U.S. medical schools to have an independent Department of Dermatology and Syphilology.

The school's Department of Neurology started in 1888 when Professor William Herdman began offering senior-level instruction in "nervous and mental diseases" (limited to several short weekly lectures, a single quiz, and a Wednesday afternoon demonstration clinic). In the 1890s a variety of elective courses, such as "physiological psychology" (taught by psychology professor Walter Pillsbury), were also available to senior students, who furthermore had opportunities for clinical experience in the field at state hospitals in Pontiac and Kalamazoo. By 1901 the Michigan legislature, having been swayed by Herdman's advocacy, appropriated $50,000 to create a psychopathic hospital at the university.[63] In his annual report for 1900–1901, President Angell noted that the ward was vital for "our medical students to study some of the problems of alienism."[64] Neurology and psychiatry eventually assumed two different, distinctive sorts of fundamental concepts and clinical practices. In 1907 the teaching and clinical functions were separated, but the two were combined into a single Department of the Diseases of the Mind and Nervous System. In 1920 neurology and psychiatry became two separate departments, reflecting growing interest in both areas, as well as an increasing tendency to form departments based on specific areas of focus and/or research.

Other innovations came from the widespread availability of new technology, perhaps most notably electricity in its many manifestations. The medical school began to offer more lessons in electrotherapeutics, initially organized by general chemistry and physics professor John W. Langley. Despite some controversy about the topic in the medical school—one of the assistants allegedly had advertised to sell an "electrical belt" to local customers—electrotherapeutics and neurology became the primary focus of the nervous and mental disease curriculum by the 1890s.[65] In 1900, electrotherapeutics was a required part of the junior year course, and the institution devoted a considerable amount of its space and budget to "apparatus for generating all kinds of electrical current." In 1902 the faculty considered renovating the anatomy laboratory to house its electrotherapeutics program, indicating the medical school's desire to invest in the technology and, by extension, the departments that utilized it.[66]

One of the school's most notable curriculum developments of this time was its transformation of clinical medical instruction, spearheaded in large part by George Dock. Dock joined Michigan's medical faculty in 1891, after training with the noted American physician William Osler and spending two years studying in Germany with distinguished scientists. Dock came to Ann Arbor with considerable experience in pediatrics, particularly infant feeding, at a time when relatively few medical schools in the United States required pediatric coursework.[67] In May 1892, the Board of Regents authorized new demonstration courses, "junior sections," for third-year students in medicine, obstetrics, surgery, ophthalmology, otolaryngology, and (after 1896) roentgenology. Over the next several years these clinical courses became mandatory for all graduates; however, the courses initially relied on hired assistants to conduct the demonstrations, rather than allowing students to have direct, hands-on experience with patients.[68]

But Dock had an even more innovative curriculum in mind. In 1899, after returning from service as an assistant surgeon in the U.S. Army, Dock introduced a clinical clerkship program as a basic requirement for internal medicine, radically transforming the course. Third-year medical students were now required to work with teaching patients at the University Hospital and to participate actively in their care. Although Osler had instituted a similar service at Johns Hopkins University, such a program was virtually nonexistent elsewhere in the United States. Other institutions recognized the value of teaching hospitals and clinical exposure, but they resisted the implementation of mandatory clerkships, noting concerns about how the public might react to medical students caring directly for patients. In Ann

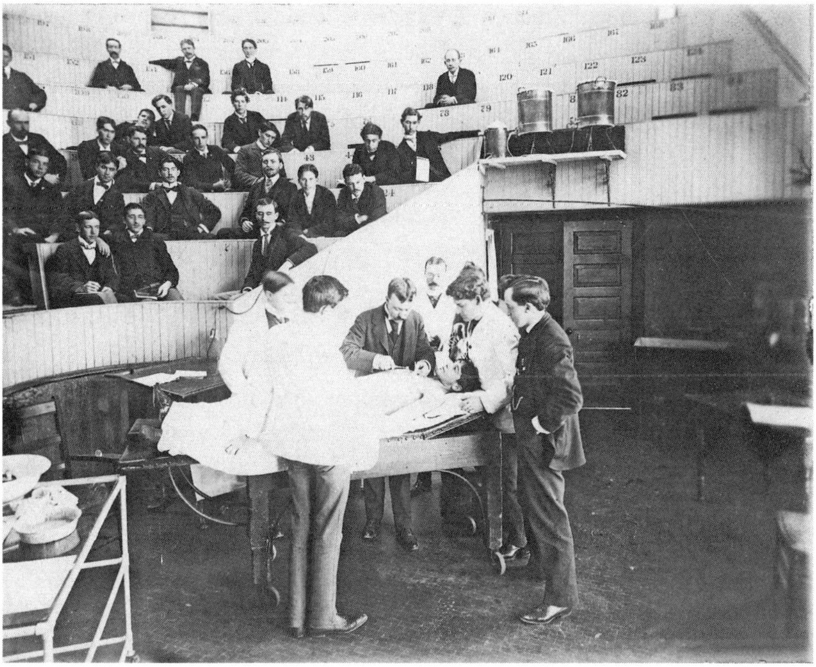

George Dock's clinic in the surgical amphitheater, 1898. G. M. Livingston. Medical School (University of Michigan) Records, 1850–2010, Bentley Historical Library, University of Michigan, Ann Arbor.

Arbor, Dock and his assistant, Aldred Scott Warthin, reached out to the local population, recruiting teaching patients with the aid of local clergy and other community leaders and relying on the good reputation (and growing patient base) of the University Hospital to provide a decent number of training cases.[69] Dock believed that "thorough study of a few patients was preferable to cursory study of many patients in a large municipal hospital."[70] This pedagogical reform, like the school's increasing utilization of laboratory science during this same time period, constituted a revolutionary shift away from passive observation and toward active learning and critical thinking both in the laboratory and on the wards. In this respect, Dock's teaching philosophy had much in common with the values of Progressive education espoused by the educational reformer John Dewey.[71]

Contemporary observers were astounded that such innovations—especially the medicine clerkship—could be implemented in a small town like

Ann Arbor. But it was precisely the medical school's direct control over the University Hospital that allowed Dock's clinical program to succeed; such control would have been much more difficult to implement in a city or charity hospital.[72] Thus, by the early years of the twentieth century, the University of Michigan was pioneering American medical education in both academic medicine and clinical instruction.

Building a Better Hospital

As the twentieth century approached, many American medical schools had followed Michigan's lead in owning and operating their own hospitals, and some came to be defined in part by those hospitals. But many, especially the smaller, proprietary schools, did not have (or have access to) a teaching hospital. While arguably important for education, hospitals continued to be marginal for most health care. Childbirth, surgery, illness, and death were seen as belonging in the home, not the hospital. Even in the late nineteenth century, popular opinion viewed most hospitals as places where people died in despair and obscurity.[73] Hospitals were simply not yet the dominant sites of physicians' practice. It was not uncommon at the time for a physician in the United States never to see, much less to enter, a hospital.

At the University of Michigan, the hospital was more than simply a physical structure. Its very existence and organization reflected its central role both for education and for patient care. The railroad expansion had made Ann Arbor's medical school and hospital more accessible for patients, students, and practitioners. Medical students regularly examined patients there, and the faculty boasted about the quality of care, claiming, "Our death-rate has been less than one-half that of any other hospitals with which we have compared [it]."[74] But the pavilion building, inarguably, was fast becoming outdated. Henry F. Lyster, a Detroit physician who served briefly as a Michigan instructor, noted in 1889 that, after more than a dozen years of operation, the Pavilion Hospital was indeed hopelessly contaminated; "all the wards are more or less infiltrated with septic material, and the hospital cannot be disinfected."[75] The only option for the school in the era of bacteriology was to erect a completely new structure.

The Pavilion Hospital was also ill-equipped to handle many types of patients, particularly in pediatrics and obstetrics. In 1887, several faculty members had appealed to Washtenaw, Wayne, and Jackson county administrators to send cases of unwed pregnant mothers to a "lying-in" ward at University

Hospital, but to little avail (and without much support from the Board of Regents). Concerns about impropriety in patient treatment also came to light that year, with accusations of "gross mismanagement" reaching a public audience.[76] Furthermore, the University Hospital was not the only care facility in the small town. Between the 1870s and the 1940s, at least seventeen small private hospital clinics with their own staffs and nurse training were housed in converted residences around Ann Arbor. Such proprietary hospitals were common in the United States at that time and constituted a considerable proportion of the rapidly expanding number of hospitals across the country. Some of those proprietary hospitals were owned and operated by Michigan faculty members, including pediatrician David Cowie and obstetrician Reuben Peterson. There they served patients (particularly women and children) from a population willing to pay for what they believed to be better service than they might receive at the university. Thus, professors at the medical school competed with the University Hospital while providing a valuable service to the local population.[77]

Given these issues, it is not surprising that a plan for the construction of a new, more modern University Hospital was approved in 1889. The project was funded by an initial appropriation of $50,000 from the state, and the city of Ann Arbor contributed an additional $25,000, signifying (yet again) the importance of the institution for the local community.[78] Although there was general agreement about the need for a new structure, there was a strong debate over its location, revealing tensions about how the hospital and medical school were to be related to the university. The Pavilion Hospital was located on the central campus, but President Angell insisted that the new facility be moved as far away from the campus as it could be, possibly because of fears of contamination. The medical faculty disagreed and in 1889 issued a statement protesting "against the location of the Hospital at a distance greater than one fourth mile from the medical building" on West University. They saw the hospital as an integral part of the university structure and claimed that keeping it on campus was in the school's best interests. As it was from the very start, the medical school was seen as an integral part of the university, both intellectually and physically. Ultimately, in 1891 a site on Catherine Street was selected, just northeast of the central campus. The new facility was ready for occupation the following year.[79]

This University Hospital reflected a new generation of hospitals in the United States. In addition to providing more up-to-date, antiseptic practices, the Catherine Street institution also introduced a more modern administrative system, one more clearly oriented toward professional training,

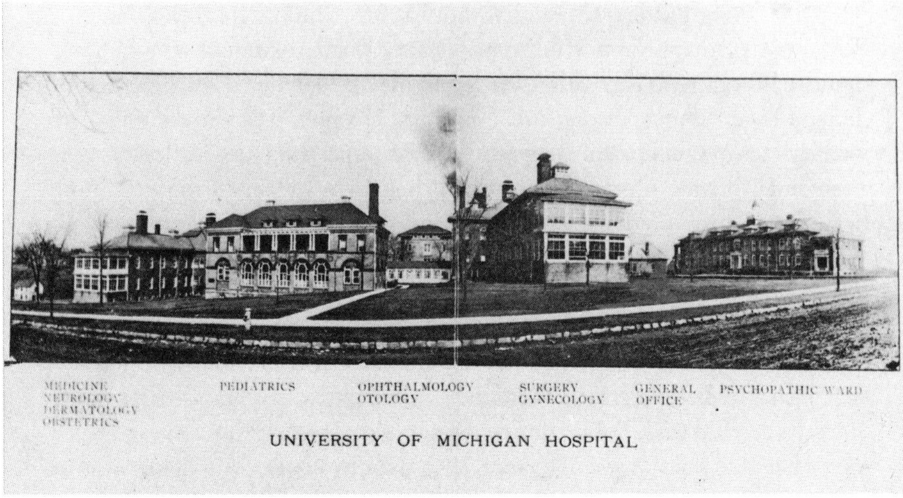

Catherine Street Hospital buildings, ca. 1906. University of Michigan Photographs Vertical File, Bentley Historical Library, University of Michigan, Ann Arbor.

which reflected similar changes occurring at a national level. For instance, the older positions of "ward master" and "ward mistress" were removed, and a hospital superintendent took over many managerial roles for hospital assistants and staff. The idea that hospitals ought to be managed systematically, with specific roles and departments, was just starting to take hold at that time.[80] The creation of a nursing service was one of those transitions. The medical school authorized a nursing school, which represented a sea change in hospital care when it opened in 1891. For most of the nineteenth century, the functions of hospital nurses had been provided by patients' family members or by patients who simply remained in the hospital after their medical issues had been resolved. When the first nursing schools opened in the United States in 1873, nursing functions started to become professionalized, and students learned their trade in hospital wards. Nursing schools not only offered education and a respectable career path for women but also provided an essential workforce for the hospital, since nursing students learned their trade on the wards. While some of their work was related to health care, a significant amount was often basic custodial services. By the end of the century, nurses had become necessary for most large hospitals (and quite a few small ones) to function. The University of Michigan's nursing students would provide essential services on the wards of the new hospital.[81]

The hospital also offered positions to medical graduates, or "internes," who worked alongside professors and advanced students on the wards. This was a shift away from the older clinical training system of solo apprenticeships. With training occurring in a medical hospital, it became possible to develop a formal curriculum and have oversight over preceptors; by training together, new practitioners developed more of a shared identity with medical students and other interns.[82] Graduate interns and senior medical students often actively cared for patients side by side. Interns' living accommodations were provided by the hospital, but they were cramped and unsanitary. In 1901, for example, five Michigan interns lived in one room "at the head of the stairs in the old surgical pavilion with inadequate toilet facilities," and a number of them suffered or even died from septic infections.[83]

Professor Albion Hewlett, for one, was concerned about the level of care provided by medical students and interns. When he came to the University of Michigan in 1908, he noted that the hospital's lack of private wards and relatively low salaries made it difficult to attract permanent medical assistants and visiting staff. Because the hospital also had a hard time recruiting graduates as interns, fourth-year students often did that work themselves—a practice that Hewlett found dangerous. Though he supported clinical instruction and active learning on the wards, Hewlett took issue with what he described as the "two classes of Internes" at University Hospital (meaning that both graduates and students were acting as interns) and claimed, "with a continual succession of students acting in this capacity, I feel that the hospital is in danger of some very unpleasant situations, possibly even of law suits."[84]

Postgraduate medical training soon started to become an integral part of specialization and hospital care at Michigan and elsewhere. Departments began offering programs in specific medical specialties that mandated one year as an intern in a general hospital setting. The Department of Otolaryngology (separated from ophthalmology) initiated one such program as early as 1906. Roy Bishop Canfield's appointment as clinical professor of diseases of the ear, nose, and throat marked a clear demarcation from the previous system, in which students had received more instruction on diseases of the eye. In 1905 Canfield was promoted to professor and the otolaryngology department was created. The following year he began hiring graduates for a three-year tenure at the hospital, with graded levels of responsibility, increased stipends, and a rotation system. This in many ways resembled what was to become a system of clinical residencies. After the ear, nose, and throat ward was added in 1913, more formal otolaryngology graduate training was implemented, and the training program lengthened to four and then to five years. Ultimately, residency programs would become standardized in a variety of specialties.[85]

Other services at the hospital became specialized in the early twentieth century. In 1903, Alonzo Palmer's widow bestowed a gift to the University Hospital to create a new ward, the Palmer Ward, intended primarily for children.[86] Herdman's brainchild, the Psychopathic Hospital, was approved in 1901 and designed to have a cooperative relationship with state asylums. Dock began sending his students there to observe cases in 1906. New equipment also entered the hospital, most notably early imaging technology. Five years after Roentgen rays were first demonstrated in Germany, surgical professors Charles B. G. De Nancrède and Cyrenus G. Darling used their own funds to purchase X-ray equipment for the hospital, and in 1903, the university allotted funds to create a Roentgen Laboratory in the basement of the Palmer Ward.[87] The equipment was initially maintained as part of the Department of Diseases of the Mind and Nervous System and Electrotherapeutics, until a new Department of Roentgenology was established in 1913. The Maternity Ward, which despite popular demand had been kept relatively small and underfunded ever since the new hospital opened, was relocated to a frame house west of the main hospital building in 1908. This move allowed for expanding its operation to include thirty beds, which enabled the hospital to house patients in earlier stages of pregnancy, rather than just perinatal cases. These women had the option of paying for their board by providing services to the hospital, such as sewing or preparing bandages. The location, however, was less than ideal, particularly after a noisy new trolley line for coal transport was laid directly between the "maternity cottage" and the delivery rooms, forcing patients in labor to cross the tracks.[88] That inconvenience notwithstanding, total patient population seen at University Hospital over the first two decades of the twentieth century steadily increased; between 1907 and 1915 alone, the total number of patients seen at University Hospital grew from 3,727 to 11,100.

The treatment of patients with contagious diseases had long been a problem for hospital care, as one sick patient could easily introduce an infection that might spread throughout the hospital. Beginning in 1902, Dock pleaded with the Board of Regents to create a contagious-disease ward, primarily for tuberculosis patients but also to be used in times of epidemics; Ann Arbor witnessed a serious outbreak of smallpox that year, which spread to a number of other Michigan towns by 1904. Dock argued that since "the hospital is always crowded to its full capacity," a separate ward for contagious disease was vital for both patients and students. Always the teacher, he pointed out that "sanatoria for chronic diseases run a serious risk of degenerating into asylums, but in a teaching hospital the many-sided criticism of students and assistants, and the repeated demonstration and investigation of each case prevent routinism." The ward would not have to be particularly large to be effective; indeed, as Dock argued, "a relatively small number of cases in various stages, carefully observed in a properly arranged hospital, can be made much more instructive than a larger number of out patients, imperfectly followed up."[89] Even a relatively small town like Ann Arbor might be an advantageous location for medical students to observe and treat infectious diseases such as tuberculosis.

After several abysmal attempts to create makeshift facilities for disease outbreaks—in 1909, during a scarlet fever epidemic, the University Hospital hastily converted two unheated summer houses into fever wards—the North Ward, or "pest house," officially opened in 1914. The city of Ann Arbor again helped fund the building, with another $25,000 contribution. The design featured a "new aseptic method . . . the second in America to adopt this plan," in which every room opened independently to the outside, and everyone entering a room was gowned.[90] Peterson, celebrating the new facility, noted that it was vital for student success in learning proper techniques for treating contagious patients, for "just as the student, drilled in surgical asepsis, is taught how to wash his hands and refrain from touching anything surgically unclean during an operation, he will be thoroughly drilled in the principles of medical asepsis, so that he neither will convey infection from one patient to another nor contract it himself."[91] Despite these admonitions, many students still came down with smallpox, typhoid fever, and other communicable diseases in the course of their studies. It is not surprising that Dock initially advised his students to observe North Ward patients through glass windows.[92]

Infection was not just limited to the hospital wards; at least one case at Michigan was a direct result of the new emphasis on bacteriology research. In 1900 a student working with Frederick Novy rolled and smoked a cigarette after handling a culture taken during an outbreak of bubonic plague in San Francisco. Shortly thereafter, the student developed the plague. He was isolated in the hospital and survived, though not before drawing intense interest from his fellow students. The American novelist Sinclair Lewis seems to have found the episode interesting. Much of his 1925 novel *Arrowsmith* was based on the University of Michigan, and the plot includes someone smoking a cigarette contaminated with plague germs (unlike the actual student, the novel's character died). Lewis likely modeled this plot twist on real-life experiences in Novy's lab.[93]

Most (but certainly not all) of the Catherine Street hospital patients were Michigan residents, many from rural parts of the state. George Dock's clinical notes indicate that he saw a number of farmers and lumbermen. In the late nineteenth century, he recruited one hundred rural patients for "an etiological study of tuberculosis in country people," a valuable data set for comparison with results gathered at Johns Hopkins in an urban population. The clinic also saw a number of immigrants and appears to have been racially integrated—in 1904, for example, Dock demonstrated "a young Negro girl from Gary, Indiana," who had been seen in both the neurology and gynecology services.[94] The primary reason for the hospital's existence was to provide students the opportunity to learn from clinical care, a priority that Hewlett warmly endorsed.[95] Thus, the Catherine Street facility (like the Pavilion Hospital before it) treated all patients free of charge, a policy that certainly helped arouse public support for the hospital. As Peterson recalled, "this idea was so thoroughly drilled into the people of Michigan that the clinical professors received letters in the early nineteen hundreds from people amply able to pay for medical services, saying they were willing to go 'before the class.'"[96] Local media lauded the university's new hospital, now impressively "on the brow of a high bluff overlooking the Huron river . . . a credit to the State of Michigan in every respect," and the medical school administration recognized that the hospital's good reputation and good deeds would benefit the medical school. As Warthin noted in 1920, "the result of the social service thus rendered to the state of Michigan by its university hospital has been a greatly increased appreciation of this service by the citizens, and a growing tendency toward a further development of this form of state medicine," not to mention better funding opportunities for renovations and expansions.[97] Within a decade the Catherine Street hospital was operating year-round. By 1908, the facility had more than two hundred beds in four main buildings, and during the following decade its services in pediatrics and contagious diseases increased dramatically, leading Hewlett to comment, "as far as size is concerned the future of the Hospital is secure."[98]

Size, however, was not the only measure of a hospital's worth, and the University Hospital continued to confront significant problems. One set had to do with the physical requirements for implementing the new scientific understandings of disease. An increasing number of laboratory studies were becoming essential for routine patient care. These included bacteriological cultures, stains for microscopy, chemical analyses of bodily fluids, and more. The studies required both space and (sometimes expensive) equipment. The

Catherine Street hospital simply did not have adequate onsite laboratory facilities. Perhaps reflecting an earlier style of medical care, the original designs for the new hospital had not included dedicated laboratory spaces, and laboratory apparatuses there had to be crammed into converted free spaces (like water closets) or hastily added outbuildings. Dock regretted the inconvenience of having student laboratories located on the main campus buildings, far removed from the hospital on Catherine Street.[99] In an 1899 letter, Peterson asked Dean Vaughan to demand better facilities at the hospital, for "without some such establishment in the near future the medical department of the University of Michigan must fall behin [*sic*] a large number of medical schools," but as late as 1908, Peterson claimed, the regents refused to acknowledge the demand.[100]

Furthermore, the university continued to resist expanding obstetric services. This frustrated professors such as Peterson, who had pleaded with the regents and the university's treasury secretary for years to open more free beds for pregnant women. The Maternity Ward that finally got approved was described as a firetrap that "constituted a serious threat to the welfare of post partum patients."[101] As before, it is likely that administrators balked at the idea of welcoming unwed mothers—the population of women deemed most likely to seek free obstetrical treatment—as teaching patients for the impressionable medical students in Ann Arbor. That was one of the reasons Peterson became such a strong advocate for state laws to provide funding for the medical treatment of needy children and adults in Michigan. Acts 274 (1913) and 267 (1915) allowed for children and adults, respectively, to be sent to University Hospital for care, including pregnant women. But the payment mechanism differed for children and adults: whereas expenses for children came from state general funds, expenses for adults came from individual Michigan counties. Many counties felt that "it was cheaper to have unmarried mothers without funds confined in unsanitary county farms."[102] Thus, the Maternity Ward remained relatively small throughout the existence of the Catherine Street facility.

The growth of the University Hospital illuminated blossoming tensions in the relationship between academic medicine and clinical practice. Dock embraced the influence of scientific medicine in practice, encouraging students to develop both their laboratory and clinical skills in parallel and to engage in their own clinical or laboratory research. However, expectations to contribute to scientific developments pressured full-time clinical instructors who had little time for or interest in academic pursuits. As Hewlett observed,

> The clinic which is not adding to the sum total of medical knowledge is already falling in the rear. In order to perform this important function two requisites are necessary. In the first place members of the clinical staff must devote a portion of their time to research; in the second place facilities for such research must be furnished by the Hospital or by the University. It is becoming evident that if the members of the clinical staff are to do research in addition to their hospital and teaching duties, there will be relatively little time left for private practice. . . .
>
> From the standpoint of the students also there is a disadvantage in bringing them in contact solely with men who devote themselves to the scientific side of medicine.[103]

The tension between clinical practice and academic research would persist.

But that clinical practice itself had inherent value. The University Hospital, although created explicitly to provide teaching cases for the medical school, served a need in Ann Arbor and the rest of the state that went beyond medical education and faculty research. The hospital had never been intended to serve as a charity, but the clinics often provided care to working-class people who could not afford to pay the usual fees, or any fees at all. Hewlett noted that a large part of the hospital's patient population were people "who are trying to husband a slender capital in the face of serious or chronic illness."[104] Some faculty members and administrators recognized that such a socioeconomic situation was mutually beneficial for the patients and the medical school. As Dock commented in 1902,

> The hospital is a great public charity. It was not founded with that aim in view, and there are some who would have the charitable aspect still less prominent than it is. But, built primarily for teaching, and in response to the demand for a shelter for those who sought aid at the hands of the medical faculty, it does a great deal of good as a secondary result of its special function. Of those who are relieved of distress in its wards, or restored to health, a large porportion [*sic*] are manual laborers and producers, that is, those whose time and health can most readily be estimated in dollars and cents.[105]

By caring for members of the working class, the University of Michigan was thus both doing good for individuals and contributing to the overall well-being of the community.

However, others saw serious problems with University Hospital patients receiving free care, regardless of their ability to pay. A Michigan member of the AMA's National Legislative Council called the practice unfair competition for other practitioners in the state, who "are taxed to help pay the expenses of an institution which is robbing us of our just dues."[106] On December 13, 1904, the Delta County Medical Society of Escanaba, Michigan, issued a statement to the Board of Regents that "the gratuitous treatment by the state of persons whose necessities do not require it is not only wrong in principle and works an injury and injustice to the profession of medicine . . . but also such gratuitous treatment will in no manner improve the situation."[107] They worried about "pauperization," a concern that "the provision of aid in any form would inevitably sap the moral capacity of those receiving it."[108]

Following the 1913 and 1915 legislation that provided state-funded medical care for children and adults in need, a decision was made to offer services at the University Hospital "at low or moderate cost," with a sliding scale based on a person's ability to pay.[109] The system assuaged some critiques; having patients pay for at least some portion of their care diminished the risks of totally free care leading to "pauperization." But this model raised concerns among the medical faculty that higher-paying patients would receive privileges and access to services denied to others. Dock had complained years earlier that "all ought to be on the same footing in the sick room," and the hospital's attention to social inequalities and material wealth could be detrimental to patient care.[110] Hewlett observed in 1916, "The remark has often been made that the very rich and the very poor receive the best medical attention. . . . The person of moderate means, however, only too frequently gets along without highly specialized services."[111] As the medical school and its hospital continued to grow and modernize, socioeconomic dimensions of patient care, and the role of the hospital in Ann Arbor and the surrounding community more generally, would become more pronounced. These concerns would play an important part in the ongoing debates over moving the medical school or its clinical rotations to Detroit, and still later the relationship between socioeconomic status and health would become the subject of intense research.

Student Experiences

In the late nineteenth and early twentieth centuries, Michigan's medical school had some of the highest standards for admission in the United States.

For example, by 1909, acceptance into the medical school required a bachelor's degree from the university's College of Literature, Science, and the Arts, or other "approved colleges and scientific schools" if those programs provided "acquaintance with Latin, and a fair reading knowledge of German or French, and . . . a year of collegiate work in Biology (Zoology and Botany), Chemistry and Physics." However, the medical school also accepted undergraduates as part of a seven-year combined degree program once they had completed sixty semester hours and could demonstrate proficiency in the required languages. Latin was a traditional requirement for many professional programs in the nineteenth century and was evaluated by students "reading four books of Caesar or their equivalent"; German and French (for nonnative speakers) necessitated at least two years of schoolwork.[112] These modern language mandates were relatively new and indicated the growing significance of European scientific research, particularly in microbiology and bacteriology. They also suggested that students might be expected to read the primary scientific literature. (Some years later the Inteflex program would also offer the opportunity to obtain an M.D. degree in seven years, albeit without the language requirements.)

Grade categories for medical student examinations included "passed, incomplete, conditioned absent, and not passed"; a student who failed an examination would have to retake the course, and any incomplete or absent conditions had to be resolved within one year, or the student would be considered "not passed."[113] In addition to achieving academic standards, students were also expected to conduct themselves with honor and discipline, a requirement that students and faculty alike took quite seriously. Student cohorts in the late nineteenth century adopted honor codes (rather than

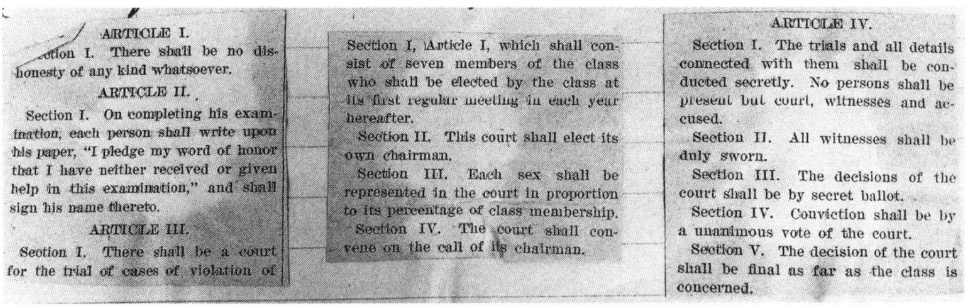

ARTICLE I.

ction I. There shall be no dishonesty of any kind whatsoever.

ARTICLE II.

Section I. On completing his examination, each person shall write upon his paper, "I pledge my word of honor that I have neither received or given help in this examination," and shall sign his name thereto.

ARTICLE III.

Section I. There shall be a court for the trial of cases of violation of Section I, Article I, which shall consist of seven members of the class who shall be elected by the class at its first regular meeting in each year hereafter.

Section II. This court shall elect its own chairman.

Section III. Each sex shall be represented in the court in proportion to its percentage of class membership.

Section IV. The court shall convene on the call of its chairman.

ARTICLE IV.

Section I. The trials and all details connected with them shall be conducted secretly. No persons shall be present but court, witnesses and accused.

Section II. All witnesses shall be duly sworn.

Section III. The decisions of the court shall be by secret ballot.

Section IV. Conviction shall be by a unanimous vote of the court.

Section V. The decision of the court shall be final as far as the class is concerned.

Student "honor plan," class of 1899. Miscellaneous, 1894–1903, Box 135, Medical School (University of Michigan) Records, 1850–2010, Bentley Historical Library, University of Michigan, Ann Arbor.

faculty proctors) to govern and monitor their examinations. These codes were determined by the students themselves (via secret-ballot voting) and presented to the faculty. For instance, the class of 1899 approved a system whereby "there shall be no dishonesty of any kind whatsoever." Each student would write and sign a pledge to that effect at the end of every examination. For cases of suspected cheating, the students convened their own disciplinary committee or "court," consisting of seven individuals ("each sex shall be represented in the court in proportion to its percentage of class membership"). Trial proceedings were conducted in secret, with only the committee and the suspected student present. Members of the court would vote by secret ballot, and a unanimous decision was required to convict; in that case, the student disciplinary chair would report the offender to the dean, but otherwise, "absolute silence shall be maintained concerning the trial."[114] Subsequent cohorts were free to modify or reject the plans, but many classes adopted similar honor codes and presented them to the faculty, where they were met with "hearty approval."[115]

Cases of student failure and misconduct occupied a considerable amount of the faculty's attention. Minutes from faculty meetings in the early 1900s noted students who were failing their courses, with brief indications of the recommendations or directives given to those students.[116] The faculty also deliberated on a variety of other issues related to student misconduct. For instance, in 1889, the instructors determined that students who were "abusive and disrespectful" to the faculty should not be granted degrees, and in 1900, two students "arrested for drunkenness" were suspended for one month in the term following their arrest.[117] Of particular concern were students who used their affiliation with the University of Michigan to advertise commercial treatments or medical services. In 1889 the faculty considered the expulsion of a student implicated for printing a "mountebank" circular (advertising quack medicines) that appeared around Ann Arbor, and in 1901 the dean barred another student from entering the school after the student advertised his services as an optometrist.[118] Furthermore, in 1903 Peterson, Dock, and others determined "that the senior class shall not accept invitations from drug firms on days on which they have regular university work."[119] The faculty was not explicit about what those drug firms invited students to do, but apparently, the temptation existed for medical students in Ann Arbor to engage in local medical commerce. The phenomenon of students presenting themselves as medical authorities was dangerous, but perhaps even more importantly, the professors in the medical school felt a need to prevent the diminution of the school's reputation by associating with commercial enterprise.

Even with the increasing demands of the program, medical students still found time to create a social community for themselves. Medical fraternities like Phi Chi had chapters at the University of Michigan by the early 1900s; the Psi chapter of that organization rented its first house, at 417 East Washington Street, in October 1906. Even with various opportunities for athletic events, "conviviality" at local bars, and the house's proximity to the Bijou Theater—in addition to "original research work with Cannibus [*sic*] Indica"—Phi Chi students maintained their good standing in the school.[120] In 1914, a group of students organized by Samuel W. Donaldson and Hubert R. John founded the Galens Honorary Medical Society (named for the legendary Greek physician) at the medical school. Initially, Galens was created to mediate issues between the students and the faculty, uphold a uniform honor system, and present grievances concerning conditions for medical students (among which were lack of locker facilities, smoking and lounge areas, and evening access to the gymnasium).[121] However, the organization's original constitution also stated the objective of "bring[ing] together for mental and social enjoyment the public-spirited men of the faculty and upperclasses." The masculine noun used in the constitution statement was not just a linguistic convention; despite the fact that women were members of the medical school class, according to its original membership rules, "no women shall be members" of Galens.[122] Most members envisioned the society as exclusive to the University of Michigan Medical School (despite some early consideration given to creating chapters at other medical schools). Within just a few years, society members were active as hosts and guides for medical school and hospital functions and even helped organize the 1916 AMA convention in Detroit. In 1918, the tradition of the All-Medic Smoker (later renamed the Galens Smoker) was initiated. The first event was held at the Michigan Union and featured refreshments and short talks delivered by professors; the name "Smoker" may derive from the widespread use of tobacco among attendees and speakers.[123]

As the class sizes at Michigan increased, so did student diversity. For instance, admissions policies under Vaughan's administration allowed for the enrollment of more Jewish students at Michigan than the national average.[124] Women also continued to find opportunities in the medical school. From 1873 to 1900 the number of women in each class ranged from eight to nineteen, and by 1900 a total of 394 women had been trained in the medical school.[125] According to an article in the *Ann Arbor Register* from 1891—when fourteen women graduated from Michigan's medical school, compared with only three from Johns Hopkins—"women and men are admitted under the same conditions and pursue the same studies," albeit not in fully integrated class sections: "they [women] work separately only in the anatomical laboratory and in certain courses where it is not deemed advisable to have the sexes together."[126] Faculty members decided which courses and demonstrations were "desirable to be presented to the combined classes" and which ones required gender separation as a matter of propriety, particularly gross anatomy. The medical faculty had voted in 1887 to hire a "Lady Assistant Demonstrator of Anatomy," May B. Stuckey, with an annual salary of $300. The school's female students were still required to conduct their dissections in a separate laboratory, even though a new facility had been constructed that same year. Before the West Medical Building's construction in 1903, women continued to sit in a separate section in the lecture amphitheater for anatomy lectures, and it was not until 1907 that a chair of anatomy, George L. Streeter, fully integrated the laboratory as well.[127] Dock addressed his female students as "Miss" or "Mrs." rather than addressing them by their

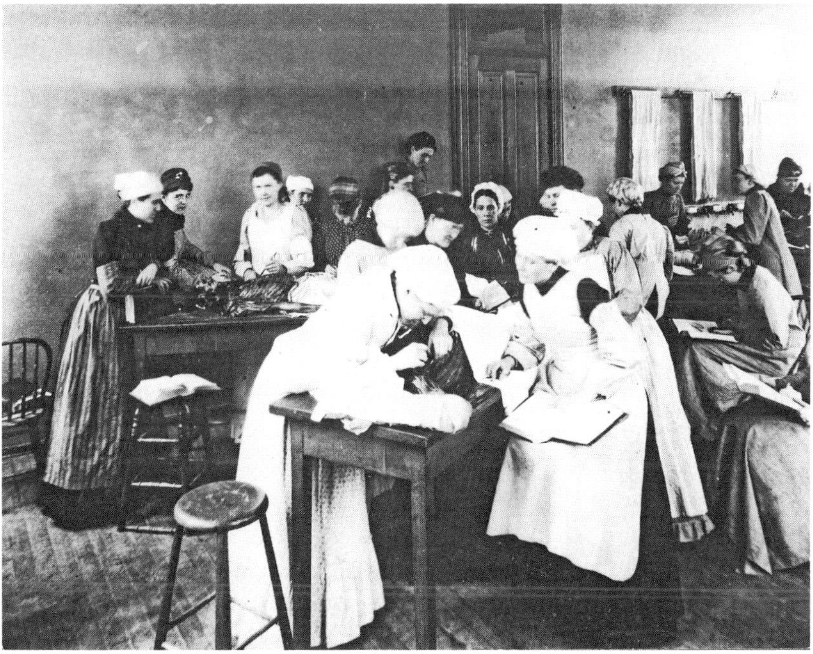

Women's gross anatomy laboratory, ca. 1893. Medical School (University of Michigan) Records, 1850–2010, Bentley Historical Library, University of Michigan, Ann Arbor.

last names, as he did with male students, but his notes reflect that he "treated the women exactly like the men . . . [and] there [was] no evidence of false modesty on the part of the women."[128] Women often exceeded the school's entrance requirements—far more female students than male came to the program with college degrees—and had higher rates of success.[129] However, the percentage of women in medical classes declined significantly in the early twentieth century. Women composed close to 20 percent of the student population in 1900 but dwindled to 2 percent of the student body in 1910. For the next three decades, between 5 and 10 percent of medical school classes were women.[130]

The first generation of female physicians had dispelled many older concerns about the effect of the profession and its training on women's bodies and minds; the fact that by the early 1900s an estimated 80 percent of female medical students in North America entered coeducational programs indicates that older assumptions about gender sensitivities were eroding.[131] In 1881, several doctors (including Emma Call, who had obtained her degree at Michigan) published a survey of female physicians for the American Social Science Association and found that "some unnecessary anxiety has been wasted" about their health. Other female Michigan graduates, such as Eliza Mosher, claimed that medicine was not only an acceptable profession for women but also a necessary one, since women "touch humanity in a manner different than men."[132] In 1898, the Board of Regents accepted a gift from the estate of New York physician Elizabeth H. Bates to establish a professorship "of the Diseases of Women and Children," on the condition that the university would continue to admit women in its medical school with the same educational advantages as men.[133] She made this gift despite never having visited Ann Arbor, suggesting that the university's reputation reached to upstate New York. (This was the first endowment for a named professorship at the university.) Despite some claims that there was little demand for female physicians in the United States,[134] female graduates from the University of Michigan went on to fulfill important roles in their communities. For instance, notable Progressive reformer Alice Hamilton graduated from Michigan's medical school in 1893. She met Jane Addams in Chicago and moved into Hull House, where she became interested in industrial leaders and pioneered a public health crusade against industrial toxins. She went on to become the first female faculty member at Harvard.[135] Katherine Crawford, an African American woman who received her medical degree at the university in 1898, served the small but steadily growing black community of Ann Arbor at a crucial point in its development.[136] Susan "Doc Susie"

Anderson, an 1897 graduate, moved to Colorado after contracting tuberculosis and spent decades in local practice before becoming the Grand County coroner in that state in 1926.[137] Women certainly stood to benefit from the educational and institutional changes at Michigan, and many of its female students graduated with success from the revolutionary program.

The Homeopathic College

After the university's separate homeopathic department opened in 1879, the homeopathic community rejoiced at their success in overcoming the institution's resistance. One initially skeptical observer was surprised and impressed by the college, its distinguished faculty, and its large patient base and noted that "doctors are not easily made in this institution." This observer's 1880 account concluded with the statement that homeopaths should "thank the people of Michigan for recognizing the just demands of Homoeopathy by establishing and maintaining on a liberal basis a department . . . in her noble University."[138] Like their "regular" counterparts, Michigan's homeopathic faculty developed a rigorous program with relatively high standards (in 1910, it was one of only five American homeopathic schools that required a high school diploma for matriculation) and clinical demonstrations in a variety of fields. A renovated and expanded homeopathic facility was included in the plans for the Catherine Street hospital project, and a training school for nurses in that facility was established in 1896. Another homeopathic hospital was built in 1900, "directly across the street from the University grounds . . . on the street car line" (it later became North Hall).[139] However, the homeopathic department remained small, and its hospital initially had trouble maintaining a sufficient patient base; as one alumnus politicly phrased it, "not until 1897 did the new hospital have any difficulty in providing comfortable accommodations for all who applied for admission."[140] By the early 1900s, the homeopathic department had eighty students (38 percent of whom came from Michigan) and twenty-six instructors, of whom fifteen were full-time professors.[141]

The apparent success of the college did little to mollify the ongoing, awkward relationship between the regular and homeopathic departments at Michigan. Some faculty members, like Vaughan and George Frothingham, did not object to the existence of the homeopathic school, claiming that the orthodox program's superior scientific fundamentals ultimately would prevail. Others wanted to limit any evidence of contact with the homeopathic school. In 1886, medical school professors determined that it "would be injurious to the good reputation of the department" to grant certification to students enrolled in the homeopathic program, and four years later the faculty issued a request to the Board of Regents "to forbid their names being used in the Homoeopathic announcement," even though homeopathic students still pursued laboratory coursework in the regular medical school.[142] In an 1895 letter, Reuben Peterson remarked that "the University had been wise in establishing two separate medical departments, and time has demonstrated the superiority of that one which has been devoted to the interests of regular medicines."[143] This grudging acceptance was predicated on the understanding that the regular medical school had nothing to do with the homeopathic college and was in no way connected to its operations or conferral of its degrees.

Tensions reached a head in the mid-1890s, when Henry Obetz, dean of the homeopathic college, supported a merger of the schools. He argued that this would better serve his school's smaller student population (at that time, there were 76 homeopathic students, compared with 375 students in the regular medical school at Michigan), but he also seemed convinced that homeopathic principles could sway the regular students to convert. Obetz's plan was met with significant opposition not only from regular physicians but also from the state Homeopathic Medical Society, which charged him "with duplicity, misrepresentation, disloyalty, conspiracy, and libel."[144] Michigan legislators proposed the dissolution of the homeopathic department (but the reinstatement of two homeopathic positions in the regular medical school) and the relocation of the entire homeopathic college to Detroit. Both proposals aroused significant opposition from both regular and homeopathic professionals, and no bills were pushed to a vote.[145] Royal S. Copeland, a Michigan graduate and homeopathic physician—who went on to a distinguished career of public service as mayor of Ann Arbor, commissioner of public health for New York City, and U.S. senator for New York—expressed strong opposition to the merger, in part through political metaphors. He claimed, "It is unwise, inexpedient, and not conducive to the best interests of the University and the people of the State to bring about this amalgamation. . . . You might just as well try to mix oil and water, to bring together the Republican and Democratic parties, or have a labor union convention in the office of the United States Steel Corporation."[146]

Despite such friction in the academy and the legislature, the local community supported the homeopathic department. With great pride, the *Ann Arbor Register* noted that "the homoeopathic college is considered one of the best of its kind in the country," and an 1895 article in the *Detroit Free Press* celebrated the growth of the homeopathic hospital population. An 1896 souvenir railroad publication claimed (somewhat defensively) that the homeopathic college "is equal to the Regular school in every way. . . . [N]o student who has graduated from this department has ever failed to be admitted to practice in any state upon his first examination. . . . [T]he principles of sound, thorough, practical, and scientific therapeutics are taught in connection with every clinical case."[147] Furthermore, the city of Ann Arbor, which had consistently provided financial support for the regular medical school, did likewise for the homeopaths. The city's voters routinely and overwhelmingly approved taxes to fund the university's homeopathic hospital.[148] Clearly, a considerable amount of the Michigan public embraced homeopathy and welcomed its presence at the university, much to the chagrin of the regular faculty, even Vaughan.

In 1920, the AMA Council on Medical Education and Hospitals invited Vaughan to chair a committee and erroneously identified him in a draft circular for the committee as "Dean and Professor of Hygiene and Physiological Chemistry, University of Michigan Homeopathic Medical School." Vaughan angrily wrote to the AMA president, "I have instructed my attorney to begin suit immediately against the American Medical Association . . . for defamation of character . . . to the extent of one million dollars."[149] The council's secretary apologized immediately, and Vaughan's threatened litigation did not proceed, but the exchange indicates the continuing animosity between homeopaths and regular physicians at the University of Michigan. Debates about which school of medical thought ought to prevail persisted well into the twentieth century.

The "Detroit Matter"

As the university's medical school grew, older debates about the wisdom of maintaining a medical school in Ann Arbor were reinvigorated.[150] In the mid-1880s, faculty members, the Board of Regents, the state legislature, and Michigan newspapers began once again to consider relocating the medical school, at least in part, to the neighboring city of Detroit.[151] Those who supported the move to Detroit at that point were certainly concerned, as Moses Gunn had been a generation before, about a perceived dearth in Ann Arbor's patient base. But the argument was now more clearly focused on the need for patients for clinical instruction, not on professors' private practice.

Despite the growing operations of the university's Pavilion Hospital, many argued that Ann Arbor was simply too small to provide an adequate number and variety of clinical cases for medical students at a "first-class medical school."

Ophthalmology chair George E. Frothingham claimed that most patients seen in Ann Arbor suffered from chronic conditions and noted that students hardly saw any pediatric or obstetric cases at all. This, he believed, had brought the medical school to a "standstill." He argued that the best way forward would be to move clinical clerkships and instruction to Detroit, and he made that argument in strong and personal terms. According to Frothingham, "Any man who advocated different views . . . would be condemned by the enlightened members of the medical profession as lacking good judgment, and this pretense would stigmatize him as a quack teacher."[152] His colleague, surgery professor Donald Maclean, claimed in a newspaper interview that without a broader patient base for medical students, Michigan's medical college would "never be more than a country school." Instead, Maclean favored students spending their first two years in Ann Arbor and their final year at Detroit's Harper's hospital.[153] Even Henry Lyster—who had been required to relocate to Ann Arbor when he joined the faculty and who supported rebuilding the University Hospital to keep clinical instruction in the town—noted concerns about Michigan's school becoming less competitive with other medical schools. According to Lyster, "Harvard and Pennsylvania colleges are at the head of the clinical procession, and if we do not wake up to the facts the university will find herself out of earshot of the music."[154] In April 1889, Frothingham appeared before a state legislative committee meeting in Lansing, Michigan, to argue against the funds appropriation for a new University Hospital. Instead, he suggested the possibility of relocating clinical instruction to hospitals in Detroit, notoriously testifying, "It was just as reasonable to expect to raise oranges in Canada as to maintain a complete clinic in Ann Arbor."[155] His striking language, as well as the fact that he traveled sixty miles to Lansing to try to persuade the legislature *not* to fund his institution, only served to escalate the underlying issue.

The question of relocating Michigan's clinical instruction to Detroit became scandalous that spring, with vociferous opposition from university faculty and officials, as well as fiery editorial comments in local newspapers.[156] Opponents of a move to Detroit argued that a dearth of teaching patients was, in fact, not an actual problem. William Herdman, for example, claimed that Ann Arbor had experienced significant growth in both of its teaching hospitals during the 1880s. Furthermore, he argued, the patient population was more diverse than supporters of the move had indicated; indeed, the University Hospital saw a wide variety of patients, not only from Michigan, and "almost every form of surgical practice."[157] Then-professor Vaughan—who admittedly had doubted the wisdom of establishing the entire university in Ann Arbor when he first arrived from Missouri[158]—agreed, arguing that not only did Michigan's students have plenty of clinical opportunities as it was, but the University Hospital's location provided advantages that Detroit's hospitals did not. He pointed out that the University of Michigan already had laboratories on campus for clinical tests, particularly urine and blood analysis, which many urban hospitals lacked.[159] Moreover, because all patients at the university expected to receive free treatment expressly for teaching purposes, any and all cases could become learning opportunities, whereas "not more than 50 per cent. received into charitable hospitals, controlled by laymen, are ever used for clinical instruction."[160] This point was demonstrated by an 1899 editorial for the *Leucocyte*, a student publication at the Detroit Medical College, in which a student complained, "Despite the 'unbounded hospital and dispensary facilities' in Detroit . . . 'half of the time [we] never get near a bedside.'"[161] Finally, the University Hospital, which was fully under the medical school's control, was in a unique position to reduce competition with other institutions in Ann Arbor and avoid conflicts of interest between faculty members and "visiting" practitioners. Ann Arbor's medical school, with its hospital dedicated to clinical instruction, was therefore much more than "a one-horse country college"[162] and derived its strength from its centralized organization. As one editorial in Michigan's *Adrian Press* colorfully explained, "To remove one branch to Detroit . . . and leave the balance in Ann Arbor would be like putting one's liver in his boot, his lungs on his shoulder and leave the heart to rattle around by itself."[163]

There were, however, more complicated factors intersecting with these surface arguments about the number of patients available for clinical instruction. For instance, opponents noted that moving clinical instruction to Detroit's proprietary hospitals would be devastating for the patients who relied on the free care they received in Ann Arbor. At a meeting of the university legislative committee, Michigan faculty members presented statistics from the mid-1880s to demonstrate that the overwhelming majority of their patient base (about five-sixths) consisted of Michigan residents, including those of "the poorer classes, . . . inmates of county houses and asylums, and such as are unable to pay for skilled medical and surgical attendance." Therefore, maintaining Ann Arbor's university hospital was useful not just for medical education but also as "a charity worthy of support . . . directly in the line of wise economy."[164]

Frothingham and his supporters did not dispute this claim but countered that in the current system Michigan medical students might be exposed to a "wrong sort" of Ann Arbor patient, particularly for cases of pregnancy and childbirth, once again raising questions about the morality of unwed mothers. General concerns about the propriety of using female patients for any kind of demonstration or instruction meant that few medical students in the United States received adequate training in women's health.[165] When the medical faculty considered devoting some of their free hospital beds to perinatal care, Frothingham called it an "outrage" and argued that "it was robbing one class of patients worthy of charity to bestow it upon a class of patients even less worthy of consideration,"[166] implicitly referring to unwed mothers as an undesirable patient population. The prevailing logic was that most respectable, married pregnant women in Ann Arbor did not visit the University Hospital to subject themselves to the indignity of demonstration. Therefore, the only obstetrical experience that medical students could get would necessarily involve dangerous exposure to local mothers of questionable morality. Frothingham's twofold implication was that a local Ann Arbor hospital should not debase itself by opening its doors to an immoral patient base just for purposes of instruction and that, at proprietary hospitals in Detroit, medical students might at least have a chance to observe the proper "class" of obstetric patients.

There were also economic considerations, in terms of both university funding and individual physicians' salaries. Opponents of the move (and the university Board of Regents in particular) worried that the university would see a steady leak of funding into the coffers of Detroit institutions and the pockets of Detroit physicians. Supporters of the move did not hide the fact that private practice opportunities were much more lucrative in Detroit, and the university's mandate that faculty members had to reside in Ann Arbor could be a financial disadvantage for potential hires.[167] There were also some concerns about the allegiance of Detroit medical practitioners to the university. Lyster, who had been hired to the medical faculty the previous year but had not yet relocated from Detroit to Ann Arbor, was suspected of conspiracy or deviousness. The *Ann Arbor Register* reported that while Lyster "favored the hospital in Ann Arbor, he indulged in a lot of vague and unsubstantial talk about the Detroit scheme, which . . . show[s] the folly and danger of having any Detroit medical men in the faculty."[168] Although these social and economic issues were not the central arguments

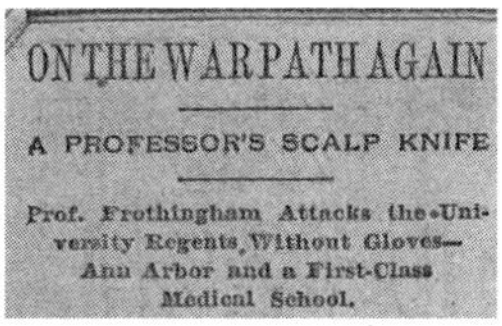

ON THE WARPATH AGAIN

A PROFESSOR'S SCALP KNIFE

Prof. Frothingham Attacks the University Regents, Without Gloves—Ann Arbor and a First-Class Medical School.

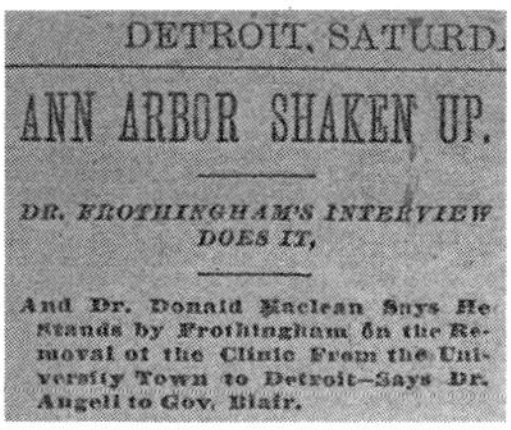

DETROIT, SATURD

ANN ARBOR SHAKEN UP.

DR. FROTHINGHAM'S INTERVIEW DOES IT,

And Dr. Donald Maclean Says He Stands by Frothingham on the Removal of the Clinic From the University Town to Detroit—Says Dr. Angell to Gov. Blair.

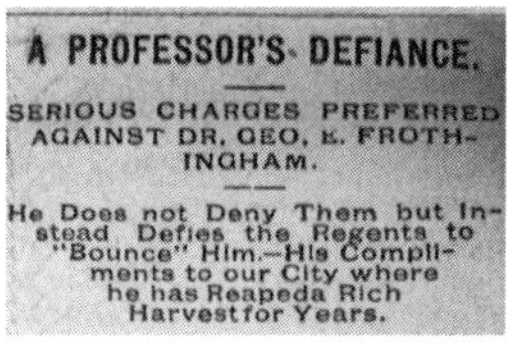

A PROFESSOR'S DEFIANCE.

SERIOUS CHARGES PREFERRED AGAINST DR. GEO. E. FROTHINGHAM.

He Does not Deny Them but Instead Defies the Regents to "Bounce" Him.—His Compliments to our City where he has Reapeda Rich Harvestfor Years.

Headlines from various Ann Arbor newspaper clippings from 1889, collected in James H. Wade's 1897 scrapbook. "Detroit, Newspaper Clippings Regarding Relocation of Clinical Work, 1889" folder, Box 135, Medical School (University of Michigan) Records, 1850–2010, Bentley Historical Library, University of Michigan, Ann Arbor.

in the 1889 Detroit matter, they add complexity to the controversy and help explain some of the urgency in considerations for Ann Arbor's new hospital. The local community stood to lose access to a valuable public service, and the university could find itself competing with a stronger medical community in Detroit.

With such passionate sentiments about keeping the medical school and its clinical instruction in Ann Arbor, it is unsurprising that Frothingham was vilified in the local press in the spring of 1889. After the professor made his inflammatory citrus analogy at Lansing, local newspapers immediately began to describe him as an unpredictable, greedy traitor. One article in the *Evening Journal*, titled "On the Warpath Again," portrayed Frothingham as a Native American savage "off his reservation . . . [with] his paint on, his quiver full of arrows, and those who know him say he will be 'bad medicine' for such of mankind as crosses his path." The *Detroit Tribune* continued the Native American "savage" metaphor (a common stereotype in nineteenth-century discourse), noting that the regents would call for Frothingham's scalp as soon as all members of the board could be present.[169] Several different papers also stated bluntly that Frothingham hated the town and people of Ann Arbor, a feeling that not only influenced his position on the Detroit matter but would also justify his removal from the university. As the *Ann Arbor Argus* reported on April 26, "There is no reason why he should remain in the employ of the university which he defies, or even live longer in the city which he damns."[170]

After Maclean expressed his support for Frothingham and agreed that a move to Detroit would be "the only thing to save the department of the university from destruction,"[171] he too became a press villain, as well as a hypocrite for having made statements earlier that decade in support of Ann Arbor's clinical instruction opportunities. The *Ann Arbor Courier* editorialized in May that Maclean and Frothingham's agenda against the medical school was "rank treason."[172] At a June 1889 meeting, the University of Michigan Board of Regents unanimously voted that Frothingham and Maclean had "placed themselves in such antagonism . . . both by their language and conduct, that . . . it is not desirable that they should longer continue their connection with the University." Both men resigned from the university the following month. At that time, Frothingham moved to Detroit, where he became president of the Michigan State Medical Society (the same organization from which he had resigned in the previous decade).[173]

The "Detroit matter," however, refused to die, even after Frothingham and Maclean were ousted and the Catherine Street hospital was completed. Fewer than twenty years after the "oranges in Canada" scandal, discussions over a potential move to Detroit once again caused friction among medical school faculty members. In 1904, Ann Arbor mayor Arthur Brown, speaking to the city council, asked that the Board of Regents "speedily dispose of this question" of relocating the university's clinical operations. Despite the regents' assurance that "the people of this state abandoned the idea of a University with separate branches in its different cities," the medical school was still considering the utility of hospital training in Detroit. Brown argued that this was a major concern for local taxpayers.[174] Vaughan, who had become medical school dean by that point, was increasingly concerned about the inadequacies of Ann Arbor's clinical facilities, and in 1906 he initiated conversations about moving some university clinical instruction to the larger city, proposing to "divide the senior class into two or three sections, and have one section at work in Detroit." This essential compromise was, in Vaughan's view, necessary to maintain the University of Michigan's reputation and standing as a premier state medical school:

> The students while working in Detroit could have all the obstetrical practice they could use, could see many more post-mortems than they do now, and see hundreds of out-patients. They practically see none of these at present, because there are none in Ann Arbor. . . . I feel very earnestly that in order to keep this school in the front rank of medical schools the clinical facilities must be improved. I am not saying one word against the clinical facilities here. They are excellent, as far as they go, and they are utilized to the fullest extent, but they are inadequate, both in quality and in quantity.[175]

At that point, professors Dock and Peterson were some of the most vocal supporters for keeping the Ann Arbor school intact. They pleaded with the state and Board of Regents to maintain and expand the University Hospital's clinical operations, particularly to provide students with more experience in obstetrics and the treatment of tuberculosis, rather than send their medical students to Detroit.[176] Several Michigan students who had participated in summer clinical rotations in the city agreed; in a 1906 letter to the editors of the *Detroit Free Press*, the students argued that such exposure (not to mention a proposed "merger" with the Detroit Medical College) was unnecessary, since the University Hospital was in fact "full to overflowing the year around," and more importantly, "the ability of the teacher and operator and not the size of the city in which a school is located, is what supplies the clinical material."[177] Dock and Peterson grew increasingly hostile toward Vaughan over the Detroit issue, which may have been a major reason why Dock left the University of Michigan for Tulane in 1908.[178] The Detroit controversy sowed discord among the medical faculty and led to several notable resignations over the course of a few decades. The resilience of this set of arguments reflected the importance of location, especially for the University of Michigan. The question of moving to Detroit would resurface a few years later with the Flexner report.

Abraham Flexner's Report and Commentary on the University of Michigan

In 1904, the AMA established its Council on Medical Education and Hospitals. Several years later the council enlisted the Carnegie Foundation for the Advancement of Teaching to study North American medical schools. To run the study, the Carnegie Foundation chose a native of Louisville, Kentucky, Abraham Flexner, who was the brother of Simon Flexner, then president of the New York City–based Rockefeller Institute for Medical Research. Abraham Flexner's charge was to visit and evaluate every medical school in the United States and Canada, observing their faculty and curriculum, facilities, budgets, and relations with colleges and universities. Abraham Flexner was not a physician, but the foundation's president, Henry S. Pritchett, chose him because he shared the foundation's views about Progressive educational reform, he was a good writer, and he had a familial connection (through his brother) to Johns Hopkins, an institution that was already held aloft as the gold standard for modern medical education.[179] Flexner's assessment of the University of Michigan's program provides an important glimpse of the medical school at a pivotal point in the school's history.

In his introduction to the 1910 study results, titled *Medical Education in the United States and Canada: A Report to the Carnegie Foundation for the Advancement of Teaching*, Pritchett claimed that unregulated medical education had "not only . . . commercialize[d] the process of education itself, but also . . . obscure[d] in the minds of the public any discrimination between the well trained physician and the physician who has had no adequate training whatsoever."[180] Despite the popularity of and support for scientific reforms in the late nineteenth and early twentieth centuries, a number of American schools—"regular" and sectarian alike—were proprietary and continued to function as "degree mills" without much consideration of responsible medical training, even as many schools began to increase both admission requirements and the length of their programs. The foundation and the AMA council agreed that regulation and higher standards for medical schools were vital for maintaining educational and professional "patriotism" and that Abraham Flexner—a layman—could provide a critical judgment of medical training without the bias of professional affiliation. Indeed, some schools believed that Flexner was visiting only as a scout for the Carnegie Foundation's philanthropic projects and were unaware, at least initially, of the real objectives of the study. Although the trend toward medical reform had already begun years before Flexner's results were published, the years following the report saw a significant change in standards, expectations, and funding at the nation's larger institutions, as well as the closure of most smaller and proprietary schools.[181]

The Flexner report (as the study is generally known) evaluated and ranked American medical schools with the following desirable qualities in mind: laboratory instruction and scientific medicine, access to sizeable hospital facilities and teaching patients, and institutional "harmony." Flexner described ideal instructors of modern medicine as "men of active, progressive temper, with definite ideals, exacting habits in thoughts and work, and with still some margin for growth."[182] Certainly, the Carnegie Foundation and the AMA council favored the model of a teaching hospital, which, the study claimed, "is as necessary to a medical school as is a laboratory of chemistry or pathology." Indeed, allowing medical students to obtain their degrees without adequate exposure to clinical experience was deemed to be detrimental to the public interest, even if those students were trained to practice within their own communities. As Pritchett indicated in his introduction, "It would mean that the sick man is better off in the hands of an incompetent home-grown practitioner than in those of one well trained in an outside school."[183] However, schools that divided their facilities into laboratory and clinical segments were viewed as problematic, since the "modern men" in charge of scientific medical education at a university medical school might have a fundamentally different theoretical approach than "the old-fashioned" clinical faculty associated with an older (and most likely urban) hospital. In Flexner's view, "There is little reason to believe that the divided school will ever function as an organic whole."[184] The only school in the study that was ranked "excellent" overall in both clinical and scientific instruction was Johns Hopkins; the University of Michigan, Harvard, Minnesota, and Columbia were rated "excellent" in one overall category, but only "good" in the other. The majority of American medical institutions were ranked significantly lower, particularly irregular or sectarian schools, and Flexner's report recommended that many of them be closed.[185]

When Flexner visited the University of Michigan in March 1909, five medical schools were operating in the state. Ann Arbor—the home of two of those schools—had a population of 14,734. Some 389 students were enrolled in the university's medical school, and each of them had earned a "scholastically honest" high school degree and completed at least two years of college work before their admission. There were sixty-three members of teaching staff in that school (of whom twenty-two were professors), and most were full-time appointees. By contrast, the Detroit Medical College had many more staff members, but fewer than half of the students.[186] Flexner lauded the university's consolidated course and claimed that its rigorous admission standards (upheld by a "vigorous, intelligent, and public spirited" state medical board) were largely responsible for the school's high student retention rate.[187] At that point, Michigan's medical school was one of only sixteen schools in the United States and Canada that required at least two years of undergraduate work, and one of fourteen institutions to provide its entire four-year course at one undivided institution.[188]

At the same time, Flexner acknowledged that increasing requirements for matriculation could be prohibitive for students in some Michigan schools—particularly the state's homeopathic institutions and the Detroit Medical College—but argued that his recommendation did not necessarily need to disadvantage "the earnest poor boy" or other deserving applicants. Indeed, compared with programs in Baltimore, Philadelphia, and Chicago, medical instruction at the University of Michigan was a bargain; according to Flexner, a six-year education (two years of undergraduate study and four years of medicine) in Ann Arbor would cost only about forty-six dollars more than the four-year medical programs available in those large cities.[189] This estimate is significant, particularly since Flexner noted that Michigan had the fourth largest medical school budget (for the medical school and the University Hospital combined) in the country. Whereas "champions of cheapness allege that large sums are needed only for research, where medicine is taught to college graduates who afterwards practise in large cities," Michigan was presented as a prime example of a successful, cost-effective establishment that would "spend these sums in behalf of high school boys who after graduation from the medical school return to the simple surroundings amidst which they grew up." Thus, the school's graduates would go on to fulfill a vital role for their communities.[190]

Despite his praise for the University of Michigan's medical school, and despite the success of University Hospital, Flexner voiced grave concerns about the institution's location and frequently described Ann Arbor's size as a "defect." Certainly, he claimed that in many ways the school had "largely overcome the disadvantages of location in a small town," and its consolidated program was one of its greatest strengths. But, he also admitted, "there is no question that, if the entire state university was at Detroit, the medical department would be better off."[191] The biggest issue was the number and variety of teaching patients available to students, which Flexner only rated as "fair" during his visit to Ann Arbor, notwithstanding reports from Vaughan and Hewlett that their hospital admissions had nearly doubled during the preceding four years.[192] Flexner seemed assured that Michigan had solved its perceived "problem" and that the school "may even turn the defect of situation to good account; for, freed from distraction, the medical [school at] . . . Ann Arbor may the more readily cultivate clinical science."[193] However, his concerns had a strong effect on the administration of the school. Vaughan later intimated to university president Harry Hutchins that the relative dearth of clinical subjects for students, and opportunities for instructors, potentially could have a damaging ripple effect on the entire school, as prospective faculty hires might be lured to other institutions.[194] Ultimately, Flexner believed that the strength of the University of Michigan's medical school far outweighed the disadvantage of Ann Arbor's size, and he took a firm stance against proposed plans to "split" the school and relocate clinical training in Detroit hospitals. Nonetheless, given Flexner's ambivalent conclusions in this report, it is unsurprising that he specifically referenced Ann Arbor as he implored his readers to "pity the small town" that needed good physicians in the 1910s.[195]

Conclusion

By the World War I era, the University of Michigan medical school had placed itself at the forefront of American medical education in a number of ways. Abraham Flexner's glowing report of the school's devotion to academic medicine, laboratory science, clinical instruction, and its modern hospital operations is clear proof that the "country medical school" of an earlier generation had grown by leaps and bounds under the leadership of Victor Vaughan and catapulted Michigan to a position of high national and international esteem. But all of these developments and debates occurred, very self-consciously, in the context of a rural town. Trailblazing faculty members like Vaughan, Frederick Novy, Henry Sewall, and George Dock not only embraced new medical theories and practices but also actively sought to demonstrate that these Progressive ideas could be implemented in a place like Ann Arbor, which despite its growth and development around the turn of the twentieth century remained a small university town.

A small homeopathic school still existed as part of the university. Concerns persisted about the environment, as Flexner was not alone in his worries about Ann Arbor's size and teaching patient population. A number of critics at the local and national levels were unconvinced that the University of Michigan could rise to the top tier of medical schools in the United States, a concern that seemed to grow only more pressing as the medical school and its hospital sought to improve and expand. By the late 1910s, it became apparent that the university would need to devote more attention to supporting its reputation and the medical school's blossoming identity as a vanguard of medical education and research, in a setting that Kenneth Ludmerer describes as "the most paradoxical in the country" for modern medical schools.[196]

THREE

The Interwar Years at Michigan

A New Era of Research

On February 10, 1927, Boston physician Henry A. Christian from Harvard and the Peter Bent Brigham Hospital delivered a stirring keynote address at the dedication of the Thomas Henry Simpson Memorial Institute for Medical Research in Ann Arbor.[1] The granite beaux arts building on South Observatory Street—complete with a walnut-paneled lobby and library, offices, laboratories, and accommodations for up to ten patients—was part of a gift to the University of Michigan from the widow of Detroit iron magnate Thomas Henry Simpson. In 1924, Christine McDonald Simpson had donated more than $400,000 to the university in memory of her late husband, who had died of pernicious anemia the previous year. Her objective was to endow a state-of-the-art clinical research facility to find a cure for pernicious anemia, which until the early 1920s had been considered an inevitably fatal condition.[2] The University of Michigan had recruited two prominent Massachusetts physicians to run the new institute. Cyrus Sturgis had studied with Henry Christian and was soon to be named to run the Department of Internal Medicine. Raphael Isaacs came from the Collis P. Huntington Memorial Hospital in Boston. In his dedicatory remarks, Christian bestowed almost spiritual reverence on the institute and the work that was to go on therein. He equated its scientific objective to the noble, "pure" search for the Holy Grail and praised the future results of the institute's scientific investigations, which would "be given freely and without price to suffering humanity." Christian also took care to point out the wisdom of having a close association between such a facility and the university. He noted that "failure to solve the problem set is not a failure in the usefulness of the institute. . . .

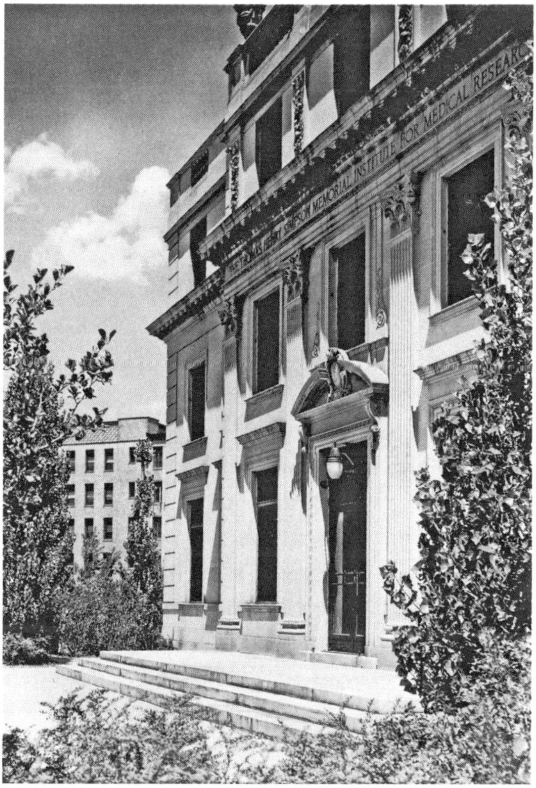

Thomas Henry Simpson Memorial Institute for Medical Research, ca. 1927. University of Michigan Photographs Vertical File, Bentley Historical Library, University of Michigan, Ann Arbor.

All research institutes are educational institutions in the larger sense of the word."[3]

Christian had good reason to be optimistic about the institute's specific research goals. Other investigators had already noted links between anemia and iron deficiency, as well as the beneficial effect of dietary therapy, but a cure for pernicious anemia remained to be found. On a deeper level, however, Christian's inference to the fundamental relationship between research and education speaks to pivotal transitions at the University of Michigan's medical school during the interwar period, as well as to the changing relationship between biomedical research and education in twentieth-century

America. When the Simpson Memorial Institute was endowed, facilities and funding dedicated to researching a single disease were rare. The Rockefeller Institute Hospital had opened the first major clinical research institute in the United States in 1910, the same year that Carnegie Foundation researcher Abraham Flexner published his exhaustive and influential report on American medical schools for the AMA's Council on Medical Education and Hospitals. Flexner's findings and recommendations marked a revolution in American medical education and research, establishing the clear priority of financial, political, and moral support for academic work and high educational standards.[4] At the same time, the primacy of the laboratory as a site of medical knowledge in the United States was growing, partly because of the successes of scientific medical practitioners and partly because it symbolically held the promise of a medicine untainted by politics. By the 1920s, many laboratory procedures had moved from bench to bedside and become standard in many American schools and hospitals.[5]

However, just as the Simpson Institute was being endowed, the medical school was facing significant challenges, some of which were related to the recently ended war. When the United States had entered World War I a decade earlier, in 1917, all medical schools felt the army's need for military personnel and medical facilities. Class sizes began increasing dramatically, and the University of Michigan, like many of the nation's larger programs, shortened its curriculum to allow students more rapidly to become physicians and enter military service. Teaching loads in some departments doubled. New courses, such as "Pathology in Relation to Military Medicine," were introduced. Investigators started to focus on questions relevant to wartime. Stacey R. Guild, a student of histology professor Carl Huber, studied the prevention of war deafness. Planning to study liquid dichlorethylsulfide, or mustard gas, faculty members in the pathology department obtained a supply from the Dow Chemical Company in Midland, Michigan, even before the substance was being produced in factories.[6] Poison gas was to become one of the most horrific features of the war. Ironically, a few years later mustard gas was found to be valuable in the treatment of some malignancies.

Some Michigan physicians and medical faculty actively served during the conflict. At times, military necessity led to unexpected changes in the faculty. Nellis B. Foster was named the new head of internal medicine in 1916. He joined the Army Medical Reserve Corps in 1917. After being sent on a medical mission to Serbia, he resigned abruptly several months later for extended military service, leaving Dean Vaughan needing to find another person to head the department.[7]

Some medical school members felt conflicted about the curricular compression. They had worked hard to create a top academic program over the previous decades and were not happy about it being abridged. In the summer of 1917, the school pleaded with the AMA to obtain furloughs for drafted medical students, noting that they had "persuaded quite a number of our medical students to remain on in the medical school, on the advice of the Council of National Defense, on this plea that their duty to the country lay in finishing their medical education."[8] The following year, the Galens Honorary Medical Society criticized the newly formed Reserve Officers' Training Corps at the university "for not allowing its medical members to resign . . . if the time involved interfered with scholastic endeavors."[9]

The war stimulated growth of southeast Michigan's newly dominant industry—automobile manufacturing. Cars and other vehicles were used to support troops in many ways, not least as ambulances. As the war ended, Ann Arbor found itself in an area that was becoming rapidly industrialized. The city was finally starting to overcome its older "country" image. In this setting, it is ironic that for several decades the medical school officially barred its students from driving.[10]

Wartime stress brought other challenges into the foreground. For almost a decade after Albion Walter Hewlett left the medical school in 1916, there was no long-term successor for his chair in internal medicine, especially after Foster unexpectedly left shortly after being hired. Relatively little funding was available for clinical research or laboratory facilities.[11] By the late 1910s the university's Catherine Street hospital building was rapidly becoming outdated and was difficult to maintain. Plans for a new University Hospital were already under way, but the building would not be completed until 1925, largely because of the interruption of the war. When the school shifted to a full-time employment plan for all faculty members in 1919, severely limiting private practice opportunities, administrators worried that potential faculty hires would be lured elsewhere by higher salaries and expanded clinical opportunities.[12] Finally, Victor Vaughan, after serving thirty years as medical school dean, retired in 1921. His successor, surgery chair Hugh Cabot, had very different ideas about the medical program and administrative methods.[13] Thus, the war threw into relief many ongoing systemic issues that had affected the school for years, and with the change of leadership in the early postwar years, the medical school found itself vulnerable to discord.

In this context, Christine Simpson's gift to the university served as a stabilizing force. It provided a much-needed benefit for the medical school and formed a significant watershed for the medical school's priorities during the

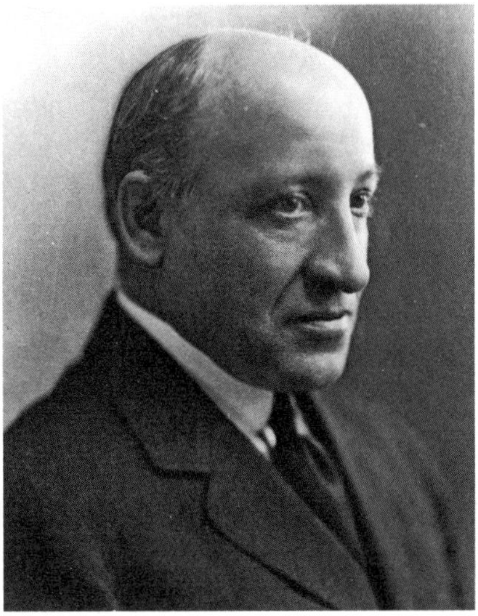

Dean Hugh Cabot. BMC Media Services Records, Bentley Historical Library, University of Michigan, Ann Arbor.

interwar years. The Simpson Memorial Institute helped elevate the prestige of Ann Arbor, the university's medical faculty, and the school's other clinical facilities at a difficult point in its history. The institute's focus also helped foster collaborative relationships with other funding sources, such as the W. K. Kellogg Fellowship Foundation of Battle Creek and the Ford Motor Company.[14] Just two years after the institute opened its doors, Sturgis and researchers at the Parke, Davis Company presented ventriculin (derived from dried and defatted hog stomach) as an effective treatment for patients with pernicious anemia (albeit one that would in a few decades be supplanted by vitamin B_{12}).[15] The importance of research, perhaps symbolized by ventriculin, extended throughout the medical school, and the partnership with Parke, Davis served as a model for collaboration between academia and industry. Not only was doing research important for those who wanted to make it their life's work in the institute, but learning about it was starting to be seen as central for all who would become physicians, at least at Michigan. As Sturgis noted proudly (and presciently) in 1928, "it should be the aim of medical schools to graduate all students with the knowledge that the practice of medicine is advancing and that some understanding of the value and purposes of research is essential to every practitioner."[16]

The focus on research, and the triumph of scientific medical thinking more generally, shaped a variety of other administrative trends during the interwar period. Individual departments began to grow and diversify, as more and more physicians chose to study specific clinical fields. Michigan was at the center of a variety of newly developing medical fields during the mid-twentieth century, including thoracic surgery, rheumatology, and anesthesiology.[17] The Simpson Institute, the opening of a new hospital in 1925 (discussed below), and the creation of other medical buildings and laboratory facilities contributed to steady expansion of the physical plant. By the mid-1930s, the university's health-related facilities had grown to the point that the Board of Regents consolidated them into a Division of Health Sciences that initially consisted of the Medical School, the School of Dentistry, the Division of Hygiene and Public Health, the University Hospital School of Nursing, the College of Pharmacy, and the Department of Postgraduate Education, all placed under the administration of a committee chaired by James D. Bruce. Critics feared that this consolidation would lead to absorption of units within the division, but the regents specifically argued that "this was not our concept" in establishing the new administrative body. Instead, they sought "to bring about the understanding that there is a natural unity in the health-science professions, and that medicine, dentistry, public health, nursing, pharmacy, and the ancillary services are but parts of the whole."[18]

Whether by intent or not, one unit was to disappear. The most significant casualty of the trend toward research and consolidation was the university's Homeopathic Medical College. Despite the controversies that had plagued its establishment, the homeopathic department had been relatively stable during the early years of the twentieth century. But Flexner's 1910 report had recommended its closure (as well as the closure of the Detroit Medical College). After World War I, the legislature voted to ask the Board of Regents to combine the homeopathic and "regular" medical schools. When, perhaps seeing no other viable option, the regents complied, the state Homoeopathic Medical Society promptly asked all faculty members to resign.[19] Detroit homeopathic physician D. A. MacLachlan complained that "the whole Faculty have been asleep at the switch." MacLachlan, himself a graduate of Michigan's Homeopathic Medical College, expressed his disgust at the administrators of "the dominant school," who would override the homeopathic program if the schools merged, and noted that "those familiar with the U.S. medical policies are not slow to recognize the velvet hands of the Ku Klux Klan of American medicine, the 'A.M.A.' behind the scenes at Lansing."[20] Another homeopathic physician, James C. Wood, stated that the move to combine the schools was part of a larger movement to destroy homeopathy more generally, or an indication of antagonisms within the homeopathic profession in Michigan.[21] The college's most illustrious alumnus, New York

Board of Health president (and later U.S. senator) Royal S. Copeland, was certainly opposed to the move, arguing that "the Regents have made a grievous mistake" in disbanding the independent program and pleading with the media to "not forget the value of the small newspapers" and local opinions, which had been so influential in creating the school in the first place. By the interwar period the "local feeling" that for years had fostered rivalries between alternative medical sects had given way to more widespread support for regular medicine and research, both in Michigan and nationwide.[22] As a consequence, the homeopathic school was gone by the early 1920s.

Rebuilding the University Hospital

Although fewer than three decades old, by the mid-1910s the Catherine Street hospital was swiftly becoming outdated. One problem was simply that of scale. The growth of the industrial economy led southeast Michigan to become a magnet for migration—particularly African Americans from the southern United States, and Southern and Eastern European immigrants—and the number of admissions to the University Hospital increased dramatically. Like American hospitals more generally, the University Hospital was becoming a place where middle-class people chose to seek health care, in part because of the promise of scientific medicine.[23] Both of these trends led to the facility becoming increasingly overcrowded. Not only did the Catherine Street facility lack adequate bed space and laboratories, but it was starting to fall apart. Reuben Peterson recalled a lecture room under the Palmer Ward that flooded after any heavy rain, so the students and faculty dubbed it the "frog pond." It is unsurprising that, as early as 1915, Dean Vaughan began requesting state appropriations to expand and modernize the University Hospital.[24] However, it soon became apparent that instead of repairing the existing physical plant, the University Hospital needed a completely new facility. The governor of Michigan, Alexander Groesbeck, was a major supporter of the project. Despite continued growth in the community's size, some of the same questions that had been raised before were raised again. People wondered about placing a large hospital in the small town of Ann Arbor, asking whether the town would ever find enough sick people to fill its proposed seven hundred beds.[25] Unlike in previous versions of the debate, this time the decision to remain in Ann Arbor was less controversial.

Because of underfinancing, construction was delayed for several years during the early 1920s, but in 1925 the brand-new hospital opened on a hill

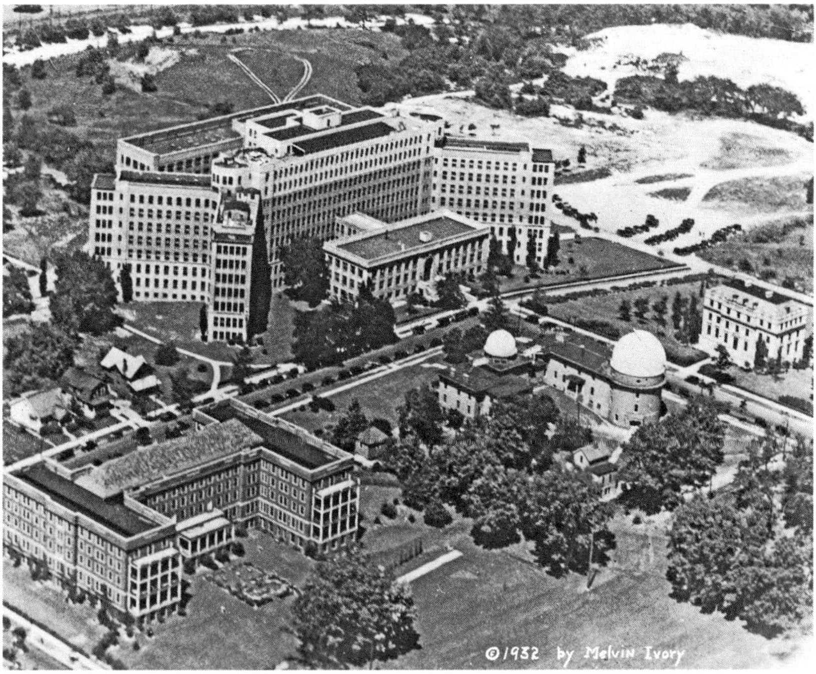

University Hospital, 1932. Photograph by Melvin Ivory. University of Michigan Photographs Vertical File, Bentley Historical Society, University of Michigan, Ann Arbor.

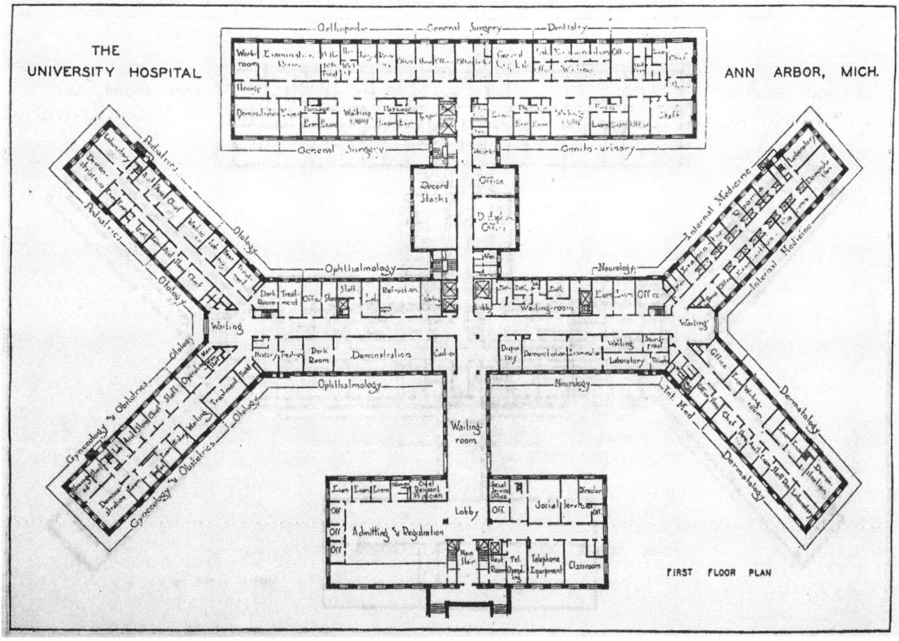

“Old Main” floor plan. From Harley A. Haynes, “The University Hospital: University of Michigan,” *Methods and Problems of Medical Education* 18 (1930): 59–74.

at the northern end of Observatory Street (southeast of the Catherine Street location), across from both the Detroit Observatory, which had opened in 1854, and the site for the future Simpson Institute. It was a dramatic structure designed by the noted architect Albert Kahn, who had designed many of the Ford Motor Company plants. He modeled the hospital on the many factories that were coming to dominate the local industrial environment and that symbolized the newest and best technology the United States had to offer.[26] Hospital director Harley Haynes described the footprint as "a double Y intersected by a double T": the main ward was located in the central part of the facility, with a surgical wing to the north and patient wards in the Y-shaped branches on either side, giving the new hospital an impressive total of 1,225 beds.[27] This massive expansion—nearly triple the size of the Catherine Street facility—required a new administrative system to handle a much larger volume of personnel; in 1930, Haynes estimated that "on an average, one and one-fifth employees are required for each bed in the hospital." The hospital director established an executive staff, made up of instructors in the medical school, "thus establishing a contact between the Medical School and the hospital administration." However, the two institutions were not subsumed into one whole: the hospital director did not serve as an administrator for the medical school, and the dean of the medical school had no direct responsibilities to the hospital. Altogether, the new hospital had nine levels, but the building was constructed on the side of a hill, so it had "three floors below the street level . . . [for] service units and certain special departments, such as those of x-ray, clinical laboratory, and physical therapy." Not only dedicated to direct clinical care, the hospital also devoted space for a social services department and occupational therapy, units that signify a broadening of the mission of the medical school.[28]

The new hospital dedicated specific spaces for scientific medical work. Onsite laboratory facilities enabled pathologists to conduct autopsies and do frozen section diagnoses more efficiently. Before the mid-1920s, all pathology work was done not in the hospital but in the medical building, and specimens had to be hand-delivered across campus. The new hospital also offered pathology consultation services to local practitioners in order to make tissue diagnosis more widely available, a procedure especially valuable for cancer biopsies. By the end of the 1920s, more than six hundred doctors had used the service, and the program handled about ten thousand consultation cases per year. Reuben L. Kahn, named director of the central laboratory and assistant professor of bacteriology in 1928, oversaw diagnostic work in chemistry, hematology, bacteriology, and serology not only for Michigan patients but also for law enforcement officials throughout the state. These outreach and public service projects grew so large that in 1932 the regents approved a Pathology Diagnostic Revolving Fund for the diagnostic service, and soon after, the hospital developed an Institute for Law-Enforcement Officers, with lectures and discussions on medicolegal issues led by medical school faculty. This was one of many ways the ideology of science led not only inward to the laboratory bench but also outward toward the larger community.

The hospital also included a specialized area dedicated to the study of heart disease called the heart station. It housed the big, bulky equipment then necessary to record an electrocardiogram (ECG) tracing, as well as serving as a location that signaled the reality (and importance) of specialized study of the heart. But the scientific mission was more all-encompassing than the rooms of the heart station. The entire hospital incorporated wiring that connected each room with the large, immobile ECG machines in the heart station. Thus, more than simply providing designated space for laboratory work, the hospital was, in a sense, itself a gigantic piece of laboratory equipment.

As before, a major objective in planning the hospital was to provide a location for education, so considerable space was set aside for lecture halls and teaching laboratories. Clinical instruction was done throughout the hospital, and once again, all admitted patients were made available for instruction. In addition, for the first time, space was available for instructing students, interns, and other postgraduates in specialties like heart disease, radiology, dietetics, and anesthesiology. The nursing school also brought its students to the wards (approximately two hundred by 1930). The presence of students did on occasion cause conflicts, since their need for attention and supervision at times interrupted the smooth operation of the hospital and put additional strain on the staff. Such problems, however, did not impede the clear pedagogical function of the new facility; as Haynes proudly described it, "The institution as a whole is very much a teaching hospital."[29]

This educational mission was not solely directed toward Michigan's medical and nursing students. Once again, the school looked outward as well as inward. Even before the new facility opened its doors, the University Hospital had started offering "clinic classes" to educate patients on the prevention and treatment of illness and to encourage them to participate more actively in their own care. The first class, offered in 1920, focused on asthma and hay fever, but the program soon expanded to include classes in infant feeding, cardiac care, and diabetes, the last especially relevant after the discovery of insulin in 1921. Some services, particularly in pediatrics, also instituted outpatient clinics in Detroit, Marquette, and other locations to provide care and education to a wider socioeconomic spectrum of patients.[30] These initiatives were related to what Naomi Rogers has described as the "New Public Health movement" of Charles V. Chapin in Providence, Rhode Island. During the interwar period many practitioners came to realize that despite significant advancements in laboratory diagnostics, surgical procedures, and pharmaceutical therapies, many patients resisted seeking treatment or following medical guidelines, particularly those with stigmatizing diseases such as syphilis or tuberculosis.[31] By expanding services beyond its walls, the new hospital was "modern" not only in its physical space and facilities but also in its outreach to the local community.

Although a marked improvement over the Catherine Street facility, the new University Hospital did not solve all of the problems the medical school had been facing for the previous several decades. For example, despite the exponential increase in patient population, the lack of space and resources for perinatal cases continued to be an issue. The assumption that only poor, unwed mothers would avail themselves of the University Hospital's free service continued to influence both lawmakers and the regents, who had hesitated to charge for maternity services until the 1920s. Even after the state legislature mandated county funding for unwed mothers in 1915 (which had allowed the University of Michigan gradually to raise charges), the University Hospital saw relatively few cases since they could be housed and treated at local hospitals or county homes less expensively. Even as late as 1936, obstetrics and gynecology professor N. F. Miller complained that Michigan students were still required to attend rotations in Detroit hospitals to receive instruction in obstetrics, a system that was "at best a poor makeshift" because "the student sees both good and bad obstetrics at a time when he is incapable of recognizing either."[32] Another alternative for patients was a private hospital for women founded by Professor of Obstetrics and Gynecology Reuben Peterson. Consisting of several houses on South Forest and South University streets, the hospital was an alternative place to care for people who preferred (and could afford) care delivered in a private, nonteaching setting.[33]

Some plans for expansion were cut short by the Great Depression. In 1929 the state had appropriated more than $300,000 to repair and rebuild the State Psychopathic Hospital, but the funding was repealed several years later because of the financial recession.[34] Broader financial issues accompanied the enormous growth of both inpatient and outpatient services in the new hospital. Older questions resurfaced about the university's responsibility to provide free care to Michigan patients and how that objective might conflict with the commercial and research interests of individual faculty members. Along with the opening of the new facility came a change in financial policy. No longer would the hospital's operations be supported by educational funds; instead, the regents determined that the hospital should impose charges for treatment and become a self-supporting institution.[35] This came at a time when practitioners and medical societies throughout the country were growing concerned about the move toward "socialized" medicine in the United States. In a 1920 speech at Indiana University, University of Michigan professor Aldred Scott Warthin noted that "the strength and significance of this movement cannot be doubted, and the medical profession cannot ignore it." In Warthin's view, state-sponsored medical treatment had been crucial to the success of Michigan's University Hospital, but he declared that the facility in Ann Arbor "is not, and has never been a charity hospital."[36] However, in the mid-1930s a significant proportion of University Hospital patients were still dependent on public funds (either from the state or from individual counties); "indigent patients" accounted for about two-fifths of all hospital registrations, whereas only about 6 percent of patients paid for both their hospitalization and professional services.[37] Furthermore, since the hospital was the site for patient care, education, and research, it was virtually impossible to make clear distinctions between which costs ought to be allocated to each unit, which could cause conflicts over budgets and personnel requirements.[38] As early as 1920, Warthin warned that this change in compensation could become problematic, asking, "Will the old commercialism . . . be replaced by another form, even more dangerous to medical teaching and research than the divided interests of the old situation?"[39]

The explosion in both inpatient and outpatient populations also strained medical personnel, including professors with duties to the medical school or research projects of their own. One estimate for pediatrics claimed that in 1935 that department's outpatient attendance was about twenty-five hundred every month, so "the teaching load of 768 clock hours had to be divided between five instructors [because] the other members of the staff were necessary to help care for the patients."[40] According to the 1939–1940 annual report, the University Hospital had two hundred doctors on staff and saw twenty-seven thousand registered patients, in addition to sixteen thousand monthly outpatient visits.[41] Full-time clinicians at the University Hospital—salaried rather than compensated for individual cases—found such a workload financially unfavorable.

Then, as now, infections in the hospital posed serious problems. While the overall incidence of tuberculosis had gone down since the nineteenth century, it continued to be a serious problem for patients and providers alike. In the medical school's 1939–1940 annual report, the dean noted that internal medicine was conducting a study on the incidence of tuberculosis among hospital employees. Horace W. Davenport claims that by 1939 there had been thirty-seven cases of tuberculosis (some fatal) among medical students alone.[42]

Students during the Interwar Years

In the years following World War I, medical educators started to reevaluate how they selected students. By the late 1920s, the medical school began devoting considerably more explicit attention to its admissions process, considering not only academic performance in traditional undergraduate premedical coursework but also a variety of personal and psychological traits. In 1928 C. S. Yoakum, a professor working at Michigan's Bureau of University Research, devised an eight-page booklet for all prospective applicants to complete that included a "Cowdery interest analysis form," intended to identify the applicant's occupational interest. Applicants also wrote a personal essay and took a reading comprehension test.[43] Moreover, all applicants now had to present themselves for a personal interview, during which they would be evaluated on such criteria as "self-possession," personal appearance, articulation, and common sense.[44] The goal appears to have been a more equitable selection process, as in 1935, the medical school claimed that "our present requirements do not allow any way for a student's background or personality to gain him admission to the Medical School. He is judged solely on his record."[45] Nonetheless, at the same time, the admissions office gathered, albeit unsystematically, some personal data on applicants' gender, race/ethnicity, marital status, home state, and premedical schools. This policy caused controversy among the faculty. While some professors (including Raphael Isaacs) supported classifying applicant races and ethnicities, others criticized using these markers as arbitrary assessments of student identity. The noted syphilis researcher Udo Wile informed Dean Albert C. Furstenberg in 1936, "I doubt the value of having on the student's record anything concerning nationality or race."[46]

Questions about race were on the minds of many medical educators. One effect of early-twentieth-century educational reforms was to create more homogeneity in medical schools across the country, in part a result of increased costs, heightened admissions standards, and at times overtly discriminatory policies. Abraham Flexner's recommendations for improving medical education—and closing substandard schools nationwide—directly increased socioeconomic and racial disparities in professional training opportunities, a trend that Flexner himself found particularly troubling.[47] In 1919, he wrote to Vaughan to inquire about the number of black students in Michigan's medical school. Despite the explicit openness of the University of Michigan to African American enrollment, the total number was probably disappointing: Vaughan replied, "There is one negro medical student in this school. He will be a Junior next year."[48] Around the same time as this correspondence, Flexner invited Vaughan to serve on a committee granting fellowships provided by Julius Rosenwald "to promising Negro graduates in medicine for the purpose of enabling them to pursue advanced work."[49]

Clearly, Flexner's missives to Vaughan suggest not only that the reformer was an advocate for increasing the numbers of African American medical students but also that the University of Michigan's program had a reputation for welcoming black matriculants. In a 1920 letter to the secretary for the AMA's Council on Medical Education and Hospitals, University of Michigan pharmacology professor C. W. Edmunds noted that the medical school had a considerable number of admissions from Lincoln University, identified as an approved arts and sciences undergraduate college "for Negro students."[50] (Established in 1854 as the Ashmun Institute, Lincoln University was the first degree-granting historically black university in the United States.) Exact numbers are difficult to verify, since Michigan did not maintain official records of student race before 1942.

Vaughan observed that African American students were more likely to suffer from the consequences of poverty, which affected their ability to succeed in Michigan's demanding program. In a letter to the president of Lincoln University, Vaughan noted that one of his black students had to wait tables four hours a day while attending the medical school. This could not have been helpful for his academic performance. Sometimes racial tensions led to suggestions of racially based improper treatment. When two students—one black, one white—were caught cheating on a pathology examination, the black student was allowed to repeat the course, but the white student was dismissed from the program, causing accusations of racial prejudice. But sometimes the racial prejudice was overt and clearly detrimental to a student's ability to learn. For example, under Dean Cabot, black medical students were prohibited from examining female patients at University

Hospital. Although that policy was rescinded in 1930, black students continued to face limited opportunities in obstetrics and gynecology clinics at Michigan for years.[51]

Other traditionally underrepresented groups—particularly Jews and women—also faced official discrimination and admissions quotas at Michigan. Although Davenport claims that the proportion of Jewish medical students at Michigan was higher than the national average before 1930, faculty members and administrators supported quotas and other restrictions on the number of Jewish students allowed to matriculate.[52] Women faced restrictive quotas (a maximum of 10 percent of the incoming class could be female) and harassment. For example, Pauline Stitt, who entered the medical school in 1929, recalled facing overt hostility from "antiwomen" faculty members, as well as prejudice from her family and community.[53] That being said, Michigan did provide opportunities for some special "quota groups," most notably

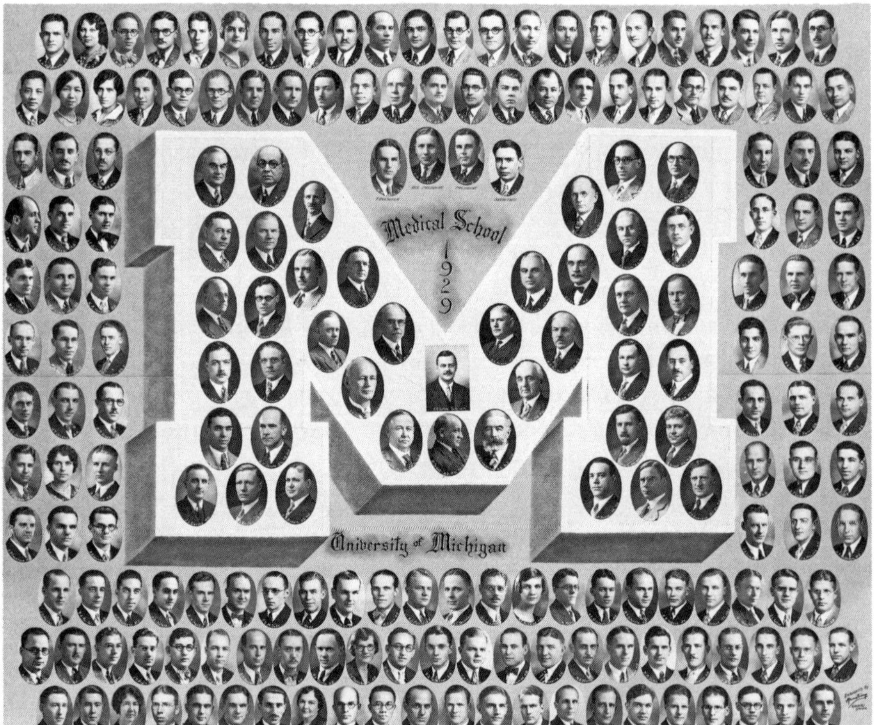

Medical class of 1929. BMC Media Services Records, Bentley Historical Library, University of Michigan, Ann Arbor.

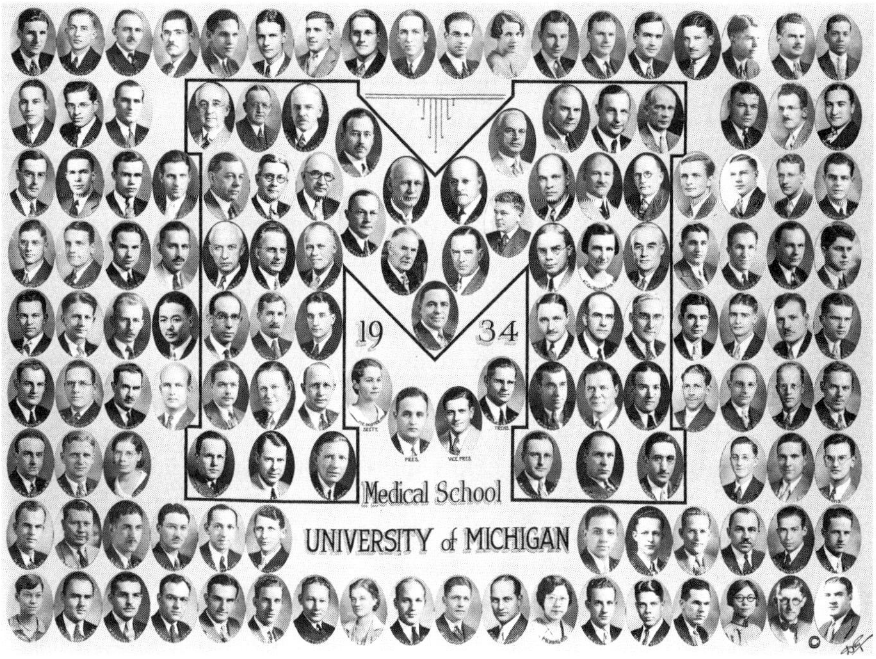

Medical class of 1934. The image includes Elizabeth Crosby, the first female professor, and more men of color than the class of 1929. BMC Media Services Records, Bentley Historical Library, University of Michigan, Ann Arbor.

through the Levi Barbour Oriental Girls' Scholarships. Inspired by an opportunity to meet three East Asian women who had trained in medicine at Michigan in the 1890s, Regent Levi Barbour established the award in 1917 to provide stipends for unmarried Asian women to receive education and training in Ann Arbor, with the intent that they would return to their home countries to better the lives of people there. In 1927, three of the twenty-nine Barbour scholars were medical school students; one was from India and two from China.[54] In general, however, the medical school was highly selective in its interwar admissions, given that it had a limited number of spaces available for each incoming class. It prioritized Michigan residents over out-of-state or international applicants; by the late 1930s, fewer than 30 percent of those accepted into the program were non-Michigan residents.[55] This factor, in addition to other quotas and discriminatory policies (both official and unofficial), determined that regional, socioeconomic, racial, and ethnic diversity would be severely limited in the student population.

The interwar period also saw significant changes in the Galens Honorary Medical Society. Beginning around Christmas 1927, the organization began its first major fund-raising campaign for children in University Hospital, which soon became an annual "tag day" to raise money for Christmas gifts and celebrations. In 1928, the first Galens Workshop opened at the hospital, providing a variety of activities for young patients. The Galens News Stand opened in the 1930s to sell a variety of goods (such as newspapers, cigarettes, and candy) to hospital visitors. In 1934, the society hosted its first Caduceus Ball, an "all-medic dance" for students, faculty, and hospital workers, which became an annual event to produce income for the Galens general fund. In the 1930s, the Galens Smoker became more elaborate (and humorous) and was moved to the Lydia Mendelssohn Theater on campus to accommodate a larger paying audience. While many members of the faculty supported the society and participated—as honorary members and Smoker performers—the administration did occasionally take offense to Galens activities. For example, in 1931 the society began printing a satirical newsletter called the "Thymico-Lymphatic Constitution," but by 1948, some of its entries apparently offended the dean of students, who discontinued the publication and put the Galens Society on a one-year social probation. However, the organization's charity functions were allowed to continue, indicating that the society had transformed itself from a relatively small social group into a service organization, with an important place in hospital operations. Galens also played an important role in curriculum affairs and the school's honor system. Before 1944, the society made annual recommendations to the dean for academic subjects and necessary teaching materials, many of which were adopted by the faculty. They also oversaw the honor council of students from all four classes.[56]

Faculty and Curriculum Changes

During the early twentieth century the medical profession in the United States in general became more specialized and more interested in research.[57] Michigan was no exception. Faculty members identified with increasingly focused areas of interest, especially in medicine, surgery, pathology, and ophthalmology subfields. Research by the mid-1930s included work on a variety of topics and with a variety of sponsors, including Kalamazoo's Upjohn Pharmaceutical Company (for the study of the Mexican agave plant), the Zonite Products Corporation of New York (for a digitalis preparation), and

Mr. and Mrs. Charles Ward Seabury (for a study of infantile paralysis).[58] In the annual report for the 1939–1940 academic year, the dean, in describing the school's major areas of biomedical investigation (which included allergies, glandular therapy, chemotherapy, arthritis, drug addiction, retinoblastoma, and trichinosis), noted that "it is gratifying to observe that nearly all of our faculty members are involved in programs of research, even though they may be carrying heavy responsibilities in the field of education and in the care of the sick."[59]

Some research projects were accompanied by public health advocacy and outreach, notably David Cowie's project to eradicate endemic goiter in Michigan with iodized salt, which coalesced into a nationwide movement during the 1920s.[60] After the development of ventriculin, the Simpson Memorial Institute broadened its scope in hematology. By midcentury researchers had conducted significant investigations into leukemia; different types of anemia; treatments using liver extract, vitamin B complex, and iron; and the use of blood or blood substitutes to treat shock.

Three major areas of interest in internal medicine—metabolism, heart disease, and microbial disease—had each coalesced by the end of the 1920s.[61] Frank Wilson acquired sophisticated new technologies with which to study the heart, including a double-string galvanometer that formed the basis for a new interpretation of the waves making up the ECG tracing. The internal medicine professor Louis Newburgh, freed from many of his clinical responsibilities, was able to do path-breaking work on diet and metabolism.

Pathology also expanded during the first three decades of the twentieth century, and by 1931 all general pathology instruction had moved to preclinical years to allow for more specialized clinical instruction in fields such as neuroanatomy and to give pathology faculty members more opportunity for ambitious research.[62] Expansions and reorganizations did not proceed uniformly across the medical school, however; for example, neurology and psychiatry were separated into two divisions in 1920, mirroring national trends, whereas pediatrics (established as its own department in 1921) remained relatively small and was administratively linked with infectious diseases until 1941, when the Kellogg Foundation gave $100,000 to the division for a ten-year reorganization project.[63]

Although support was undoubtedly strong for such research initiatives, some faculty members were ambivalent about focusing so much on research. They worried about how such priorities might conflict with both instruction and patient care, particularly after the new hospital opened to serve a much larger number of cases. Sturgis was concerned that narrow specialization and concentration on research could lead to professional tunnel vision; as he later reflected, a "physician may be preeminent in his own chosen field but conspicuously deficient or disinterested or both in other aspects of medicine."[64] When he became chair of internal medicine in 1928, Sturgis rearranged the general medicine service to balance the research and teaching demands of the department, allowing his more productive (and lucrative) researchers, such as Wilson and Newburgh, reduced service commitments to conduct investigations while assigning other senior faculty members to increasing work as attending physicians.[65]

The university's adoption of a full-time employment requirement led to tensions, particularly for those medical faculty members who were less engaged in research and did not have outside sources of funding. Many American medical schools had already adopted full-time plans for their basic science instructors, but clinical faculty found such plans disadvantageous, since university salaries could not compete with private practice income. When Michigan first considered full-time appointments for its medical school, the idea was immediately controversial and inconsistently applied, leading several junior faculty members to resign to take positions at competing local institutions, such as the Henry Ford Hospital.[66] Even before assuming his position as dean, Cabot acknowledged that full-time professorships were necessary for the good of the students, since part-time faculty members (supplementing their incomes with private patients) were much more likely to shirk their educational duties. But university compensation alone was inadequate to maintain some high-quality faculty members, many of whom expected to earn large salaries through private practice.[67] In 1926, Dean Cabot and University Hospital director Harley Haynes pleaded with the Board of Regents to reconsider full-time medical faculty appointments at Michigan, where "economic and professional difficulties are highly peculiar." To recruit and keep the "thoroughly first-class clinicians" that the medical school desired for its faculty, the university should devise "some plan which is both economically sound and appeals to the proper desires of men in their position." The dean suggested a base academic salary for teaching and additional compensation from a private patient fee "pool," which would be lower than "commercial" doctors earned but enough to make the position competitive and worthwhile. In Cabot's view, "We must retain some of the atmosphere of the practicing physician and . . . we cannot succeed if we try to put these positions on a truly academic basis."[68]

The issue of medical faculty salaries was probably the largest, though not the only, contributing factor to Cabot's relatively short tenure as dean.

He was also concerned with social class issues of health care, and by the end of the 1920s he seemed to lend support to the controversial notion of compulsory health insurance for the middle and lower classes. Furthermore, Cabot had a reputation for being "domineering, arrogant, and tyrannical," according to a headline article in the *Washtenaw Tribune*.[69] In a 1921 letter to university president M. L. Burton, Royal Copeland had stated, "If you have ever applied a muffler, for goodness sake put one on this Dean. . . . [I]f any man in the world needs to be instructed in psychology and tactfulness, Dean Cabot is that man."[70] In February 1930, the Board of Regents (having received a request from several department heads in the medical school) voted to demand his resignation as dean and advised the creation of an executive committee to manage the medical school in Cabot's stead until a permanent successor, A. C. Furstenberg, was named in 1935. Soon thereafter, Cabot left Michigan for a position at the Mayo Clinic in Minnesota.[71]

Even with significant organizational and priority changes in the school (not to mention faculty turnover), the medical school curriculum changed relatively little from the 1910s to the 1920s. In the 1910–1911 academic year, freshmen students studied anatomy and histology/embryology for six days each week in their first term, with laboratory components for both courses. Physiology, regional anatomy, neuroanatomy, and bacteriology were added in the second. Sophomores during the first semester had daily morning lectures in physiology, physiological chemistry, or pathology, and they had physiology and physiological chemistry laboratories in the afternoon; during the second semester, lectures were offered in pathology, pharmacology, hygiene, diagnosis, and surgical anatomy, and afternoon laboratory sections were occupied with pathology and pharmacology. Juniors and seniors received lectures, laboratory or demonstration/recitation sections, and clinical exposure in a variety of subspecialties, including ophthalmology, otolaryngology, dermatology, pediatrics, obstetrics/gynecology, psychiatry and "nervous diseases," surgery, pharmacology, and medical jurisprudence. All seniors were also required to attend autopsies, and "optional laboratory courses" were available in a variety of subjects. A decade later, in the 1921–1922 schedule, the program remained mostly unchanged, except for the additions of preventive and internal medicine, neurology, and roentgenology for the upper classes. Professor Aldred Warthin also hosted a monthly history of medicine journal club, inviting students to present articles on topics related to the history of medicine into the 1920s.[72]

However, the program did begin to change significantly later in the interwar period, particularly once Vaughan retired. By the mid-1920s, faculty members had expressed concern about admissions standards and requirements. Both Cabot and Furstenberg were worried that the emphasis on undergraduate coursework in sciences as a requirement for matriculation at the exclusion of liberal arts courses meant that, as Dean Furstenberg complained in a later annual report, "the opportunity for a liberal education is no longer given the student who contemplates the study of medicine."[73] The highly selective admissions process undoubtedly helped reduce student attrition rates, which had been almost 50 percent before the war,[74] but high premedical standards could also be a disadvantage for recruitment. The executive committee of the medical school argued that there was a discord between "cultural education" and "training specifically preparatory to the study of medicine" in Michigan's undergraduate program and wondered, "Is it possible that we are asking the Arts College to give a course of training which really lies within the province of our Medical School?"[75]

The requirements for matriculation were even more problematic for applicants coming from outside the University of Michigan. Some came from undergraduate programs with reputations for grade inflation, which did not inspire much confidence in a prospective student's ability to succeed. Michigan offered remedial summer courses, but many good students did not want to take them.[76] In a 1935 letter to Dean Furstenberg, department secretary A. C. Curtis complained that "our requirements are at present so high that . . . we have lost many of the good students from other universities located outside of the state of Michigan because those students were accepted by other class A schools, and they have not wished to attend the University of Michigan Medical School enough to spend an extra summer session or year to meet our requirements."[77]

Concerns were also growing about imbalances in the program's subject matter and the division between preclinical and clinical courses. Because of the prestige of faculty members in fields like ophthalmology and otolaryngology during Vaughan's deanship, Michigan students received a disproportionately high number of hours devoted to those subjects. Thus, some parts of the "curriculum called for more knowledge of the subject than seemed necessary for the general practitioner."[78] Moreover, Michigan's medical school—in deference to Vaughan's and Frederick Novy's research interests—maintained a significant bacteriology component, leaving less time available for pediatrics, physiology, and "newer developments in endocrinology and related subjects," not to mention elective courses.[79] The program's emphasis on laboratory experimentation—one of its most cutting-edge features in the late nineteenth century—was called into question as well. In 1935, Professor

F. J. Hodges argued that "it is not only impossible but inadvisable to attempt to teach technical details to the undergraduate student of medicine."[80] The executive committee of the medical school worried that the four-year curriculum had an even larger systemic flaw in its "divorcing" of basic sciences and clinical courses. A survey of medical school graduates between 1931 and 1933 asked students, "Wherein do you believe you failed to get full benefit from your work at the University?" Many graduates claimed that they had too much preclinical work and wanted more "friendly and helpful" faculty assistance to find internships and private practice opportunities. This may have reflected the fact that while faculty members were becoming more focused on science and specialization, the overwhelming majority of graduates were going directly from medical school to general practice. Such feedback led the executive committee to wonder, "Is it true that medical education is organically defective?"[81]

Clearly, a major assessment and revision of Michigan's program was needed. In October 1935 the executive committee described the four most important criticisms they had received from alumni, the proceedings of the Association of American Medical Colleges, and individual practitioners:

1. The current premedical curriculum was too narrow and stereotyped.
2. The medical courses were too crowded.
3. Seniors and young graduates did not retain knowledge about the fundamental basic sciences taught to them during their first two years.
4. The time required for students to complete undergraduate study did not reliably measure their acquisition of medical training.[82]

The faculty was presented with other concerns as well, particularly the dearth of both adequate space and personnel for clinical instruction at the university (even a decade after the hospital's reconstruction). At that time, the first-year classes admitted about 130–140 students (out of 800–1,200 applicants). An AMA inspection committee had recommended limiting the freshman class to 100 students "to avoid placing a burden upon the limited facilities in equipment, personnel and budgets."[83] Many faculty members supported lowering the cap on matriculation. Newburgh recommended a maximum of 60 students, even while admitting that was "practically out of the question." But the school recognized that reducing class size would cause problems in the relationship with the larger community. In its 1936 report on curriculum revisions, the medical school observed, "We must not overlook our responsibility to the state as a huge state-supported institution.

. . . [I]f we were to limit the number of Freshmen to 100 and likewise give full recognition to . . . the taxpayers of this State, our problem of selection would become a difficult and embarrassing one."[84]

Faculty members also voiced serious concerns about the medical school's inadequacies in clinical instruction, another hallmark of modern medical education for which Michigan had played a leading role. There were significant disagreements about when and where clinics should be offered and whether it was appropriate to expose first-year students to clinical encounters. Relationships with busy clinicians did not always go well. According to Hodges, "There is a distinct tendency to regard the student as a necessary nuisance, one interfering with the speed with which patients may be routed through the various clinical departments."[85]

This discussion culminated in a set of proposed revisions for the admissions process and curriculum that the medical school executive committee sent to the faculty in 1936. According to the proposal, class sizes would be capped at 125 students, with Michigan students composing about 80 percent of that number. In terms of matriculation requirements, the committee recommended "more cultural work in premedical years" and instructed admissions officials to give higher priority to an applicant's "family history" than other stated criteria, such as scholastic average, personal interview (in which "some form of psychiatric anamnesis should be used in the selection of students"), and geographic location.[86] The revision also called for a less demanding schedule for students, with more opportunities for "reading time" during the first years. Although there were still disagreements about prioritizing "cultural" and "scientific" work, the committee recognized that bacteriology should be deemphasized in the curriculum to allow for more focus on industrial medicine and psychiatry-related subjects (including psychology and neuropsychology). Despite the criticisms about separating preclinical and clinical coursework—and despite Newburgh's suggestion that basic science subjects could be combined with clinical subjects—the committee maintained the division, arguing, "It is not the student who forgets his basic sciences but the clinician who fails to emphasize them."[87]

Dean Furstenberg invited faculty members to comment on these changes, and the individual responses provide a fascinating glimpse into the culture of the medical school, and the Michigan community more generally. One unsigned letter to the dean claimed that family history "greatly outweighs all others" in criteria for admission to Michigan's medical school, because it is "a biological rather than an environmental concept." This correspondent advised the school to consider "integrity, intelligence, honesty, local community standing of the parents on the constructive side, and insanity, anti-social behavior, ne'er-do-wellism and low intelligence . . . on the unfavorable side," as well as to conduct physical exams of each candidate "for appearance, general health, [and] stigmata of degeneration."[88] This commentary probably reflected ideas about eugenics, which were widespread within the medical community during the 1930s.

Several faculty members advocated for a more "cultural" approach to premedical coursework as an effective way to create more civic-minded doctors in the state. The distinguished neuroanatomist Elizabeth Crosby, the first woman to be named professor at the medical school, argued that "the general practitioner should be an important factor in the social, educational, intellectual and the political life of the community in which he will practice his profession" and thus "should have a background of general knowledge and culture which will enable him to be a leader."[89] Newburgh agreed but believed that courses like U.S. history and democracy should be mandated for all Arts College students; for prospective medical students, the sciences should remain paramount in the undergraduate program, but perhaps with more emphasis on psychology.[90]

There was also considerable support for a closer pedagogical connection between preclinical and clinical subjects, but the division between the two was not just a curricular issue. Howard B. Lewis suggested it was instead a "geographical problem" and noted that "if the preclinical subjects were taught in the same building as the clinical . . . the students would refer their problems of the clinical years to the preclinical men more frequently."[91] Others suggested that the problem lay with individual clinicians who failed to emphasize the scientific basis for their practices, which could be alienating for medical students and patients alike; as Newburgh claimed, "If we could make the future physician understand what he is dealing with, the patient would not in desperation go to the Christian Science healer or the chiropractor."[92]

Furthermore, several faculty members, like Lewis, supported decreasing "congestion of the courses" and the medical school's "undue emphasis on laboratory work," because "for the average medical practitioner, who is not going into research work, the laboratory work could be decreased very materially without seriously handicapping the student's background."[93] Such comments again recognized the difference between the worlds of the academic professor and that of the general practitioner and suggested differences in the type of training each required.

There was also a call for reducing more outdated subjects, such as materia medica and hygiene, in favor of more modern courses, such as biochemistry, psychiatry, and industrial or occupational medicine. But there were limits on how much to add. Even research specialists like Newburgh addressed the problem of introducing too many subfields in the clinical years, with the earnest plea, "How can a specialist really appreciate his position until he has a thorough knowledge of the human being as a whole?"[94] Clearly Newburgh was concerned primarily with how well the program would train Michigan's general practitioners, rather than academic physicians or research scientists, and actively participated in the discourse about modifying medical instruction to suit the needs of both aspiring doctors and the people of Michigan in the early twentieth century.

One significant remedy for concerns about curriculum limitations was to expand postgraduate education requirements. Many professionals at Michigan recognized that four years of medical training were no longer sufficient, particularly with the rise of specialization during the 1920s. However, when the AMA's Council on Medical Education and Hospitals pleaded with the medical school to adopt the fifth-year internship as a requirement for the M.D. degree in 1919, the faculty unanimously denied the proposal, arguing, "The School should not grant its degree for work which it does not supervise."[95] Furthermore, Dean Vaughan maintained that a rotating internship was largely unnecessary. In these internships the intern would rotate among the services, typically spending three months each on medicine, pediatrics, obstetrics/gynecology, and surgery. Vaughan in essence advocated a quicker route to specialization, arguing that "if a man has decided when he graduates that he is going to be a surgeon or an internist or a specialist in some line, he will waste less time and be a better man if he takes a long time special service in the hospital."[96] Nearly a decade later, the editor-in-chief of the medical fraternity newsletter *Phi Delta Epsilon News* asked Dean Cabot his opinions about compulsory fifth-year internships, and the dean claimed he could "see no method by which the University can adequately control and oversee the opportunities and supervision which the interne will receive." Certainly, internship programs in earlier years had been successful, but in 1928, Cabot doubted "whether there are in this country enough hospitals which I should regard as thoroughly firstclass to accommodate all of the fifth year students, should this practice become general."[97] In the 1920s training after medical school remained distinctly uncommon.

By the early 1930s, however, internship and residency programs were becoming more prevalent for U.S. medical graduates in a variety of institutions. During the Great Depression, many Michigan alumni had a difficult time finding jobs or internship placement and wanted to receive more assistance from the medical school. Moreover, expanding internship programs could help alleviate staffing pressures at new hospitals and help Michigan maintain its competitive place among other top-ranked medical schools in the United States.[98]

The university was selective about its interns, dissuading applications, for instance, from married doctors; and, as at many medical schools and hospitals in the early twentieth century, there was evidence of discrimination against Jewish and Irish interns in the hiring process.[99] In 1939, a new Interns' Home was completed on the hospital campus, connected with the main buildings via an underground passage. The new dormitory could accommodate sixty-one people and provide them attractive amenities, including single rooms, private toilets, and marble showers. Interns living in the home also enjoyed "a photographic darkroom, a recreation room covering 2,000 square feet and adjoined by a kitchen, and a handball court." Recreational facilities were thoughtfully located far away from sleeping quarters, in order to allow house staff the opportunity for a peaceful rest. There was also "a lounge room with paneled walls and built-in bookcases, . . . [and] a magnificent view of the Huron River and surrounding country." Such pleasant living arrangements may have contributed to Michigan interns' reputation for decadence during the early 1940s.[100]

Education did not end after internship. The medical school also began adopting continuing education programs for community practitioners in the late 1920s, an idea that Vaughan had started to implement on a small scale early in his tenure as dean.[101] In 1926, the Michigan State Medical Society council invited representatives from the state's medical schools to consider an effective way to address the need for professional development among Michigan practitioners, and the following year that committee recommended that the university (and its state funding) should assume control of a postgraduate education system. The new Department of Postgraduate Medicine, led by James D. Bruce, was the first of its kind in the United States. It would organize courses both at Michigan and in extramural centers around the state, such as the Detroit College of Medicine and Surgery, the Detroit Receiving Hospital, the Herman Kiefer Hospital, and the Children's Hospital of Michigan in Detroit. When the program began admitting students in 1929, only forty-four doctors registered for its first offerings (internal medicine and surgery). Within a decade, however, the program grew exponentially, in terms of both size and scope. By the 1939–1940 academic year, the department had more than two thousand registrants and hosted fifteen intensive courses in Detroit and Ann Arbor, as well as offered a variety of programs in other places throughout the state, such as Saginaw, Battle Creek, Flint, Grand Rapids, Jackson, and Traverse City. The department estimated that postgraduate students represented about one-half of all cities and towns in the state of Michigan, but physicians from other states also enrolled in the program.[102] Such staggering growth is a clear indication that the medical school was serving an important function in the Michigan medical community, providing state-of-the-art instruction for medical students and professional development opportunities for the state's doctors at a time when the culture and practice of medicine in the United States was changing dramatically.

Conclusion

The interwar years saw momentous change at Michigan's medical school, from the influx of new money and space for biomedical research to the administrative turnover in the dean's office. In many ways, Victor Vaughan had represented an older ideal of the medical pioneer, and many policies that he had implemented or supported remained in place throughout his tenure as dean. During the 1920s, however, the school was faced with a different academic landscape and new people in positions of leadership. The population of Michigan was changing, as the state became more industrialized and its residents demanded new kinds of health care. Faculty members and administrators during the 1920s and 1930s grappled with fundamental questions about the future of medical education, and what would characterize the profession in the coming decades, as their students had to learn more and more in increasingly limited space. The expansion of the medical school and its research enterprise, as well as the encouragement of specialization and postgraduate training, would continue into the years of World War II and beyond.

FOUR

Expansion and Consolidation

The Watershed of World War II

World War II started in 1939. When the United States entered the war in 1941, medical education throughout the country was already transforming. Just as had been the case during World War I, the conflict had a profound effect on medical schools and hospitals. All types of health-care personnel joined the military, leaving behind shorthanded and stressed staff, faculty, and student bodies. Demand for new medical procedures and technology forced revolutionary changes in U.S. health care and research—changes that would persist long after the war's end. People around the country and at Michigan reflected on the war's widespread impact on medical schools, and in 1942, graduates heard Colonel Grover Cleveland Penberthy of the U.S. Army Medical Corps deliver the University of Michigan Medical School's convocation address, titled "Contributions of War to Medicine."[1]

This was a world war, one that affected everyone, whether formally in the military or not. All able-bodied people were expected to contribute to the war effort. More doctors were needed to care for the rapidly expanding army. To allow for the training of the thousands of doctors needed in the conflict, the federal government granted military service deferments to all U.S. medical students for the duration of medical school and one year of internship.[2]

Physicians, nurses, staff members, and students—even those who had been deferred from the draft—left Ann Arbor to serve in the military, often overseas. Many staffed the 298th General Hospital in France, Belgium, and the United Kingdom, which treated some forty-three thousand patients. Hospital staff sometimes found themselves delivering care under intense enemy fire.[3] Other university physicians served in noncombat roles, but

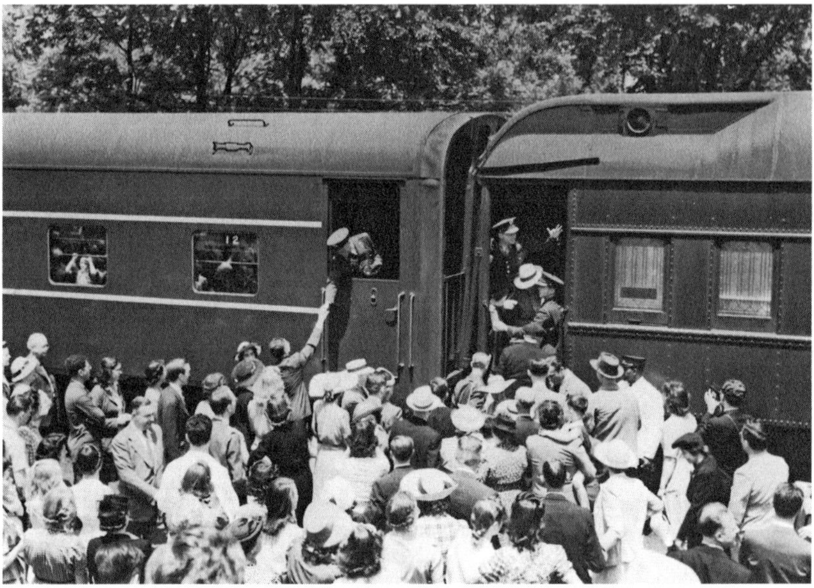

The 298th General Hospital departing from Ann Arbor, ca. 1942. Harry A. Towsley Papers, Bentley Historical Library, University of Michigan, Ann Arbor.

they were no less important. The noted heart specialist Frank Wilson was invited to visit South America by the U.S. State Department in 1942, in the middle of the conflict, to speak on his research on electrocardiography. While the physicians in Brazil and other countries were doubtless happy to learn more about the intensely technical research Wilson was doing in Ann Arbor, the impetus for the State Department to send him on his 1942 visit may also have been to spread U.S. goodwill to strategically important parts of the hemisphere and to encourage them to join the United States and the Allies in the war effort (which Brazil did).

Back home, schools did what they could to support the rapidly expanding medical corps. Beginning in 1942, to get young physicians more rapidly into the field, sixty-six of the seventy-eight medical schools in the United States and Canada began offering an accelerated, three-year program of study. This plan was implemented at Michigan as well, even though teaching staff had already been reduced by 40 percent. The decision generated concern. Could high standards for medical education be maintained in such accelerated pathways? In his 1943–1944 annual report to the university president, Dean Albert C. Furstenberg described the shortened curriculum as

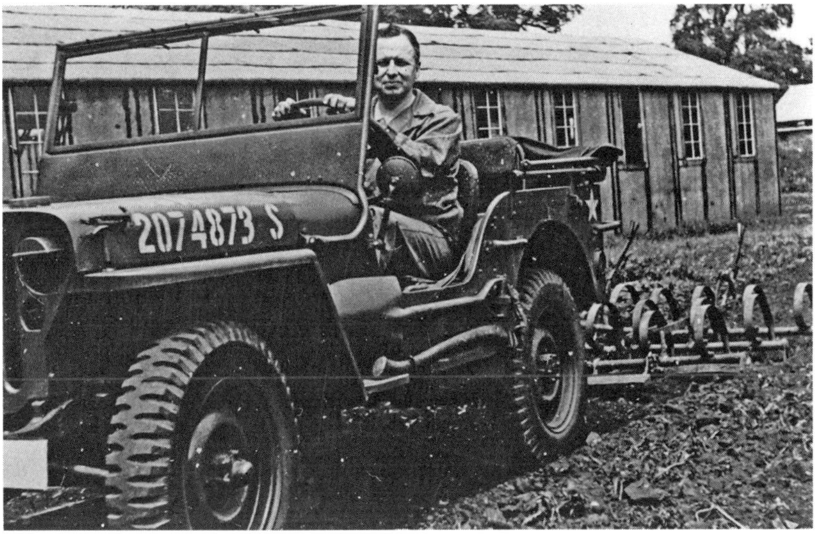

Faculty member Harry Towsley in France, ca. 1944. Harry A. Towsley Papers, Bentley Historical Library, University of Michigan, Ann Arbor.

"one of education's decadent trends," which "we view with anxiety," fearing that such a curriculum could have an adverse effect on the profession even after the war.[4]

However, once the war ended, so did the accelerated program. But the military concerns did not. Following the end of World War II, the United States entered the Cold War, a war marked by occasional very hot periods, such as the Korean War. President Harry Truman had characterized the physician work force as an important element in the Cold War, and when the Korean War started in 1950, some U.S. medical schools went back to a three-year curriculum. While Michigan did not resurrect the accelerated curriculum of World War II, it increased its enrollments, which grew rapidly. In 1940, the school had 131 first-year students (out of 472 in all four years). A class size that had grown to 165 just before the onset of the Korean War expanded to 200 freshmen in 1951; by 1954, Michigan's medical school had a total of 775 students—the largest enrollment in North America.[5]

The changes at Michigan and elsewhere were not merely those of scale. Physicians returned from World War II military service to usher in a fundamentally new era of American medicine. The war had been at its heart a science-based war, and from its beginning U.S. leaders knew that science could well determine who would win the war. They had to invent new mechanisms for using federal funds to support wartime scientific research being done in nonfederal institutions, often universities. The best-known scientific developments may have come in the realm of physical sciences, such as radar and the atomic bomb. But also critical were medical advances, such as the mass production of penicillin, malaria treatment, and blood banking. After the war ended in 1945, the mechanisms that had been devised to fund wartime scientific research were transformed into a system for supporting research during peacetime, leading to unprecedented funds—especially from the National Institutes of Health (NIH) and other branches of the federal government—being made available for the construction and renovation of medical facilities, new faculty appointments, and, most of all, more biomedical research. During the second half of the twentieth century, the medical school embraced the research enterprise as a primary goal for medical schools even more than it had during the interwar decades. Investigators studied a long list of subjects. They worked on combatting and preventing major endemic health problems and on developing revolutionary procedures and therapies, such as antibiotics, anticoagulants, effective treatments for syphilis and tuberculosis, chemotherapy, angiography, and renal dialysis.[6] The influx of NIH research funds allowed for a rapid expansion of medical schools. More and more investigators obtained funds to do research. This explosion of so-called soft money was the underpinning for many (if not most) of the incremental research projects that were becoming ever-more central to the mission of the academic medical school during the latter half of the twentieth century.

At the University of Michigan in 1940–1941, total extramural funds, both private and federal, amounted to only $137,000. By 1950 that number exceeded $500,000, and five years after that, it had reached $1 million.[7] Many administrators welcomed this change and expressed the popular idea that advances in research (and financial support) would necessarily help improve teaching and patient care. The university-affiliated hospital was the ideal location for such research, and Michigan had already established itself as a frontrunner in American academic medicine.

If research were to become a dominant part of the school, the question arose: How were the educational, clinical, and research functions to be related? Longtime faculty member Reuben Peterson had considered the mechanism of this consolidation even before World War II, as he applauded in 1939 the cooperation between scientific medicine and clinical instruction at the medical school in his history of the University Hospital:

> Today the greatest harmony and co-operation apparent exist between those who administer and teach the so-called basic sciences and the clinical teachers. As one who was serving the School when the West and East Medical Buildings were erected and who used, unsuccessfully to be sure, what little influence he had to have the last building placed in close proximity to the clinical teaching unit, so that both types of teachers might benefit, is it too much to hope that the next step in advance will be a complete medical unit situated ideally on the bluffs overlooking the Huron?[8]

This hope for physical proximity was soon to be realized. As early as 1950, the Board of Regents started to develop ambitious plans for a consolidated medical center, initially to comprise the medical school, the University Hospital complex, and the School of Nursing. These plans included a new medical science building to house preclinical classes for the medical school, a library and administration wing, new hospital facilities and outpatient clinics, and an Institute for Clinical Medical Research. Between 1940 and 1970, fifteen new medical buildings were constructed, and the total square footage of building space devoted to medical education, patient care, and research more than doubled. By the 1960s, the University of Michigan Medical Center—frequently described as "sprawling"—was celebrated as an innovative physical plant ideal for the pursuit of medical knowledge.[9]

The postwar years also saw a profound change in postgraduate education and medical specialization. Before the 1940s, many medical school graduates went directly into general practice, often without completing any sort of formal internship or residency program. Those few young doctors who completed internships did so in community hospitals, and few went on to specialize in a residency. However, the war did much to change all that. For one, doctors in the military were exposed to specialty training and practice and saw what additional skills specialized training could offer. In addition, general practitioners saw advantages offered to those physicians who had received formal certification as specialists from newly formed private boards (such as the American Board of Internal Medicine or the American Board of Surgery). When the war started, the medical corps expanded rapidly, reaching a peak size of seven hundred thousand—more than three times the size of the entire army in 1939. To organize the medical corps, the army used what markers they had. This meant that physicians with specialty certification entered the military at a higher rank and higher pay. Many of those who had entered military service as general practitioners returned home wanting to complete further training and become specialists.[10]

As Dean Furstenberg pointed out, "medical students no longer can expect to gain all of their knowledge in school," and postgraduate instruction was fast becoming critical for success in the modern profession.[11] The availability of research dollars and funding for new faculty positions enabled medical schools like Michigan to rapidly expand their postgraduate education programs. Interns fulfilled vital hospital staffing positions, and community and academic hospitals sometimes competed to recruit interns. By and large, the academic hospitals won out, because they were able to provide more state-of-the-art programs and technologies. In many places, such as Michigan, academic institutions began to expand their affiliations with community hospitals to decrease competitiveness, accommodate a growing number of students, and increase their outreach to a broader community.[12] Michigan's medical school created or strengthened existing relations with a variety of other Ann Arbor institutions, particularly the new Veterans Administration (VA) Hospital (dedicated in 1953) and St. Joseph Mercy Hospital, as well as Wayne County General Hospital in Detroit.[13]

Along with formal residencies, the medical school's "extramural" course offerings also continued to grow, expanding its postgraduate education to

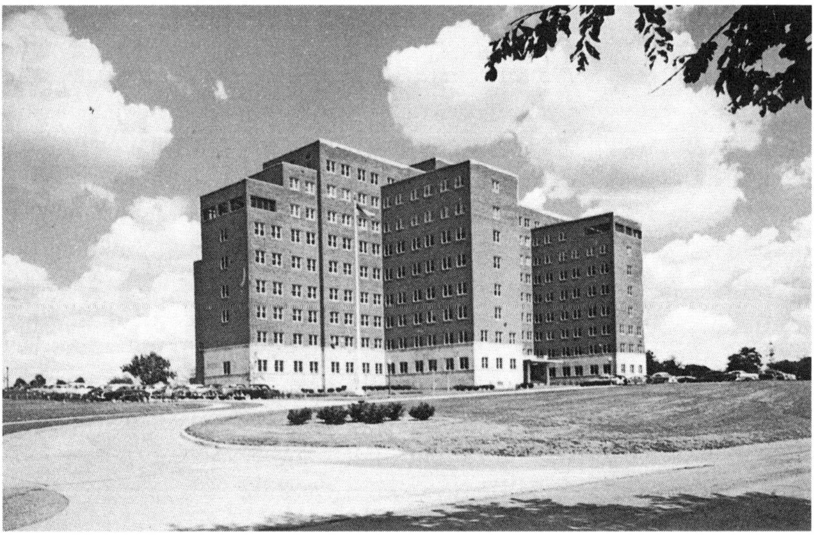

Veterans Administration Hospital, Ann Arbor, mid-1950s. Postcard Collection, Bentley Historical Library, University of Michigan, Ann Arbor.

physicians and other health-care professionals outside the university and, by 1958, to nineteen other institutions in the state. Michigan faculty members provided instruction at the Ann Arbor facility and oversaw medical staff members in their own hospitals; they also maintained a close relationship with the Michigan State Medical Society for clinical conferences and other continuing education opportunities. Individual departments also began creating projects for outreach to a broader professional community; in 1966, for instance, anesthesiology organized a School of Respiratory Therapy at Washtenaw County Community College.[14] This continued commitment to postgraduate education was exceptional among U.S. schools and helped strengthen the University of Michigan's relationships with other state institutions and practitioners in the mid-twentieth century.[15]

Along with the rapid rise in NIH research funding, science and research became seen as the touchstones for excellence in medical training and care. This trend to emphasize scientific medicine is reflected in the printed brochure used to provide prospective students with information about the medical school. In 1955, the brochure included a photograph of two male physicians transferring radioactive cobalt into "the 'theratron,' which is a new instrument used in treatment of cancers and deep tumors." By placing the image in a prominent position in the brochure the school was stating that one of the most important things about going to school at Michigan was the opportunity to learn about the very latest and most modern science and technology. The brochure also noted the growing importance of postgraduate training. It stated that "one more year of study and apprenticeship is still necessary . . . before a young doctor can sign a prescription or enter into practice on his own," a year that is described as "fascinating to the young physician." The text goes on to say that "three to five more years of supervised practice in a hospital at a relatively low salary" (as an intern or resident) were necessary because, "increasingly, medical services in this country are being given to doctors who have specialized in one area of medicine." In 1958, the format and text of the brochure were unchanged, but the photograph of the theratron had been replaced with an image of "two [male] surgeons . . . performing an operation with the aid of a new 'heart pump' which University medical researchers have developed." Clearly, the school was proud of its research accomplishments and firmly dedicated to the rise of specialization that had, in part, enabled the growth of Michigan's prestige during the postwar years.[16]

Members of the American medical profession viewed these transformations as largely positive; however, some observers began to recognize potential disadvantages of medicine's new priorities. There was not universal agreement that federal support of research was necessarily a good thing or that it was always desirable to obtain as much funding as possible. Former dean of Harvard Medical School Robert S. Ebert noted, "It became a matter of faith, rather than reason, that only good could come from the support of biomedical research and that more was inevitably better. . . . [M]edical schools welcomed the change, but with almost no realization of how profound the change would be."[17] Michigan chair of internal medicine Cyrus Sturgis once turned down the offer of additional funds from NIH on the grounds that all research projects were fully funded.

The effect on patient care was also questioned. Ebert was concerned that "the generalist . . . could no longer compete with the full-time specialist" in the midcentury profession, and that trend was becoming increasingly evident in American medical schools. By the 1960s, some physicians and medical professors worried that the growing focus on research, expansion of specializations, and reliance on new medical practices and technologies could have a deleterious effect on patient care.[18] National reports such as the "Coggeshall Report" of 1965, chaired by University of Chicago vice president for medical affairs Lowell Coggeshall, emphasized the importance of improving the training of medical students, and doing so in ways that reflected the health needs of the population.[19]

Michigan physicians also began to be concerned about what focusing on research might mean for the future of medical education. Michigan pediatrics professor E. H. Watson warned in 1953 that the "understandable desire on the part of medical schools to capture 'big names' for faculty positions and department heads" resulted in hiring conventions that favored research excellence and publications over clinical and teaching experience. Nonetheless, most faculty were expected to care for patients and to teach. This, in Watson's view, "is unfair to the members and students of the department," as well as to such a candidate for hire, since that candidate must "function in areas in which he has no special skill and no longer has time to do the things for which he is best fitted."[20] While it is unclear just how widespread agreement with Watson's opinion might have been, it should be noted that Watson was board certified in 1937, before certification was usual (or expected), and he held leadership positions both locally and nationally.[21]

Postwar Faculty Developments

The growing primacy of research and clinical specialization had started at Michigan before the war. Albert Carl Furstenberg discovered a way to manipulate water metabolism to help treat patients with episodic vertigo, tinnitus, and hearing loss, known as Meniere's disease. The Department of Pharmacology had partnered with the Rockefeller Foundation and the National Research Council to study mechanisms of drug addiction. The school's 1939–1940 annual report boasted that nearly all of its faculty members were involved in some form of research, particularly concerning allergies; malignant disease and chemotherapy; nutrition, vitamins, and metabolism; glandular therapy; arthritis; infantile paralysis; drug addiction; retinoblastoma; and trichinosis.[22] But after the war, the increasing availability of funding from federal sources, the university's Horace H. and Mary A. Rackham Fund for graduate students, and other university foundations encouraged the growth of research enterprises in many different areas, and important work was conducted in several different schools on campus. For example, renowned virologist Thomas Francis, Jr., the first scientist to isolate the influenza virus, arrived at Michigan in 1941 to found a School of Public Health on the invitation of Henry F. Vaughan (Victor Vaughan's son). During the years of World War II Francis began recruiting Michigan students and U.S. Army corps members for epidemiological research, exemplifying an important trend in the study of disease that focused more on large populations than on individual cases. In the 1950s, Francis developed the first large-scale community study of endemic disease, which involved ninety-five hundred residents in the village of Tecumseh, Michigan. He then took the lead on one of the most important studies of the mid-twentieth century, one aimed at control of the then-dreaded disease of polio. On April 12, 1955, Francis took the stage at Rackham Auditorium in Ann Arbor and announced to an anxious world the good news that the Salk poliomyelitis vaccine was "safe, effective, and potent" after an unprecedented study that had involved more than a million participants and became the gold standard for prospective, double-blind clinical trials.[23]

The university benefited from Cold War government investments in technological development, especially nuclear technology. World War II had been marked by the use of two nuclear weapons, and the postwar political environment saw such weapons (along with the science that had created them) as being key to the nation's survival. But nuclear techniques were not only used for bombs; nuclear power also looked promising. And clinical care, too, could benefit from the new world of the atom. In 1954 Michigan received a major research grant for radiology and cancer treatment from the U.S. Atomic Energy Commission. This came four years after the agency's director of information services, Morse Salisbury, had delivered the medical school centennial convocation speech "The Atomic Energy Program of the

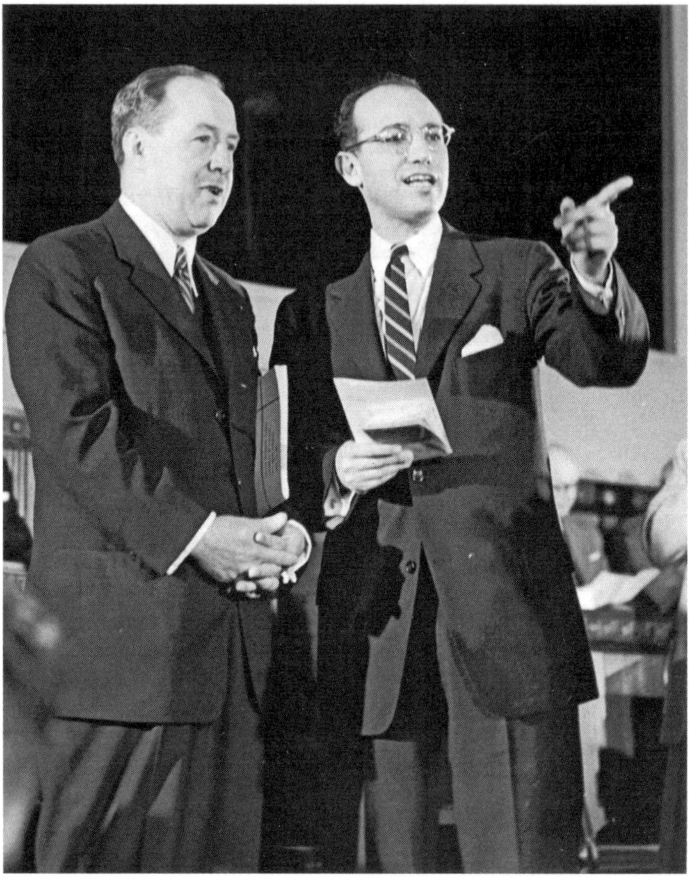

Thomas Francis, Jr. (left), and Jonas Salk (right) at a press conference on April 12, 1955. Photography by Eck Stanger, *Ann Arbor News*. School of Public Health (University of Michigan) Records, Bentley Historical Library, University of Michigan, Ann Arbor.

People of the United States" and four years before the University of Michigan received "a powerful new charge of radioactive cobalt . . . equivalent in power to $75,000,000 worth of radium" for study on its campus.[24]

The medical school saw a wide range of research achievements during the postwar era. Like the School of Public Health, the medical school utilized Michigan students as experimental subjects, particularly to test an influenza vaccine during World War II. Soon after the war it found itself at the forefront of a number of important medical developments, including the use of corticosteroids for inflammation, enzyme identification, a refined design for "iron lungs" to treat respiratory failure in acute poliomyelitis cases, electrophysiological studies of anesthesia, and fundamental research on ketamine.[25] In the spring of 1954, the Kresge Research Building—financed by an endowment from Detroit's S. S. Kresge Foundation—opened to house the first otophysiology research laboratory and, after 1962, the Kresge Hearing Institute. In the 1950s Basil Hirschowitz, a gastroenterology fellow, collaborated with colleagues in the physics department to invent the first fiber-optic endoscope. Also in the 1950s, in the Section of Cardiac Surgery, Cameron Haight worked with Dick and Norma Sarns to improve the new technology of cardiopulmonary perfusion machines (and in so doing demonstrated how academic research could effectively collaborate with the biomedical industry). A major discovery in endocrinology came in 1954 when Jerome Conn described primary aldosteronism, a curable form of hypertension later named "Conn's Syndrome." In 1964 Stefan Fajans helped elucidate the nature of diabetes by studying seven generations of a Michigan family who had come down with the disease but who did not require treatment with insulin. They had developed the disease at an unusually early age. Fajans termed this syndrome "maturity onset diabetes of the young," or MODY.

The explosion of biomedical research was based in part on scientists' increasing use of animal models of human disease. Inbred mouse strains became a powerful tool for understanding the underlying science. Proper care of laboratory animals was once the responsibility of each investigator, but the rapid growth of animal research at the medical school led to the creation of a specific laboratory animal medicine unit in the 1950s, originally located in the Kresge Medical Research Building. This unit was expanded into the Animal Care Unit under veterinary direction in 1962.[26] In 1968 the unit was renamed the Unit for Laboratory Animal Medicine.

Outside observers noted the high quality of Michigan's faculty and facilities. In 1958, during a survey visit to the medical school, Northwestern Medical School assistant dean John A. Cooper and his team lauded the considerable amount of research funding and activity in Ann Arbor, as well as the "impressive" number of scientific publications that resulted from this activity.[27] The "sudden and seemingly unlimited availability of federal funds in support of research and education" at Michigan allowed the medical school to recruit more faculty members with full-time salary compensation while allowing them to devote their major energies to what one historian describes as "a frenzy of research activity" in the 1950s and 1960s.[28]

This activity was accompanied by rapid growth in the overall number of faculty members, residents, interns, and other employees. Between 1940 and 1971 the number of all employees associated with the University of Michigan Medical School and hospital—including emeriti faculty—grew from 164 to 578. A few specific examples give a sense of scale: the anatomy faculty at Michigan tripled, and the neurology and physiology departments experienced fourfold increases between 1950 and 1970. The seven microbiology faculty members, six of whom had full-time appointments, of 1940 grew to twenty-six by 1970, including thirteen full-time positions and six postdoctoral fellows.[29]

The growth of the school led to the reorganization of some departments and the invention of others. The expanding microbiology department was removed from its auspices in the Pasteur Institute in the 1950s and became its own department in the medical school in 1963. Urological and thoracic surgery were founded as distinct, separate divisions in 1940, sixteen years before the first open-heart operation was performed at University Hospital. The urology chief, Reed Nesbit, acquired an international reputation for his clinical skill. In 1961 he was asked to fly to Taipei to operate on Chiang Kai-shek. The trip required him to spend six weeks abroad, but it had a successful result.[30] Thoracic chief Cameron Haight had in 1933 performed the first total removal of the left lung for bronchiectasis in two stages. Anesthesiology became a distinct department in 1949. The anatomy department created separate areas for developmental, microscopal, neural, and gross anatomy, as well as research concentrations in neurosurgery and comparative neuroanatomy, largely conducted by Elizabeth Crosby's team.[31] In 1950 the physical medicine and rehabilitation department was removed from roentgenology and over the next several years developed a division of vocational rehabilitation and an orthotics research division. Human genetics, which began at the university as a "heredity clinic" in 1941 to collect data and provide genetic counseling, became a separate department under the leadership of James V. Neel in 1956 (the first such department in the United States) and received new research facilities in 1964, funded primarily by the Detroit civic leader Lawrence D. Buhl. Around the same time, the Upjohn Pharmaceutical Company of Kalamazoo established an institute for clinical pharmacology research at Michigan to investigate drug addiction and dependence. By the early 1970s the medical school's research facilities were among the most extensive in the country.[32]

Although this expansion gave Michigan's faculty an impressive, and well-deserved, reputation for productivity, it introduced a number of admin-

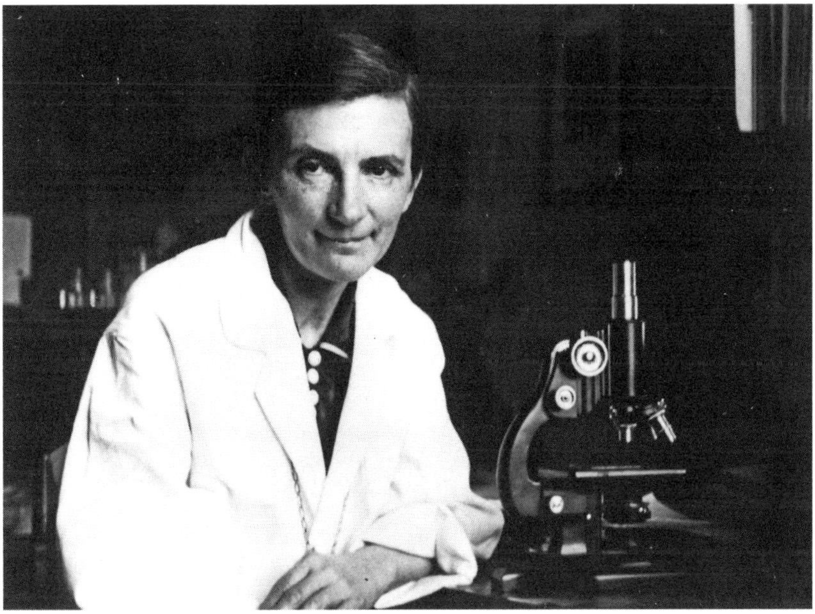

Neuroanatomist Elizabeth Crosby, the first woman to receive a full professorship at the medical school. Elizabeth Caroline Crosby Papers, Bentley Historical Library, University of Michigan, Ann Arbor.

istrative problems. When Furstenberg was preparing to retire as dean in the late 1950s—"the last of the deans to combine chairmanship of a department, private practice, and medical administration"[33] the institution's size made some wonder about the feasibility of effective communication, not to mention a coherent medical education program. The 1958 outside review recommended that the new dean, William N. Hubbard, Jr., take the opportunity afforded by a transition in leadership for "a thorough and critical self appraisal" of the school's operations. It advised the creation of a small group of faculty, meeting as an executive committee, to advise the dean's office more effectively, as the senior faculty as a whole had simply grown too large to serve that function.[34]

"Growing Pains" in the Curriculum

In the school's 1939–1940 annual report, Dean Furstenberg quoted a description from the AMA's Council on Medical Education and Hospitals of the basic medical course as "relatively simple and unified. Its chief objective is to prepare the student to pass the state licensing examination," noting that "the undergraduate student is like a galley slave, chained to his bench."[35] But rapid postwar changes in the medical profession had a strong effect on medical education, which soon became neither simple nor unified.

One set of issues had to do with scale and space. Medical schools felt "a great deal of pressure . . . to accept more students and turn out more physicians. Additional facilities and increased budgets [were] the order of the day."[36] At Michigan, the price of expanding the medical school program was certainly steep; Professor Rollo McCotter claimed in 1947 that "any projected building to house adequately preclinical sciences in the next ten years is going to cost about four times that of the East Medical Building, or in round numbers, between $3,000,000 and $4,000,000"[37] (approximately $32 million and $43 million in 2017 dollars). Nonetheless, new facilities for preclinical, basic science education were absolutely necessary, as class sizes grew in tandem with the expansion of the medical center. Planners worried that the "sprawling" physical plant would isolate preclinical education from clinical personnel, technology, and practices. In 1950, as the medical school celebrated its centennial anniversary, its curriculum committee began to consider strategies to modernize its program and narrow the growing gap between basic sciences and clinical studies and faculty.[38] One strategy was to build new facilities so that the various parts of the medical school could be close to each other. The Medical Science I Building, ready for occupation in 1958, was located adjacent to the School of Nursing and connected via a bridge to the main hospital. This allowed the medical school administrative offices and departments of pathology, biochemistry, and pharmacology to relocate from the old West Medical Building on the university's main campus, "in the best interest of close cooperation of the departments in their educational and research programs." The new building was certainly more comfortable—visitors praised its fully air-conditioned classrooms—and though its lecture halls were not as large, they provided better views for students. Just over a decade later, the completion of Medical Science II brought the departments of anatomy, microbiology, and physiology to the medical center complex from their older home in the East Medical Building. The Department of Human Genetics, which originally had been located in the 1910 ear and eye ward building on Catherine Street, was also given space in the new structure.[39]

But the physical plant was not the same as the curricular structure. Dean Furstenberg had described Michigan's postwar four-year medical curriculum as "cumbersome and unwieldy," as it reflected the growing diversity and research interests of the school's faculty and its autonomous departments.[40] Freshmen at Michigan were exposed to a particularly large amount of study in anatomy (including gross, microscopic, and neurologic), as well as biochemistry, bacteriology (idiosyncratically, offered before physiology), and a "personality growth and development" psychology class. In addition, first-year students were expected to complete a first aid course and observe in a freshmen clinic. Sophomores focused mainly on pathology and physiology and also took courses in pharmacology, the history of medicine, "applied" anatomy, psychiatry, and human genetics, in addition to learning about physical and clinical laboratory diagnosis and taking a surgical clinic course.

The third and fourth years were dominated by clinical education in the form of lectures, small sections, ward rounds, and rotations. The "juniors" were exposed to the four major clinical fields of general medicine, pediatrics, surgery, and obstetrics and gynecology but also took clinical courses in psychiatry, neurology, syphilology, and radiology. "Senior" students continued rotations in the four major fields but also had electives in otolaryngology, ophthalmology, neurology, and outpatient clinic, as well as coursework in medical jurisprudence and required attendance at surgical pathology conferences. Successfully passing national board examinations was required at the end of the second and fourth years, and "the entire school participate[d] in the California Cancer Knowledge Examination," a set of questions designed to assess knowledge of cancer given to students at forty schools across the country in 1950.[41]

Michigan's crowded course load aroused some concerns, as did the issue of just who was to do the teaching. As early as 1953, Watson (echoing the sentiment of Pennsylvania medical school dean John McK. Mitchell) argued that Michigan's emphasis on research for promotion, rather than excellence in instruction, was "one of the greatest weaknesses of our present . . . system" and that "too little is heard about improving the quality of medical teaching by a program of selection and training."[42] Furthermore, there were clear tensions between the basic science and clinical faculty members, often manifest as condescension or hostility toward the students. At that time the assumption was prevalent (at least among the basic sciences instructors) that clinical coursework early in medical school could be detrimental to students—they might be "seduced by the taste of the clinic and will not then want to return to the laboratories." However, some of these same instructors felt they "have other jobs to do than to teach medical students" and resented their educational obligations.[43] Several students claimed that their preclinical courses were too lecture-heavy and that the "emphasis placed upon examination and grades . . . was deleterious to the development of a mature attitude towards studies."[44]

While praising the facilities, the April 1958 survey team delivered a strong critique of Michigan's educational program, arguing that the medical school faculty relied too heavily on "passive" modes of learning, particularly didactic courses and short-answer assessment tools (mostly multiple-choice and true/false examination questions).[45] The team was particularly concerned about third-year clinical lectures, which "are not received with enthusiasm by the students" and were widely considered to be outmoded. Instead, the team recommended that Michigan consider more of a "clerkship" or preceptor model for its third-year clinical courses—ironically, what George Dock had implemented many decades earlier—as well as small discussion groups or seminars.[46] The visit summary also noted that the curriculum and administration of the school would benefit from an awareness of the "necessary interdependence of the disciplines" in medical education and suggested better communication and cooperation between the school's departments. In all, the team concluded that despite the laudable and impressive record of research at Michigan, they had to agree with "the feeling expressed by many of the faculty that a searching and thorough consideration of the entire curriculum for medicine is urgently needed."[47]

The medical school reacted to the site visit team's report with a bit of defensiveness—pathology professor D. L. Hinerman avowed, "We have one of the outstanding medical schools in the country . . . [and] our product is a fine one, whether due to or in spite of our influences"—but it did take Cooper and his team's critique seriously. That summer, the curriculum committee "worked tirelessly" to develop a new plan involving more integrated courses and a less demanding schedule for the students.[48] As part of that process, in June 1958, Michigan hosted the nation's first teaching institute for medical education at the Michigan Union, bringing together 215 University of Michigan faculty members as well as administrators, professors, and education experts from outside the university. As Furstenberg observed at the meeting, "It would be a sad commentary if, as a leading apostle of medical education in this country, the Medical School of the University of Michigan were compelled to admit its inability to tackle this job."[49] In his welcome address, University of Michigan president Harlan Hatcher praised the attendants at this historic meeting "for taking the problem of teaching medicine as seriously as you take the problem of research in medicine," emphasizing that, while instruction and research were both important dimensions of the school, there were fundamental differences in how those dimensions were prioritized.[50] Attendants discussed what they considered to be the most pressing issues in medical education, including the inadequacy of noisy, hot, and poorly lit or ventilated classrooms; the necessity of effective communication between departments and divisions; and the importance of bringing more clinical instruction into the first two years of medical school.[51] The most persistent theme of the institute, though, was the importance of active learning for medical students. As George E. Miller, professor and director of the University of Buffalo's Project in Medical Education, pointed out,

> Our actions suggest that our major goal is to stuff the medical student with information. He seems almost like a barrel into which we run a constant infusion of rather intoxicating material and we are terribly pleased, when we tap the bung at some future time, to have what we put in flow out again. . . . The behavior of most medical faculties indicates that what we really believe is the more facts we can put into the student the better educational program he will have.[52]

To make sense of an ever-increasing body of knowledge was virtually impossible for passive, "vegetated" students. Medical faculty members needed to make students more responsible for their own learning and to provide them with opportunities for active learning and participation, even in research. Conversely, many attendees argued, medical faculty members needed to be less concerned with their students' perceived failures and weaknesses and stop complaining about how students were annoying or irresponsible with their free time (which, many instructors believed, or perhaps suggested tongue in cheek, was spent mainly on the golf course).[53]

While the teaching institute appears to have been intended as a single (not an annual) occurrence, the medical school's investment in the event clearly indicates its recognition of the scope of the problem and the importance of Michigan maintaining its historical reputation as being in the vanguard of modern medical education.[54] It inspired increasing attention to curriculum revision. The medical school began to apply significant pedagogical reforms in subsequent decades, including a shift toward a more disease-specific model of course design. Faculty member Richard D. Judge, a cardiologist, took the lead in using new technology for the educational mission. He coordinated a closed-circuit color television system to deliver lectures, demonstrations, and conferences to a variety of Michigan's affiliated hospitals "by microwave." This technological development foreshadowed the creation of the school's audiovisual library of teaching aids, available for students and professionals at other medical centers.[55] It also presaged the creation of massive open online courses (MOOCs).

Several pressing issues for Michigan's medical instructors remained unsolved, particularly those arising from the relatively large size of the student body. After the Korean War ended in 1953, much of the pressure to grow the school came from the state legislature, which feared a shortage of doctors.[56] Michigan continued to enroll an "unusually large medical student class" (206 in the 1958 class), and even with a low student-to-teacher ratio (due to the school's growing faculty), that translated into a comparatively high teaching load for its instructors. The site visit team warned that "if teaching demands become too heavy, the faculty may not have the energy or interest in providing stimulating and challenging courses for the medical students." Moreover, the team recognized that larger class sizes made it more difficult to implement the active learning curriculum reforms advocated by many educational reformers.[57] In the mid-1960s, as class sizes continued to grow, students criticized the didactic focus of Michigan's medical courses, particularly in the first two years. One anonymous student's letter to the editor of the student paper, the *Paeon*, criticized the quality of the teaching: "In the first two years of lecture-based teaching . . . we do not see real live physicians and medical scientists. We, see *lecturers*. Although they have spent many years learning their fields, many have spent little time learning how to be lecturers."[58] This student observation reflected in part a misapprehension among the faculty about what was required to be a good teacher. As George Miller argued at the 1958 teaching institute, "We operate under a tacit assumption that if a man is skilled in his subject matter, he is a good teacher. I believe one could accumulate a massive body of data to deny the accuracy of this assumption."[59]

As Michigan class sizes continued to swell, some observers argued that the state needed another medical school. In the late 1960s, Michigan considered once again creating an accelerated curriculum track to accommodate medical school expansion, which school department chairs roundly denounced as an "inadequate" plan because of the pressures such a move would place on staffing and space and, most importantly, its threat to the quality of the overall program. M. H. Seevers, the chair of pharmacology, sarcastically advised Dean Hubbard "that expansion of a class could always be done and that it would mean that the faculty and staff should become very skillful in the use of space"; he also recommended that teacher salaries should be raised to reflect the new demand, reasoning that "if we are to sell our souls, get a good price for it."[60] This resulted in a stalemate between increasing faculty responsibilities and the impetus for significant curricular and pedagogical reform, a stalemate that would continue at Michigan for decades.

Postwar Medical Students

In the mid-twentieth century, applicants to Michigan's medical school were required to have completed at least ninety semester hours of undergraduate work, with specific courses in chemistry, biology, physics, English composition, and a foreign language, maintaining at least a 2.5 grade-point average. Aspiring medical students also needed to complete the Medical College Admission Test (MCAT), supply recommendation letters, and present themselves for interviews.[61] Dean Furstenberg continued to argue that applicants should have a broad general undergraduate education, but most Michigan faculty members believed that "science courses are still paramount for medical students." These differing emphases on what was important could create a dilemma for the admissions office and sent mixed messages to premedical students at the university.[62] Nonetheless, the school (along with the Michigan state legislature) was clearly dedicated to its tradition of prioritizing Michigan residents for admission and began to restrict the number of out-of-state admissions by enforcing quotas and raising nonresident tuition rates.

The school supported the inclusion of minority groups relatively early in the United States. Before 1960, for instance, Michigan's medical school was said to have had more African American graduates than all other U.S. medical schools combined, excepting the medical schools of Howard University and Meharry Medical College—both historically black institutions. However, the school's percentage of students from underrepresented groups still remained quite small and certainly did not come close to reflecting gender and racial balances in the state of Michigan. In 1960, only five first-year medical students at Michigan were classified as "black." Two years earlier, only eleven women were in an entering class of 206.[63]

Socioeconomic diversity was also a goal, but it was made difficult to accomplish because financial aid was not always easy for students to obtain. Although loans were available from a variety of sources (including Galens and local medical societies), the medical school discouraged first-year students from relying on loans, and most scholarships at Michigan (up to $500, around $4,260 in 2017 dollars) were reserved for junior and senior students.[64]

This posed a major financial problem for students during their first few years. Furthermore, according to Michigan Health Council president Herbert Estes, many students preferred not to incur debts through loans and so paid for their education with summer jobs, part-time work, or (for more advanced students) "externships" in local hospitals, sometimes working up to forty or fifty hours a week. Many medical students were married and relied in part on spousal income for their educational expenses, but they also needed to supplement that income to support their families.[65] The administration certainly did not recommend employment for its students but acknowledged the necessity of "activities that are unprofitable from an educational point of view." As professor of pediatrics Harry Towsley described extracurricular work in 1958, "At least 50 percent of our Senior students have families of from one to four children. It is not only that students like to eat—they have to feed their families . . . [and therefore] take jobs which are probably detrimental to their ultimate education, but economically I don't know what we can do."[66]

All of these obstacles meant that embarking on a career in medicine was not an easy path. The new emphasis on specialization led to an increased length of time required to become a successful, fully trained practitioner or established researcher. This made medicine a field with a daunting financial and time burden for many aspiring doctors, who still would have to face competition for jobs and grants when their training was complete.[67]

Although the program was strenuous and many Michigan medical students were forced to work during their education, the school did offer a variety of extracurricular activities to make student life more enjoyable. A new student dormitory, the Victor Vaughan House, had opened in the fall of 1939 with 109 male occupants. It provided space for 149 altogether, as well as social functions and a place to live in "clean, pleasant, and cheerful surroundings [which] create an atmosphere conducive to health and study."[68] Medical fraternities offered housing, social events, and intramural sports like football, handball, and basketball. The school's history of medicine journal club (which had originated years earlier with the support of Aldred Scott Warthin) continued in the meetings of the Victor Vaughan Society. A number of other student organizations originated (or continued to operate) during the mid-century years, including the Christian Medical Society, the Committee for Student-Faculty Relations, the Student AMA, the Victor Bond Medical Society, and the local chapter of the Student Health Organization.[69] The Galens Honorary Medical Society expanded its activities during the postwar decades, including giving freshmen tours and orientations. Starting in 1931 it organized free X-ray tuberculosis tests for medical and nursing students. By the late 1950s the program had become extremely successful. Previously, three to seven students had been hospitalized at any given time, but by 1957 it was noted that only one medical student had contracted the disease in the past five years.[70] Galens also sponsored guests and speakers. In July 1965, the society hosted forty Swedish medical students on their national tour of American medical schools, and in the spring of 1968, Galens sponsored an Ann Arbor speech by Christiaan Barnard, the South African surgeon who had the year before performed the first human heart transplant. The group also took on the responsibility of providing audiovisual projection for all medical classes and assisted foreign and low-income students with their scholarship and loan funds.[71] They also continued the tradition, started in 1937, of giving a faculty teaching award dubbed the "Silver Shovel," complete with a shovel of the type used to clean out barn stalls. As a charity organization, Galens raised thousands of dollars to fund hospital facilities, such as the Galens Workshop and Multi-Purpose Room in the C. S. Mott Children's Hospital in the late 1960s. The organization's annual Christmas

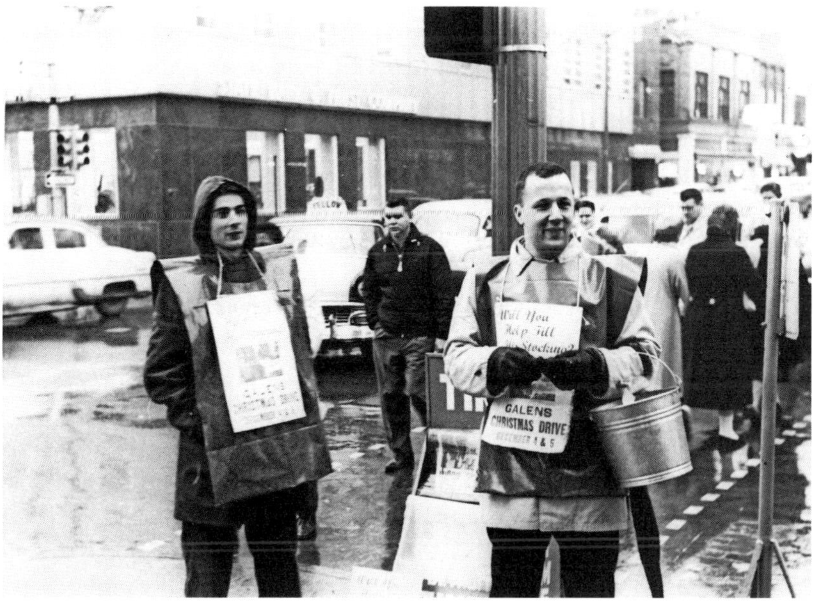

Galens Christmas drive, downtown Ann Arbor, ca. 1960s. Child and Family Life Department (University of Michigan) Records, Bentley Historical Library, University of Michigan, Ann Arbor.

bucket drive for 1967 brought in a remarkable sum, a record of $14,500 (more than $100,000 in 2017 dollars), which then–Galens president Lee R. Britton claimed was "a real tribute to the members, but most of all to the many fine friends that Galens has in the city of Ann Arbor."[72]

As the school felt political pressures to enlarge its medical class sizes in the mid-twentieth century, some faculty members worried that along with such expansion the average quality of the student body would deteriorate. The admission rates would seem to support that fear. In 1956 the medical school accepted every state citizen making application who met the minimum entrance requirements. Dean Furstenberg observed two years later that fewer college students seemed interested in medicine than other professions (such as law or engineering) and that medical schools were not attracting as many top-tier applicants as they had in previous years. He also noted that many aspiring medical students could not afford the time and expense necessary to become a physician, which along with "the depression drop in births a generation ago" contributed to a decline in applications.[73] Between the 1940s and the late 1960s, however, rates of student attrition—which some may have expected to rise—actually fell significantly in those enlarged classes. In 1948, for example, the freshman class had 146 students enrolled at the start of the year (of 468 total), and 9.58 percent of that class dropped out. Two decades later, there were 210 freshmen (out of 797 total), and their class attrition rate was only 1.95 percent for 1966–1967. President Hatcher wrote to Michigan governor George Romney to report the "good news" of the medical school's increased size, noting that "the shortage of doctors has, of course, been a matter of great concern, and our Medical School has been working to extend its capacity," apparently with great success.[74] The 1971 class of 202 was the school's largest graduating class to date.[75]

Despite decreasing attrition, some faculty members at Michigan voiced increasingly negative opinions about medical students and their attitudes during the postwar years. Watson observed "two deplorable changes . . . as the student proceeds through his clinical courses. He loses much of his eagerness to study and learn, and he becomes overly self-confident and arrogant." Miller agreed, noting that students "enter enthusiastic, curious, and eager, yet when they get to the final year they have become blasé and are inclined to look upon the patient to whom they are assigned not as a challenge or an opportunity to learn but simply as a burden." The problem did not lie solely with the students. Overall, in Miller's view, "there is really not very much respect for the student body at Michigan. . . . [T]he faculty does not really regard the students as mature, adult, and responsible individuals but instead as rather petulant and retarded children who have to be driven to achieve the goal."[76]

This negativity was not lost on the students themselves, who were growing more disillusioned with the simultaneous pressure and tedium they experienced in the medical school's program. In 1966, when the student paper, the *Paeon*, was launched, editor-in-chief Glenn W. Geelhoed described the title's origin as "a delightfully abstruse pun. . . . [A]lthough M1's through M4's [first-year through fourth-year medical students] have known themselves to be 'paeons' for some time in the sense of the term's popular parlance equating it with 'serf,' the term has a medical heritage that ideally fits it for the descriptive role it will now serve as the printed voice of the medical student." Geelhoed went on to explain that Asclepius, as physician to the ancient Greek gods, was described as a "paeon," meaning helper, but the editorial betrays the defiance of Michigan's medical students in adopting the term—a defiance that is echoed in letters and articles published over the next two decades.[77] That defiant spirit is also evident in the changing culture of the Galens Smoker, which by the mid-1960s had evolved into more boisterous satire. Parodying popular theatrical shows such as *My Fair Lady* and *The Music Man*, the annual Smoker allowed students to vent their frustrations and poke occasionally quite pointed fun at faculty members. In 1965, Galens president Terry Bergstrom described the event as "the real 'equalizer' of the year," assuring Dean Hubbard that "our object is not vulgarity but entertainment—and, from time to time, a 'suggestion' to the appropriate people."[78] These trends, though seemingly minor, foreshadowed a period of significant medical student alienation and dissatisfaction at Michigan in the coming decade, which former faculty member Horace Davenport described as "disastrous."[79]

"Old Main" Hospital and Its Effect on Clinical Teaching

The Ann Arbor hospital population shifted notably during World War II. The Michigan state legislature had decreased its state appropriations to provide for children with disabilities and chronic medical conditions, and the university saw a precipitous decline in its state-sponsored hospital revenue. In 1942, for example, only about 51 percent of patients were classified as "indigent," down from 80 percent only five years earlier. Thus, by the end

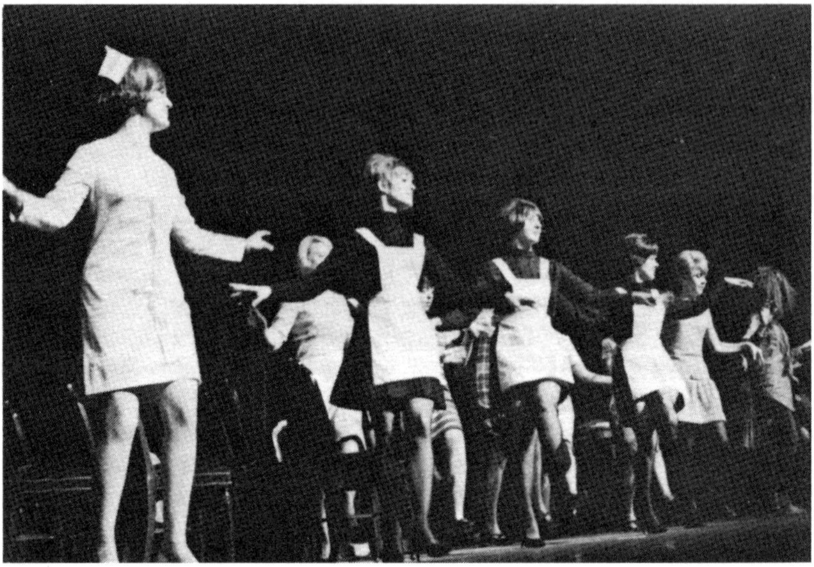

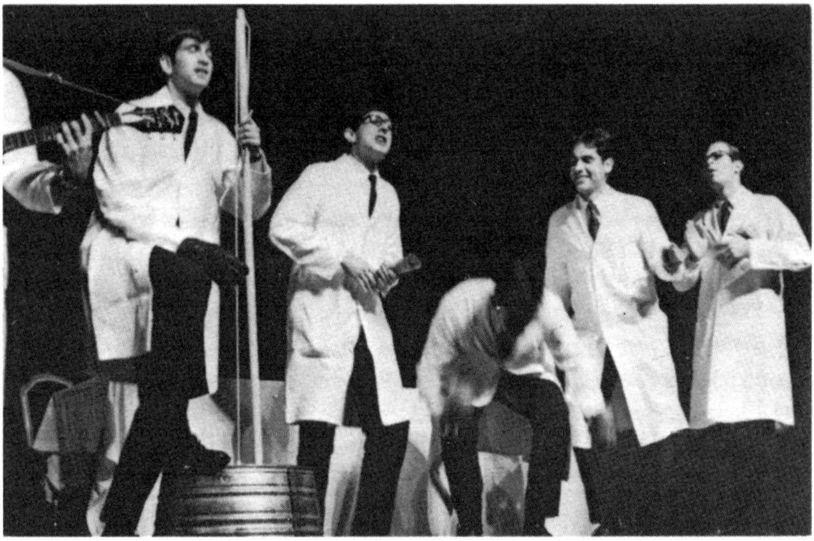

Galens "variety show" photos, printed in the *Paeon*, March 1968. Box 5, Medical School (University of Michigan) Publications, Bentley Historical Library, University of Michigan, Ann Arbor.

of the war, "almost 50 percent of patients were paying the hospital directly for care."[80] Meanwhile, the growing influx of medical students put more pressure on the availability of clinical services and space for teaching. Nevertheless, the University Hospital continued to focus on providing the most advanced and effective care available for all of its patients.

The medical school increased its cooperation with outside funding partners and arrangements with other local health-care institutions. In 1941, for example, Michigan (with support from the W. K. Kellogg Foundation) instituted the country's first program of routine tuberculosis screening, offering chest X-rays to all hospital registrants upon admission. A Rapid Treatment Center for sexually transmitted infections opened in the old hospital building on Catherine Street and was soon the site of a fourth-year medical student elective in the Department of Dermatology and Syphilology. In the fall of 1947 a newly constructed Veterans Readjustment Center was opened, the first in the United States to be operated by a teaching institution. The March of Dimes funded a polio respirator center at Michigan—the third in the nation—in 1951. The new outpatient clinic building opened in 1952, and, most importantly, the VA Hospital quickly became an important partner for the medical school after 1953.[81] Thus, by the mid-1950s, the medical center was experiencing significant growth.

In 1958 Dean Furstenberg noted the vital significance of maintaining and expanding clinical services as part of the school's responsibility to the citizens of the state:

> This medical school has a huge state service responsibility. Few medical schools in the country share the obligations which we have to the state in which we reside. When you take into consideration that we admit approximately 15,000 patients a year . . . and handle some 20,000 to 21,000 patient visits monthly in the Outpatient Building, one realizes the extent to which we must serve the taxpayers of Michigan.[82]

In his annual report for the 1959–1960 year, Dean Hubbard claimed that "this faculty will face an unprecedented demand for its services to both patients and the community" in the coming years, a clear recognition that postwar Michigan would need a reliable supply of practitioners and, by extension, adequate clinical space to train and employ them.[83]

However, despite the expansion of the medical center, it was becoming evident that the medical school simply could not provide enough clinical instruction at University Hospital for its postwar students. The 1925 "Old Main" building was still the primary hospital structure, and by the early 1960s it was becoming rapidly outdated. The building lacked air conditioning and other modern conveniences and provided little room for new machinery or services. Very little space was available for nurses, administrators, and house staff, who were forced to share that space with a growing number of students. According to the 1958 site visit, "If all the beds in the University Hospital and the VA Hospital were filled and used for teaching medical students, the number of patients would be barely adequate for clinical instruction."[84] The university and state legislature had already initiated their plans for the medical center's eventual renovation and expansion—in 1965, buildings near the observatory were demolished to allow for rerouted traffic patterns and the construction of a large parking structure[85]—but it would be years before a new University Hospital would replace "Old Main."

As had been the case for decades, clinical services for obstetrics and pediatrics patients continued to be problematic. To be sure, the changing postwar patient census in the hospital wards had allowed for the creation of more semiprivate rooms and other designs to increase patient privacy, which helped pave the way for a new Women's Hospital to open in early 1950. But that initial facility was not designed for "cutting-edge" maternity care. One long-standing nurse, Hazel M. Avery, had attempted to incorporate an innovative rooming-in program into the hospital design, arranging for mothers and newborns to share a room. Early studies had shown that this system encouraged breastfeeding and enhanced the mother-child relationship. But developers denied her proposal and instead allowed for nurseries between two-bed wards.[86] Even after the Women's Hospital opened, for years afterward the school was still forced to rely heavily on clinical partnerships with other hospitals, particularly Wayne County General, to provide obstetrics and gynecology instruction. As class size expanded, outsourcing clinical education to the school's affiliated hospitals was absolutely necessary.[87] While the pediatrics service did experience some notable advances during the postwar years—the state's first pediatric neurologist Richard Allen arrived at Michigan in 1957 and instituted universal neonatal phenylketonuria screening in Michigan eight years later—a general pediatrics hospital still did not exist at the medical center despite "the long-standing desire . . . to have separate and adequate hospital facilities for the care of children." There was no specific pediatric wing in "Old Main," and child patients were most often hospitalized in the contagious disease unit for common illnesses such as diphtheria, meningitis and encephalitis, pneumonia, pertussis, tetanus,

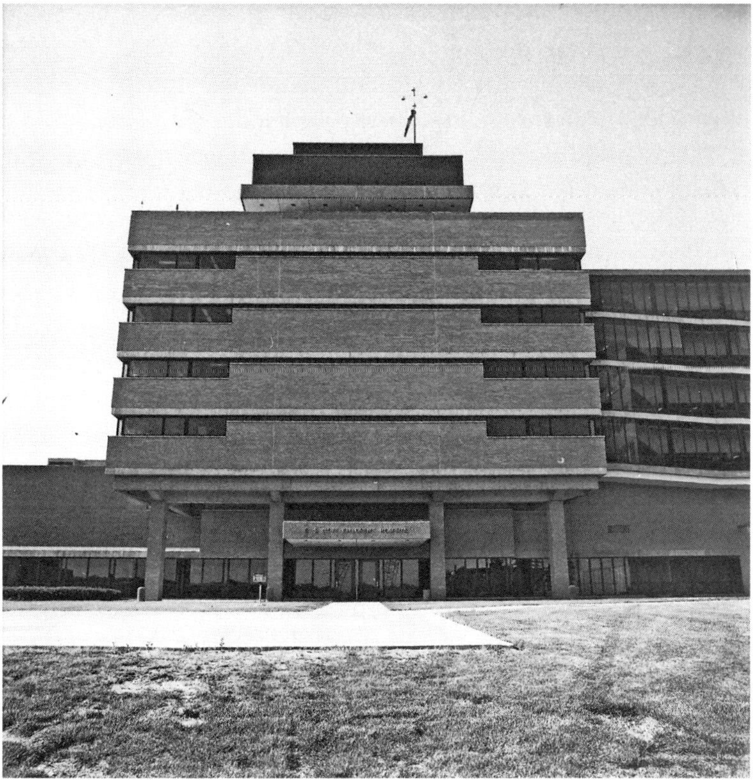

Front view of the C. S. Mott Children's Hospital, opened in 1969. BMC Media Services Records, Bentley Historical Library, University of Michigan, Ann Arbor.

polio, and diarrheal infections.[88] But this was to change with the C. S. Mott Children's Hospital, made possible by a $6.5 million gift from the Charles Stewart Mott Foundation in Flint. (Mott was one of the largest shareholders in General Motors.) This was arguably the university's first general pediatrics hospital facility since the Palmer Ward. Its 1969 opening came fourteen years after the opening of a children's psychiatric hospital and eight years after the creation of a rehabilitation facility for children with polio and cystic fibrosis.[89] But clinical expansions were not happening equally across all departments, and some parts of the medical school faced a perceived dearth of "clinical material," just as had been the case nearly a century before.

Just as undergraduate medical education faced challenges, so, too, did postgraduate programs. Physicians came home from the war aware of the advantages to be gained by specializing in a clinical field, and they increasingly did so in hopes of becoming board certified. Internal medicine professor and graduate medical education coordinator Charles F. Wilkinson believed that the speedy advancement of medical knowledge in the mid-twentieth century made an effective postgraduate program not only useful but necessary. Wilkinson also argued for an increased educational component. Rather than being seen merely as someone necessary to do work, "the intern should no longer be considered a slave" on a hospital house staff. Wilkinson argued that internships should be lengthened to two years and provide basic professional development opportunities, such as journal clubs, academic conferences, and teaching rounds on the wards.[90] In the late 1940s the University of Michigan and Wayne State University in Detroit housed the only medical schools that sponsored internships and residencies. Branching out to affiliated hospitals, both in and outside Ann Arbor, seemed like an effective solution to the problem of creating better internship and residency programs and maintaining a sufficient patient base for a growing number of postgraduates.[91]

By the early 1950s, the medical school had started to implement graduate training programs in thirteen hospitals in Michigan, overseeing those programs for quality control and providing their interns and residents with basic science supplemental instruction at the medical school in Ann Arbor. This also helped elevate the prestige of residencies in fields like pediatrics, whose Ann Arbor facilities were less than ideal. For instance, after the Kellogg Foundation's $100,000 grant to reorganize and expand Michigan's pediatrics department in 1940, the pediatric postgraduate program involved an internship and year "abroad" in accredited hospitals or clinics, rather than mandating that all of the postgraduate work be conducted at the university. Wilkinson claimed this was useful not only for students and residents but also for the population of Michigan, which was at that point still predominantly rural. While the departments and residency offerings at the university were becoming highly specialized and more research-oriented, internships and residencies at community or voluntary hospitals were more encouraging of full-time clinical practice, which could serve a need for the people of the state.[92] By 1958, the University of Michigan had one of the largest internship programs in the country, and individual residency programs had developed clinical relationships with the VA Hospital and St. Joseph Mercy Hospital in Ann Arbor, the Henry Ford Hospital in Detroit, Wayne County General Hospital, the Ypsilanti State Hospital, and the Southern Michigan State Prison in Jackson. Thus, the medical school's tradition of providing its instruction in university-owned facilities within the city limits of Ann Arbor was no longer practical, particularly as "Old Main" aged and crumbled under the growing student population and the rapid advancement of medicine.[93]

Conclusion

In 1967, President Hatcher commended the consolidation that had occurred on Michigan's medical campus during the previous several decades, proudly noting, "the traditional fields of scholarship are no longer little islands—or perhaps they might more aptly have once been called little kingdoms—each separate and at war with all the others."[94] The medical center seemed to be a shining example of innovation and prestige, bringing an unprecedented number of students and faculty members, as well as research grants, to the university. In July 1969, the Board of Regents' vision for a medical center was fully realized when Dean Hubbard took on a new administrative title as dean-director of the medical school and medical center. That year, for the first time, all facilities associated with the medical school and the hospital were located on a single campus ("north of Ann Street, east of Glen") and the clear links between instruction, clinical service, and biomedical research seemed firmly in place.[95]

Yet "medical schools, often incorporated into so-called academic medical centers, were becoming parts of large far-flung empires,"[96] which led to a paradox of simultaneous expansion and growing insularity in the second half of the twentieth century. As funding for research and physical plant development skyrocketed, and as medical departments became larger and more complex, it became more difficult for administrators to divide resources between research, teaching, and patient care. The medical profession had changed from an older standard of general practice—family physicians, house calls, and "free" treatment at teaching hospitals—to more specialized knowledge and practice. Meanwhile, people in industrial cities like Detroit were increasingly dealing with the deleterious health effects of poverty and discrimination. By the late 1960s medical schools and their faculty members had seen the support they traditionally had received from the public begin to weaken.[97] In 1966, Michigan's informational brochure changed its text to reach out to aspiring physicians on a more personal level, asking "Do You Want to Be a Doctor?" and offering explanations for "some popular misconceptions" about the medical profession.[98] In this climate of both prosperity and pressure, it is unsurprising that in 1964, the University of Michigan Medical School's class day ceremony address—delivered by Joseph C. Hinsey, director of the Cornell Medical Center in New York—was titled "Medicine in Our Changing Order."[99]

And the order of American medicine was indeed about to change, and change drastically, in no small part as a result of an initiative announced elsewhere on campus only a few months earlier. When President John F. Kennedy was assassinated in November 1963, he was succeeded by Lyndon Baines Johnson. Both had made significant announcements in Ann Arbor. As a presidential candidate, Kennedy had stood on the steps of the Michigan Union in the early morning hours of October 14, 1960, and asked students whether they were willing to contribute one to two years to serve some larger purpose, thus introducing the idea of what was to become the Peace Corps. His first example was of medical students going to Ghana, an interesting choice of an example, given the strong relationship the medical school was later to adopt with institutions in that nation.[100] After Kennedy was assassinated, Johnson set out to remake American society. On May 22, 1964, he became the first sitting president to offer a commencement address at the University of Michigan. Johnson stood before around eighty-five thousand people in the football stadium, the "Big House," to propose a plan to improve the quality of our American civilization and create what he called a "Great Society."[101] A key element of that society lay in the provision of health care, and Johnson laid out the ideas for what were to become Medicare and Medicaid. He signed those programs into law in 1965, and enrollment started in 1966. By offering a means to pay for health care for millions of people, Medicare and Medicaid transformed the provision of health care across the country and at the University of Michigan.

FIVE

Weathering Change as a Bellwether

The View from 1969

The year 1969 marked a particularly celebratory period for Michigan's medical school. Not only was that the year of the centennial anniversary of University Hospital, the first university-owned and -operated hospital in the United States, but the geographical and administrative consolidation of the University of Michigan Medical Center also heralded an important shift in the school's identity. For the first time in the school's history all formal medical activities for the university were situated on fifty-three acres of contiguous space overlooking the Huron River. Two brand-new facilities, the Medical Science II Building and the Towsley Center for Continuing Medical Education—endowed by the Margaret and Harry Towsley and Herbert H. and Grace Dow foundations—provided state-of-the-art facilities for medical education and research. The passage of Medicare and Medicaid would provide full or partial compensation for thousands of new patients. Looking forward, the medical center was dedicated to developing or continuing strong relations with diverse schools throughout the university, such as dentistry, engineering, public health, pharmacy, social work, and the University Health Service.[1] Administrators applauded this consolidation as a logical culmination of the medical school's mid-twentieth-century growth and prosperity. In his remarks on the medical school during the University of Michigan's sesquicentennial commemoration, university president Harlan Hatcher looked forward to the expansion of interdisciplinary programs and "cooperative work by medicine, public health, and business administration" that he anticipated would be supported by the medical center.[2]

The celebration, however, was somewhat short-lived, as academic medicine began to experience what university historian Alexandra Stern describes as late-twentieth-century "tectonic shifts."[3] Once-solid sources of support started to slip away. Although the U.S. Senate's Committee on Labor and Public Welfare had determined in the early 1960s that the nation was suffering a shortage of doctors and offered legislation to provide funding and other incentives for expanding programs at schools and teaching hospitals such as Michigan's, that support waned by the early 1970s. Economic recession and inflation threatened government spending for education, Great Society health-care programs (like Medicare and Medicaid), and biomedical research. In 1971, surgery chair Charles G. Child III reported a significant decline in federal research funding for the Department of Surgery, estimating a reduction of nearly 25 percent over the following three years. At the same time, the cost of health care in the United States was rising precipitously, by more than a third from the previous year (although the actual percentage of gross domestic product, from 5.0 percent to 6.9 percent, seems quite small from the perspective of several decades later). The state of Michigan, the center of the nation's automotive industry, was hit particularly hard by economic downturns. While the University of Michigan's researchers continued to receive federal and private grant money for biomedical and clinical investigations, the university's financial support from the state plummeted.

These economic changes coincided with a broader general mistrust in and criticism of U.S. institutions in general.[4] The civil rights movement

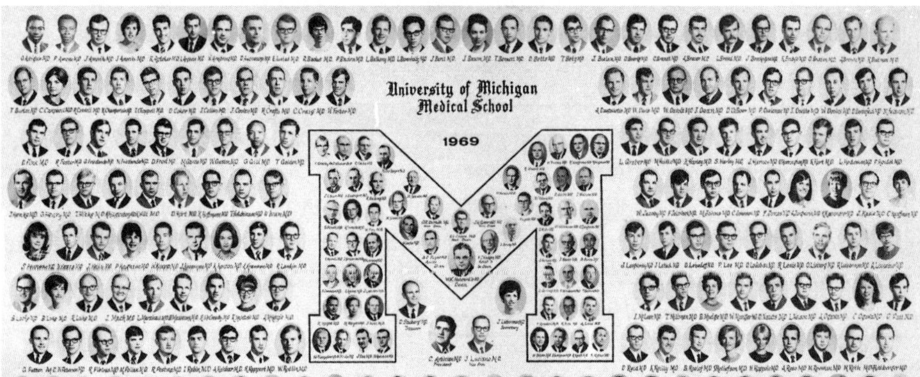

Medical school class of 1969. BMC Media Services Records, Bentley Historical Library, University of Michigan, Ann Arbor.

was reshaping the United States, including the world of medical education. Recognizing the pernicious effects of structural racism, national leaders created federal affirmative action policies to increase the numbers of medical students from minority populations. In a January 1969 letter to university president R. W. Fleming, Dean Hubbard reflected on the "Negro physician problem" in the United States, claiming that a dearth of black physicians across the country had led to a general health-care crisis for African Americans, since "Negro physicians are most likely to distribute their efforts within the Negro community."[5] At that point, only twenty-one African American medical students were enrolled at Michigan. Even so, the University of Michigan had the fourth-highest enrollment of black students, other than at historically black medical schools, of all 1969–1970 first-year medical cohorts in the country.[6]

But the difficulties in recruiting and supporting a more diverse group of students were not captured in a mere listing of numbers. While Hubbard did "not believe that there is any evidence of discriminatory practices against Negro medical students," he insightfully described Michigan specifically as a "white" university with a "white" medical school. Moreover, he noted that to increase the low application rates in Michigan's African American community, the medical center needed to change its reputation for exclusivity and privilege. Later that year, the medical school engaged in a "concerted effort to recruit minority group students from outside the State of Michigan," particularly students at historically black colleges, as well as prospective applicants from inner-city Detroit.[7] Notwithstanding these efforts, citing "strictly confidential" Association of American Medical Colleges statistics on the rate of black medical graduates, Hubbard was pessimistic about the medical school's ability to recruit more African American medical students, residents, and faculty members.[8] Both administrators and medical students gathered to discuss these issues. In 1973 Ann Arbor hosted the first national symposium addressing the problems of black medical students. There, David Satcher (an African American physician who was later to become director of the Centers for Disease Control and Prevention and Surgeon General of the United States) frankly addressed the difficulties black physicians faced when seeing patients in predominately white institutions such as the University of Michigan.[9]

In addition to debating who ought to go to medical school, people were wondering how many physicians there ought to be, and what kind. Despite earlier encouragement to increase class size, by the early 1980s some analysts claimed that increased numbers of medical school graduates in earlier decades had produced a "glut" of doctors in the U.S. marketplace. Not only were there too many, but they were not always the type of physician most needed. Reflecting concerns about the maldistribution and type of physicians, the AMA, the Michigan State Medical Society, and medical school administrators acknowledged that the rise in specialization had accompanied a shortage of primary care practitioners, particularly in rural areas and inner cities. One solution might come through a new specialty. Family medicine is a (perhaps the) prototypical primary care specialty; it is also one of the youngest medical specialties, having been approved in 1969. Initiatives to increase diversity dovetailed nicely with plans to develop a family practice residency program.[10] The politics of Michigan medical students also transformed as aspiring doctors entered medical school more often wanting to enter primary care than they had in previous decades, and they voiced more support for national health insurance and a more equitable distribution of health-care resources.[11]

The school began considering plans to trim the size of its entering classes. On the one hand, a smaller number of students required a smaller clinical base for their education. On the other hand, diminished enrollment could threaten patient care and reduce the number of interns available to fulfill vital functions in local hospitals. It might also alienate prospective clinical faculty. In 1983 the school deferred a plan to cut 13 percent of its class. According to Acting Dean Peter Ward, the school needed subsidies from research contracts and patient income to survive with increasingly constrained government funding, and limiting student enrollment could potentially threaten income from those sources.[12] Furthermore, the school recognized its obligation to train doctors who would deliver health care in Michigan, a task made more difficult by skyrocketing tuition rates and fewer opportunities for federal student loans, especially for students who came from limited financial means (and a set of circumstances that might encourage students to go into more lucrative specialties).[13] As an institution historically poised on the leading edge of medical innovation, Michigan's medical school thus found itself revisiting some older problems to maintain its position in a rapidly shifting world.

Faculty and Research

By the early 1970s, both the location and structure of the medical school were in flux. Governance was becoming more complex; expanding leadership included a dean, several associate and assistant deans, an executive committee for the faculty, a registrar, an administrative associate, and many more clerical staff. Growing pains of the new administrative structure were obvious not only within the institution but also to outside observers. During a 1982 accreditation site visit, the Liaison Committee on Medical Education (LCME) survey team noted the absence of "a workable structure to unify the health sciences units in the decision-making processes of the university."[14] In response, the Board of Regents created the position of vice provost for medical affairs to manage a more integrated health system at the university.[15] Eight years later, this did not appear to have solved the problem. Another accreditation team remarked on "continuing anomalies in governance" that resulted from the complex "matrixing of organizational relationships" between the vice provost, the dean, the provost, the hospital director, and the vice president for research.[16]

In 1973, the Board of Regents implemented changes in how physicians billed for patient care by endorsing the creation of coordinated practice plans, also known as medical service or "practice" plans. These would eliminate the previous system of private practice, in which physicians had offices and billings (termed "P numbers") that were separate from the university. Instead, under the new system, the practice plans would establish the basis for salaries for clinical faculty by determining how revenues from patients would be divided between physicians and the university. Such payment schemes were certainly neither new nor unique to Michigan; the first medical service plan in the country was implemented around 1910, and the number of such plans at American medical schools had increased from five in 1950 to sixty-six by 1978. In some ways, this seemed to be a way to address long-standing concerns about how experienced clinicians could provide high-quality care for patients in the University Hospital. Decades earlier Hugh Cabot, even before he became dean of the medical school, had envisioned "a system of full-time, hospital-based group practice where patients would pay according to their means and where all would receive the same high-quality care."[17]

However, when applied to a late-twentieth-century academic health center, the system proved to be a two-edged sword. The earlier system at Michigan had allowed some faculty members to earn income from billing private patients being seen at university facilities. That plan's critics dubbed it a "two-class system" and argued that it forced most of the faculty to accept salaries that were comparatively low among academic medical schools.[18] Now, in the 1970s, faculty wishing to avoid a salary cut felt increasing pressure to focus on clinical practice rather than research, pressure that one chair described as "the most important and potentially destructive current issue within the Medical Center."[19]

Institution of the medical service plans had a positive effect and helped some areas (particularly surgical subspecialties) recruit new physicians. But while some departments saw benefits from the medical service plans, others faced significant hurdles. Radiology, for example, had to change the work assignments of more of its faculty so that they spent increasing amounts of time doing clinical procedures, which led to a decline in the department's research and teaching activities.[20] In obstetrics and gynecology, some faculty left for other hospitals because their service plan "effectively prohibited members from maintaining private practices with their attendant incomes." Department chair J. Robert Willson had warned about this in 1969, claiming that "unless we can provide jobs which make it possible for our faculty to teach, do research and practice and unless income approaches that for private practice, we will not only lose important faculty members but will be unable to recruit replacements."[21]

Even those departments that prospered with the plan were wary of its long-term consequences. A survey of medical school chairs and section heads in the late 1970s noted that "the potential for a negative impact does exist," particularly if patient care mandates affected faculty research.[22] Some were concerned that funds from the plans would be limited and possibly vulnerable to third-party vendor restrictions and fluctuations in patient volume. Moreover, the university's medical service plans might lead to strained relations between full-time clinical faculty and community practitioners, not to mention non–tenure-track physicians.[23] But these concerns notwithstanding, the plans were here to stay. A 1977 study conducted by the Association of American Medical Colleges found that "medical practice plans have become an essential element in the structure of medical schools."[24]

More and more money was in play. Medicare and Medicaid brought in more patients, and the expanded use of new technologies for diagnosis and treatment drove up the cost of health care. New tools such as CT scanners had to go somewhere, which created new demands for space in the increasingly crowded and outdated medical center physical plant. Furthermore, the growing influence of third-party vendors like Blue Cross/Blue Shield led to increasing competition between University Hospital and community hospitals and caused conflicting interests between the policies of insurers and the policies of the university. Thus, Michigan found itself in a bind, trying to balance "the brisk growth and widening scope of clinical programs against fiscal and space constraints."[25] These challenges were taking a toll. Some departments, even large ones like internal medicine, were becoming "inbred and . . . declining in terms of accomplishments and reputation" during this period.[26] The implementation of practice plans came when some departments were facing significant state and federal funding cuts, faculty losses, hiring freezes, and "rock bottom morale."[27]

Despite the "dispirited mood" of academic medicine in the 1970s and concerns about medical service plans,[28] the Michigan medical faculty continued to grow and remained dedicated to its missions of teaching, research, and clinical service. Some departments aggressively recruited new, younger faculty members, including internal medicine chair William N. Kelley, a rheumatologist from Duke University, whose appointment led to a rejuvenation of the Department of Internal Medicine. The internal medicine faculty expanded from 148 to 233 members during the 1980s alone, while the average age of its faculty decreased from forty-five to forty years.[29] By the end of the twentieth century the internal medicine department had nearly 500 faculty members and had almost doubled the number of endowed chairs it had in 1970. The obstetrics and gynecology faculty, while small compared with internal medicine, also increased exponentially in the late twentieth and early twenty-first centuries, from fewer than 10 faculty members in 1964 to 83 in 2015.[30]

Compared with other medical schools in the United States, Michigan had long maintained a large number of individual departments.[31] New departments were organized, including the neurosurgery department (headed by Karin Muraszko, the first woman to chair a department of neurosurgery) and the urology and orthopedic surgery departments in 2001, cardiac surgery in 2012, and the Department of Biomedical Engineering, created in 1996 as a joint department in the two schools after decades of collaboration with the university's College of Engineering.[32]

But the creation of these departments was not inevitable. The history of nuclear medicine may provide insight into the contingent nature of medical specialization. The field had its origins in post–World War II interests in the applied uses of radioactivity. The original Michigan nuclear medicine program was led by William Beierwaltes, who traveled to Oak Ridge, Tennessee, in the early 1950s to work on the newly available radioactive substances. He then studied the role of radiopharmaceuticals in the diagnosis and treatment of endocrine disorders. At Michigan he founded one of the earliest nuclear medicine fellowship programs in the country. As a program dealing with both hormonal disorders and radioactive materials, it could have legitimately existed in radiology or internal medicine, but it was founded as part of the Department of Internal Medicine in the 1960s. When MRI scanners became commercially available in the early 1980s, there was more debate over who should control the new technology—radiology or nuclear medicine (which would have put control of MRIs into the Department of Internal Medicine). MRI machines went to radiology. When Beierwaltes retired in 1983, a committee was appointed to consider the administrative status of the division. The committee recommended that it stay in internal medicine. Another committee in 1989 saw the location as detrimental to radiology, but no changes were made. The Division of Nuclear Medicine was eventually moved to the Department of Radiology late in 2000.[33] This brief history illustrates that while the current system of specialization may appear to make sense, dividing lines had to be drawn, and those lines could be (and in some cases were) drawn differently from the way they are drawn in the current system.

Research excellence remained a high priority for the school. Research expenditures in the later decades of the century grew from $35 million to well over $100 million, particularly in the fields of biotechnology and bioengineering, oncology, genetics, neuroscience, and aging.[34] The dominant source of funding was the federal government, mostly through the National Institutes of Health (NIH). Some research initiatives followed population needs. By the late twentieth century diabetes had become an epidemic, and in 1977 the medical school was one of the first institutions in the nation to receive funding for a diabetes research and training center. Six years later, the center participated in a decade-long study of diabetes control and complications, "the largest, most comprehensive diabetes study ever conducted."[35] At the same time, the U.S. population was getting older, and the field of geriatric medicine began to grow. Michigan's Division of Geriatrics was founded in 1984, and five years later the first geriatrics research and training center in the United States was founded with considerable philanthropic support, including from the Ministry of Health and Welfare of the government of Japan and from the pharmaceutical company Tanabe.[36]

Another major source of research funding came from the Howard Hughes Medical Institute, for molecular genetics, whose University of Michigan unit, established in 1983, quickly became a "hot bed" for investigations in the blossoming field of gene therapy.[37] In 1989 Francis Collins was part of a team that used an innovative technique called chromosome jumping to identify the gene responsible for cystic fibrosis. (Collins left Michigan in 1993 and is now the director of the NIH.) Some departments saw particularly dramatic increases in funding during this period: internal medicine's research funding nearly doubled between 1985 and 1990, radiology research expenditures tripled over the course of the 1990s, and pathology's total funding from the NIH expanded from about $400,000 in 1980 to $27 million by 2013.[38] Another marker of the institution's status was the decision in 1995 to move the editorial offices of the prestigious *Journal of Clinical Investigation* to the University of Michigan for a five-year term.[39]

The school's reputation as a center for research and innovation was recognized in a variety of other ways as well. One was the movement of educational and clinical activities beyond the boundaries of Ann Arbor, or even of the United States. For instance, the Department of Obstetrics and Gynecology launched a postgraduate training program in Ghana, part of an international collaboration funded by a Carnegie Foundation grant.[40] This project expanded and thrived. It has not only anchored an extremely successful program in Ghana but also served as the model for many subsequent international collaborations. (Recall that John F. Kennedy's original remarks about the Peace Corps specifically referenced Michigan medical students and Ghana.)

The income generated from grants contributed to faculty expansion and the institution's prestige and was seen as contributing to excellence in the educational mission. According to the school's 1990 accreditation report, "it is believed that medical students derive an appreciable advantage from a research oriented faculty." However, support for research and faculty expansion existed alongside controversies and tensions that had been present for more than a century. The 1990 report also identified "a favorable problem" resulting from such exponential growth, namely, the limitations placed on the school's physical plant. The site visit team observed that "there is virtually no unutilized research space in the Medical Center,"[41] echoing much older space pressures that the school had faced. Some departments continued to have a particularly difficult time maintaining sufficient space for administrative, clinical, and research purposes.[42] More concerning to some was the conflict of priorities created by increased research funding. There are a limited number of hours in the day to devote to teaching, research, and patient care. A 1984 medical education task force reported problems of conflicting demands on professors' time and resources and suggested that a solution to this problem should privilege teaching duties over research.[43] Twelve years later, as the school continued to expand, an article in the *Ann Arbor News* noted that medical "faculty members are being stressed by an increase in clinical duties, a decrease in the availability of research funds and a decline in patient care reimbursement."[44]

The inappropriate use of research funds also became a source of controversy. When former chief of urology Joseph Oesterling resigned in 1997 after pleading guilty to charges of expense account abuses, including double and triple billing for trips to medical conferences, the school's reporting of research-related expenses, particularly travel, came under increased scrutiny. Administrators pointed out that such travel expenses—for the likes of conferences, seminars, and professional board activities—were necessary to maintain the school's productivity and prestige. At that time the University of Michigan Medical School was ranked tenth best in the nation, according to *U.S. News and World Report*, and the school's spokespeople said that such rankings "rely heavily on visibility and reputation . . . in attracting students, grants and patients."[45]

Around the same time some University of Michigan faculty members were concerned that the rapid expansion of the health system was leading to the replacement of tenured and tenure-track faculty by a growing number of nontenured clinical physicians, who were not members of the instructional track and for whom the academic expectations were different. In 1998, internal medicine and pharmacology professor William Ensminger warned that untenured clinical faculty could "dilute the academic flavor" of the school, and "'one could end up with a medical school faculty where the majority of physicians live and work as far away as Sault Ste. Marie.'"[46] Ensminger's comments are reminiscent of much older tensions between research and clinical interests at the medical school, as well as long-standing concerns about the school's physical space and faculty presence in Ann Arbor.

But in the latter part of the twentieth century, different types of concerns about the composition of the faculty started to be raised. Just as was the case for medical students, increasing attention started to be paid to faculty diversity. In 1970, the medical school had 481 male instructional faculty members and only 64 women (two-thirds of whom held positions at relatively lower levels, such as instructor or lecturer).[47] According to internal medicine professor John M. Weller, the major reason for "a limitation on the availability of qualified women physicians" was the relatively low percentage of female medical school graduates.[48] At that time, 9.5 percent of the medical school's most recent graduated class had been women, and the current class was 7.4 percent female. Some fields, particularly surgery, had an even more significant gender imbalance. Surgery chair Charles G. Child III claimed in 1971 that "for many years American surgeons have anguished over what to do about women who wish to become surgeons." The problem, he said, was that the department saw "few women applicants and those who do apply are usually of very modest accomplishments." Moreover, raising essentialist arguments that harkened back to thinking of several decades before, Child doubted that women were "peculiarly fitted" to be surgeons, since "surgery seems to be a man's world and those women who do enter it are converted to male behavioral patterns as rapidly as possible." Michigan was hardly unique in having few female faculty. Child also pointed out that even in the nation's only remaining women's medical school (in Pennsylvania), the surgical department chair, all surgical division heads, thirteen other department chairs, and the dean were all men.[49] Some other departments had a better record for gender diversity and more clearly prioritized the status of and opportunities for female employees in the late twentieth century.[50] Yet there, too, the senior leadership remained generally male.

Despite efforts to increase faculty diversity, the 1990 LCME accreditation site visit report listed "inadequate numbers of under-represented minorities on [the] faculty" as a "weakness" of the medical school, a problem Michigan shared with most other major medical schools.[51] Later that decade, the medical school experienced several widely publicized cases of reported racism and sexism in a variety of departments. After a policy of rewarding departments for minority faculty recruitment failed to produce the desired results, Dean Giles G. Bole, Jr., initiated a cultural diversity assessment in 1996. The results are worth noting. There were twenty-six African American faculty members (out of twelve hundred), and 85 percent of those agreed that "the environment is cold and unwelcoming." Women also reported gender discrimination, with 83 percent of female instructors reporting that "men faculty are taken more seriously by the administration than women faculty."[52] Joyce C. Mitchell, a member of the pediatrics department and assistant dean for student and minority affairs, claimed, "I actually feel on firmer ground here as an African American than I do as a woman," but acknowledged that both racism and sexism were problems at the school.[53] Thus, tensions over diversity and inclusion continued to affect the University of Michigan—along with most other academic medical centers—despite Michigan being a frontrunner in the medical education of women and members of racial minority groups.

Modernizing the Medical Curriculum

Into the late 1960s university leaders recognized that in order to accommodate sweeping changes in knowledge, health-care costs, and expectations of graduating medical students, the medical school curriculum and environment needed a significant overhaul. As President Harlan Hatcher remarked in 1967, "Medical education is caught between a population which wants and needs more medical care and a system . . . which requires more time from the student."[54] During the late 1960s, the program introduced more clinical and interdisciplinary coursework in the first two years of its curriculum, provided more elective opportunities, and started to eliminate some older "formal" coursework in fields like radiology.[55] It formalized an arrangement with Detroit's Henry Ford Hospital in which third- and fourth-year medical students would experience medical education with a different patient population. However, "in spite of the knowledge explosion in the sciences and the vast changes in the health care delivery system in this country," the school did not implement any major curricular revisions for at least a decade after the early 1970s.[56]

Instead, the University of Michigan focused its attention on expanding access to its medical school, most notably with its Integrated Premedical/Medical Program, commonly called Inteflex, which began in 1972. The program had a number of goals. It was not only intended to increase diversity and the number of students entering primary care disciplines; it also rationalized the curriculum by reducing redundancy between the undergraduate and the medical school curriculum. By eliminating premed competition, it was hoped that the program would reduce attrition, especially of women and minorities. Initially, the Inteflex track admitted students to the medical school directly from high school for a six-year simultaneous undergraduate and medical degree program. Priority was given to Michigan residents—only 20 to 30 percent of Inteflex spots were open to out-of-state applicants—and the school encouraged the enrollment of "qualified underrepresented minority students, and qualified students from small communities and rural settings."[57] Over time, the program grew in length, to seven years in 1982 and eight years in 1994, and admissions requirements increased. By the early 1980s, the school required a grade-point average of 3.8 or a position in the top 5 percent of an applicant's graduating high school class. By the mid-1990s, the program also required applicants to submit MCAT scores.[58] Inteflex students spent their first years at Michigan taking a combination of undergraduate and medical school courses and then completed their basic sciences during their fourth and fifth years. The final years were nearly identical to the clinical coursework of other upper-class medical students. The university's outreach to local high school students, initiated with Inteflex, was enhanced in the mid-1990s when the medical school received

NIH funding to create the Minority High School Summer Research Apprenticeship Program.[59] The program graduated many physicians, including the television correspondent Sanjay Gupta, but it eventually came to an end. The last class of students entered in 1998.

The Inteflex program was generally lauded as a success, not just for its outreach to traditionally disadvantaged communities but also because of its liberal arts emphasis. Program director Alphonse Burdi noted in 1988, "Two outstanding national studies over the past two years have clearly called for a strengthening of the liberal arts education of our physicians. . . . Society now demands more compassion from the medical world. Inteflex continues to be a pace setter or model program in meeting this demand."[60]

Most Inteflex students did well, but the program was not free from controversy. In the early 1980s an Inteflex student, Scott Ewing, was dismissed from Michigan after failing part I of the National Board of Medical Examiners test. He sued the university, claiming that he was the only student ever removed after a single failure of that examination. Lower courts upheld his dismissal, ruling that academic freedom gave the university the right to set the standards by which students would be evaluated. The case was eventually appealed to the U.S. Supreme Court, which unanimously agreed that the state did not have a right to overturn the university's decision.[61] Even so, the lawsuit was concerning to the medical school faculty and undoubtedly influenced the curriculum revision committee's 1991 assertion that "the academic review process is increasingly adversarial and litigious."[62]

Another program that sought to offer a flexible educational program for medical students was the seven-year Medical Scientist Training Program for the combined M.D. and Ph.D. degrees.[63] This program was established in 1979 and had its first NIH grant approved in 1980. Medical students would typically attend the first two years of medical school. They would then pursue a Ph.D. program and after finishing that degree would return for the last two years of medical school. The clear majority of students receive their Ph.D. training in the natural sciences, taking advantage of the strong basic science departments. The program continues to exist, and in recent years an increasing number of students have elected to cross Washtenaw Avenue to study in the social sciences and humanities.

Beginning in the early 1980s the school had begun to adopt important changes in course delivery, recognizing that becoming an excellent physician requires more than merely the mastery of a set of facts.[64] As "the largest supplier of future M.D.'s in the U.S.," the University of Michigan felt a strong obligation to reform its educational system, particularly after the

1982 LCME accreditation team reported that the "overall direction of the curriculum appears to be inadequate."[65] Pedagogical reform continued to be strained by class size. In the early part of that decade the incoming class size was capped at 217 students, with 44 spaces available for Inteflex students. By 1991, the school recognized that the large number of students "[impaired] implementation of a flexible educational program" and forced instructors to rely on outmoded class formats as well as crowded lecture halls and clinical demonstrations. In addition, the school's 1991 curriculum report noted that "there is no orientation for faculty to prepare them for their teaching roles."[66] Under pressure to apply for research grants and increase clinical income, many faculty members felt little incentive to improve their instructional delivery or contribute to educational innovations. Although curriculum decisions were solely the responsibility of executive faculty committee members, individual departments controlled their own course offerings. But with such a large and diverse faculty, it was difficult to maintain centralized leadership, relevance, and regulation of course content as well as to balance the needs of students against department and faculty interests in order to create a well-rounded curriculum. The faculty emphasis on research was palpable to medical students, and not always welcome. One student had commented as early as 1978 that she was afraid of "Michigan's research-oriented reputation," although she noted that she was satisfied with her education regarding how best to communicate with her patients.[67]

The 1991 curriculum report stressed the need to broaden the educational focus and provide more emphasis in other areas, including primary care, disease prevention, and nutrition.[68] Although the first two years of study continued to focus on basic sciences and were "organized largely by traditional disciplines," the medical school created two new courses: Introduction to Clinical Sciences and an interdisciplinary course, Neural and Behavioral Sciences, both of which constituted 43 percent of scheduled time for the basic sciences phase of the medical curriculum. The school also implemented a four-week "interphase" between the basic sciences and clinical years, "designed to provide a relevant, practical clinical problem solving experience for students about to enter the clinical phase." The latter two years of the curriculum were divided into required clerkships (in medicine, surgery, pediatrics, neurology, psychiatry, and obstetrics and gynecology) and elective rotations offered at five "core" community hospitals and approved medical facilities.[69]

The school also began a major shift toward digitized systems in clinical care and instruction. In 1990 the ILIAD pilot program initiated the university's first digitized medical information system. By the end of the decade, the medical school had a virtual reality–enhanced "Medical Readiness Trainer" to simulate the emergency room. One of the largest plastination laboratories in the nation was established in 1989. Plastination involved replacing the water and fat in tissues with plastic, enabling organs to be more easily used for training. The lab provided specimens that could be used to enhance anatomical instruction, even though the school regularly received hundreds of cadaver donations for gross anatomy students each year.[70] The plastination laboratory made organs available for study not only in Michigan but also around the United States. Clinical courses also introduced new methods for teaching preventive medicine. For instance, hypertension specialist Andrew Zweifler received a grant from the National Heart, Lung, and Blood Institute to develop new pedagogical approaches to teaching students about preventive care.[71] Additionally, third-year clerkship students attended required weekly conferences that addressed ethical, cultural, and economic issues of clinical practice, including issues around death and dying.[72]

When the LCME survey team visited again in 1990, they found much to praise. The report commended the school on its faculty's excellence, its successful recruitment of more minority students, and its new facilities and planned expansions; they accredited the program for another seven years. However, the team noted that plans to reform the first two years of the medical program had not been fully implemented, again in large part because of the particularly large class sizes at Michigan. The curriculum still remained focused on traditional fields, lecture-based instruction, and passive methods of student learning. Furthermore, "many faculty and students observed that minimal or no incentives exist to encourage participation in or achievement of excellence in teaching."[73] This LCME critique was an important factor in the school's decision to reconsider many parts of the curriculum.

In 1991 a curriculum revision retreat gathered eighty-six faculty members and student representatives to consider how and where to enhance critical thinking, provide rigorous systems of evaluation, and create "room for innovation and diversity."[74] The school decided to end the formal separation of the curriculum into two-year preclinical and clinical phases. It would include both clinical subjects and basic sciences in all four years. Rather than having primarily discipline-based courses, the creation of several second-year interdisciplinary organ system–based and disease-based sequences with lecture and laboratory components helped facilitate the inclusion of basic science learning into clinical contexts and diminished the traditional focus on departmental coursework. Finally, the program also instituted courses to emphasize professional ethics and awareness of patient issues, including the rising cost of health care.[75] An article in the *Ann Arbor News* lauded this change, noting that "there will be more attention to the human side of medicine—issues such as bedside manner, medical ethics and how illness affects the family."[76] A course called Introduction to the Patient not only emphasized patient-based clinical experiences at an earlier point in the curriculum, but it also included information about alternative healing practices such as acupuncture and herbal medicine.[77]

To some extent, the planned revisions were a reaction to outside criticisms of Michigan's "old curriculum," but an effort was also made to craft changes specific to the local environment. As Associate Dean Wayne K. Davis noted in 1993, "Michigan problems require Michigan solutions. . . . [W]e did not want to look to other schools for solutions to problems." Interestingly, though, the problems Davis and others identified in the late twentieth century bore remarkable similarities to earlier concerns and controversies.[78] Although faculty and students agreed that traditional methods of lecture delivery and "killer" exams were unsatisfactory, opinions remained divided about how to prioritize social and behavioral sciences, as well as humanities, in the curriculum, just as they had been in the earlier part of the twentieth century.[79]

Furthermore, as it had for more than a century, the school faced concerns that clinical instruction was insufficient at the University Hospital. In the 1990s, the problem was not an inadequate number of patients, but rather the type of clinical training that the hospital provided. According to the 1991 curriculum revision retreat report, "Most medical student training in the clinical phase [at University Hospital] occurs in an acute, tertiary care hospital setting, [but] most clinical practice does not." This restated the existing tension between what sort of physician the medical school was intended to train. The report went on to say that "there are limited opportunities for students to observe or be part of actual clinical decision-making," restating the problem that the clerkship of a century ago was intended to solve.[80] These echoes of the medical school's past show how even as the school continued to reshape its identity as both a local institution and a national trendsetter—and to provide students with "the professional attributes of compassion, *honesty*, integrity, and social and *professional* responsibility in the context of a diverse and changing society"—some fundamental issues remained from long ago.[81]

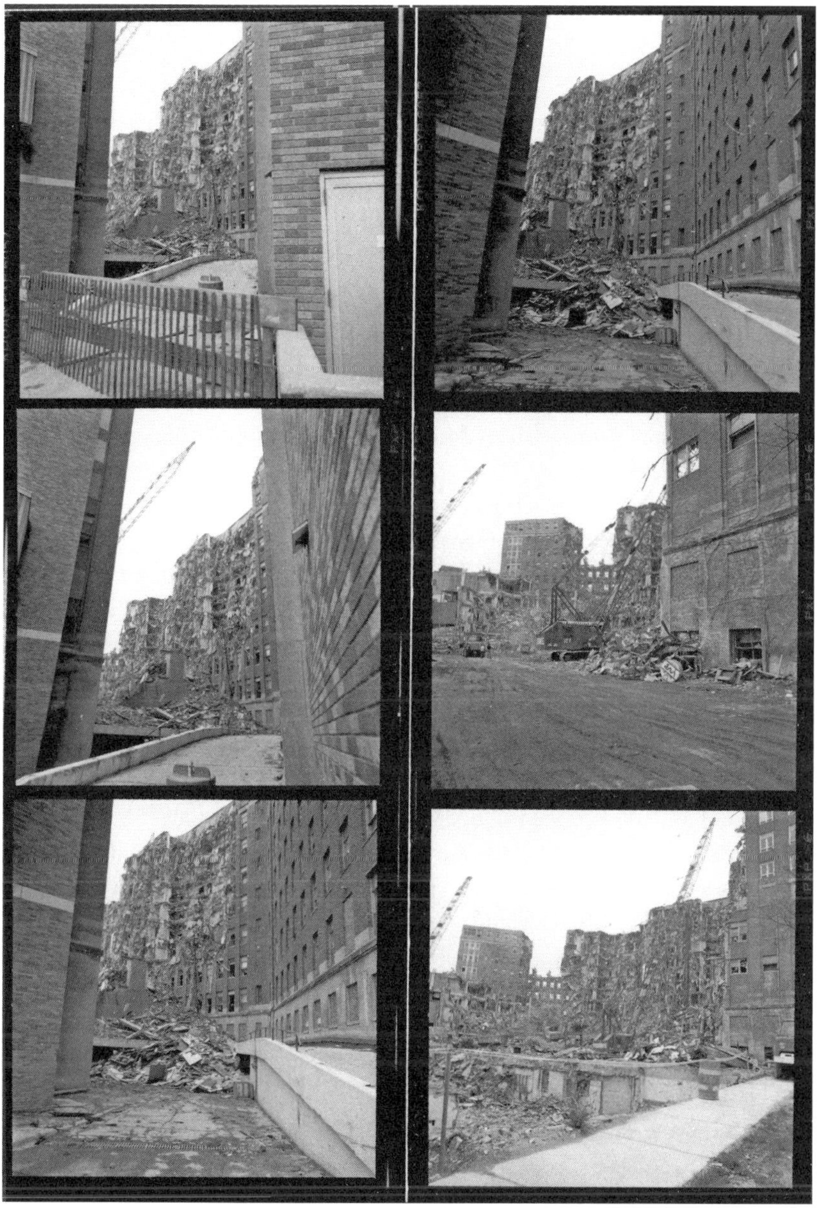

"Old Main" hospital demolition, 1989. BMC Media Services Records, Bentley Historical Library, University of Michigan, Ann Arbor.

The Replacement Hospital

During the 1970s the number of patients being seen in medical school hospitals increased across the country.[82] In Michigan, patient visits at the University Hospital went up significantly despite nursing shortages, as well as blackouts and power surges caused by the outdated electrical system of "Old Main."[83] Even in this constrained physical plant, new subspecialty fields began offering postgraduate programs and training for innovative procedures. For example, the cardiology division at Michigan helped create the coronary care unit as a "new concept in clinical care delivery" and began to implement new techniques, such as echocardiography.[84] The pathology department's services also expanded; pediatric pathology was introduced after the C. S. Mott Children's Hospital opened in 1969, and the number of clinical pathology laboratory test results for the university as a whole grew steadily over the next several decades, almost doubling between 1981 and 1993.[85] Other new clinical facilities were constructed during the 1970s and 1980s, such as the James and Lynelle Holden Perinatal Hospital (now called the Holden Newborn Intensive Care Unit) for high-risk obstetric patients and the James and Lynelle Holden Research Laboratories. This unit became the first in the United States to directly and intentionally link an obstetrical hospital with a children's hospital, thus facilitating a multidisciplinary approach to the care of very vulnerable infants. Ophthalmology benefited from the creation of the Parkview Comprehensive Eye Center (formerly an extended-care nursing home) and W. K. Kellogg Eye Center, completed in 1985.[86]

While the expansion of medical center services was beneficial for some departments, it put pressure on others, such as radiology, which depended on the availability of space and specialized personnel for its equipment. In some cases, radiology students, residents and fellows, and faculty members relied on affiliate hospitals to use new and innovative equipment that the university lacked. The VA Hospital in Ann Arbor, for example, obtained a full-body computed tomography (CT) scanner in 1977, three years before the University Hospital. During the 1970s, the department suffered low morale and staffing problems as a result of such constraints. One external review committee went as far as to say the situation threatened "the tertiary mission of the entire medical center."[87]

Other clinical departments continued to rely on affiliations with community hospitals to provide an adequate patient base for rotations and clerkships. The cooperation of the medical school with the VA Hospital continued to be an essential element of its mission. The internal medicine department created an associate chair for veterans' affairs to help provide access to research centers and clinics, as well as support for physician-scientist positions in VA facilities. However, other affiliations could become unstable. Wayne County General Hospital (a significant partner for many departments) had financial and accreditation problems during the 1970s and was privatized in 1984, ending its relationship with the medical school.[88] The lack of space on the Ann Arbor medical center campus forced some services to move offsite at great inconvenience. For instance, Michigan was one of the earliest participants in the national Breast Cancer Detection Demonstration Project conducted between 1973 and 1980, which studied the utility of mammography. But the original imaging facility was located on West Washington Street. Since this was some distance from the operating rooms, until the mid-1980s women with nonpalpable lesions had to cross town from West Washington Street to the hospital to have their biopsies.[89]

All of these issues made the case for a new hospital clear. In 1981, the state legislature approved a $285 million replacement hospital project, not only to update the university's services for patients but to help support its academic enterprise. University president Harold Shapiro claimed that the new hospital would help the university increase sponsored medical research from $30 million to $50 million a year.[90] The "replacement" University Hospital opened in 1986 with 550 patient beds.[91]

The Michigan health system continued to expand its outreach for patients and community institutions through the 1990s. In the middle of that decade, the pathology department took over forensic pathology services for Washtenaw and Wayne counties on a contractual basis, continuing a tradition of medicolegal work that had begun at the university more than a century before.[92] Other departments also extended their outreach, with affiliations throughout Michigan (such as nuclear medicine services in Saginaw, Flint, and Battle Creek) and other states (including VA outpatient clinics in Toledo, Ohio, and Ft. Wayne, Indiana). In 1999 the school partnered with the Ford Motor Company to provide care for asthmatic employees of the automotive industry and created sinusitis and specialty care centers in Livonia, Michigan.[93]

Other new departments reached out into the community. Emergency services were originally part of the Department of Surgery, with accompanying intense debates over just who was to be in charge. In 1982 one of its key innovations was the Survival Flight system, the first medical flight service in Michigan, which established a tangible connection with the community. Emergency medicine followed the national trend toward departmental status, becoming in 1999 the Emergency Department of the medical school. Since 1991 the residency program has been coordinated with St. Joseph Mercy Hospital. The department also staffs a site at Hurley Hospital in Flint and had one at Foote Hospital in Jackson, Michigan, until 2009. These community sites serve to move the department past the boundaries of the Ann Arbor institution. And since the field became a mandatory rotation for medical students in 2006, all medical students are able to see the importance of this larger vision of care.[94]

After the 1960s the obstetrics and gynecology department sought to provide a more comprehensive focus on women's health and family planning, rather than on only childbirth and pathology. The department implemented more obstetrics and gynecology coursework in the second and third years of the curriculum and started to teach students how to perform gynecological exams in the Introduction to Clinical Sciences course using training teaching patients, people who had received training in helping teach medical students to do the examinations.

But the department also found itself in the middle of several controversial areas. Department chair J. Robert Willson became a target because of his influential textbook *Obstetrics and Gynecology*, first published in 1958, which was then a required text for medical students. On April 11, 1973, the organization Advocates for Medical Information labeled the book as misogynist and held a demonstration on the main campus to burn Willson's book as a "tool of sexual oppression." From a different political direction, the department attracted attention for its advocacy of women's sexual and reproductive rights, support for unwed teenaged mothers in Washtenaw County Intermediate School District, and affiliations with Planned Parenthood. In 1969, after the Ann Arbor Planned Parenthood clinic was destroyed by fire, the organization temporarily moved to the university's obstetrics and gynecology outpatient facility.[95] In the early 1990s, the new department chief, Timothy Johnson, decided to teach his residents to perform abortions in cooperation with Planned Parenthood. Johnson, an advocate for abortion rights, believed that "when medical schools neglect to teach abortion, they limit availability of the surgical procedure because fewer doctors will know how to perform abortions safely and legally."[96] In many respects, Johnson's position resonated with Reuben Peterson's mission to provide comprehensive gynecological services at University Hospital nearly one hundred years earlier.

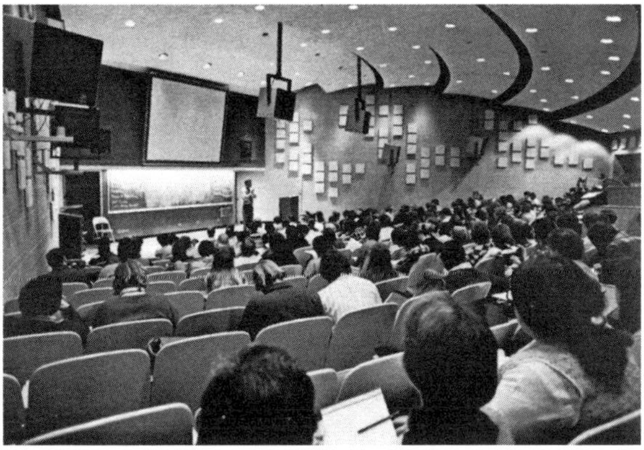

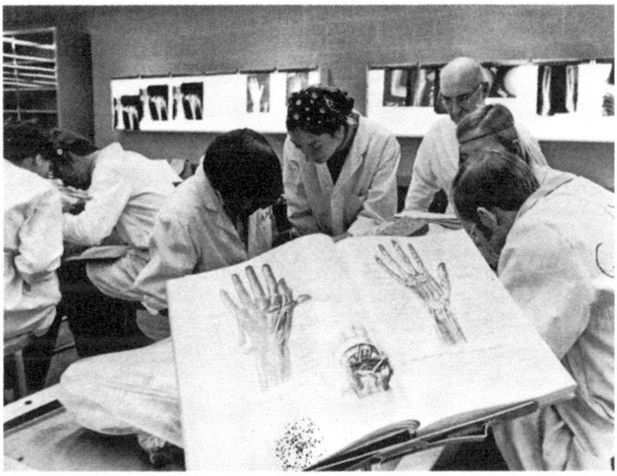

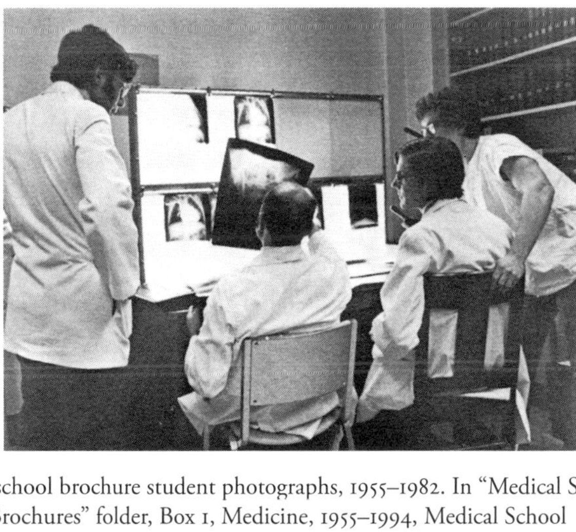

Medical school brochure student photographs, 1955–1982. In "Medical School Printed Brochures" folder, Box 1, Medicine, 1955–1994, Medical School (University of Michigan) Publications, Bentley Historical Library, University of Michigan, Ann Arbor.

The Students

At the start of the 1960s, Michigan's medical school had one of the largest enrollments in the nation, but the steady growth began to taper.[97] The student body at the medical school changed dramatically beginning in the 1970s. The school introduced initiatives (beyond Inteflex) designed to attract and retain students from disadvantaged backgrounds and minority groups, supported by a grant from the Health Careers Opportunity Program (which later evolved into the AIMED grant project) and the Robert Wood Johnson Foundation Student Aid Program, both implemented in 1972.[98] The photographs chosen for the medical school's brochure reflect the changing demographics of Michigan's medical students during the later decades of the twentieth century. Stock photographs of single students that had appeared in the brochure for years were replaced with group images that eventually included more women and students of color. For example, in 1970, the brochure kept the same text and basic format it had in the 1960s, but a photograph of a white female student that had first appeared in 1955 was replaced with an image of three male students, one of whom is African American. In the 1978 brochure, a photograph of a woman sitting with two male students and a male professor is placed next to a statement about the school's Title IX policy regarding sex discrimination, and in the 1982 brochure, a photograph of several women of color was placed directly above the school's Equal Opportunity/Affirmative Action clause.[99]

The rising costs of medical education contributed to a national trend of medical student dissatisfaction in the later decades of the twentieth century, and Michigan was not immune. In 1978 a group of students, dressed in their white coats, attended a meeting of the Michigan Board of Regents, where they made the regents aware of the effect of tuition payments on their lives. One second-year student had already accumulated $14,000 of debt ($51,000 in 2017 dollars). Another student blamed financial anxieties for causing distress among his fellow students, noting that 50 percent of students were getting psychological counseling. A few years later, in 1982, the state proposed a massive increase in medical school tuition rates. Had the proposal been adopted, University of Michigan medical school student tuition would have jumped from $5,000 ($13,000 in 2017 dollars) to more than $20,000 ($53,000 in 2017 dollars) a year.[100]

Although Michigan's admissions costs rose more slowly than the national average, by the late 1980s about 60 percent of its students received financial aid, and on average, its graduates incurred a total medical school debt of more than $30,000 ($67,000 in 2017 dollars).[101] Even with financial assistance, just as in previous decades some students were forced to work while going to school, which threatened their success and raised concerns that medical school would become "the exclusive domain of the rich" in the state.[102]

The 1974 "Medical Students Guide to Life in Ann Arbor," a handbook for new matriculants produced by students themselves, provides an interesting glimpse into student perspectives and experiences. The guide suggests that new students might feel overwhelmed by the amount of required work; in a section titled "Some Thoughts on Enjoying Yourself," the handbook recommends, "Try to meet people who are not medical students. . . . Try to read things that are not medical books. Try to get some exercise, you will be more nearly alive."[103] The guide also includes recommendations for family resources (including schools and child-care facilities) and suggestions for community involvement and service, including crisis and women's shelters, organizations for people involved in relationships with members of the same sex, and the Free People's Clinic on East Liberty Street, where "fourth year students may work as 'doctors' without further training sessions. The Free Clinic sees itself as a model for patient oriented free health care."[104] The handbook also supplies advice on buying alcohol (the legal drinking age in Michigan at that time was eighteen years) and smoking marijuana, which was decriminalized in Ann Arbor in 1972 but could lead to arrest by state or federal officers outside the city limits.[105] This handbook may have helped students deal with problems that continued to confront them—a 1984 education task force report found that anxiety, competitiveness, and the school's "failure . . . to foster the development of compassion in future physicians" remained top concerns for Michigan's medical students in the 1980s.[106]

Medical school administrators did pay attention to the environment in which students learned. In June 1974, the Furstenberg Student Study Center was dedicated. It held student health services, places for academic and personal counseling, and "a carpeted, computerized student study complex" with audiovisual carrels, microfiche reader stations, individual study rooms, and an "unusual . . . conversation pit with colored cushions scattered around its steps."[107] The "design-oriented" study center went on to win an award from the American Institute of Architecture. Clearly, Michigan was trying to provide spaces and resources to help students succeed in the medical program.

The school continued to accept about 80 percent of matriculants from the state of Michigan, as dictated by the state legislature. With the national

The FREE PEOPLE's CLINIC

The Free People's Clinic begân operation in January, 1971, to provide an alternative for the many people who were not receiving adequate health care either because of lack of money, because of the general bogueness that exists with most doctors and hospitals, or both. It was hoped that the Free Clinic would not only provide an economic alternative to the established institutions, but would also be a model of the way that health care should and could be delivered to people.

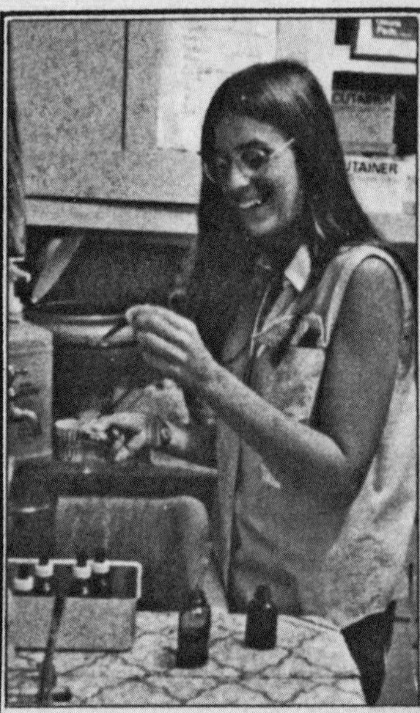

A Free Clinic worker in the lab.

The Free People's Clinic believes that health care is a human right, and not a privilege to be based on **how** much money a person has or anything else; that health care means caring about people, not just treating their diseases; that an emphasis on health education, preventative medicine, demystification and deprofessionalization of medicine must underlie all interactions between staff and patients; and that no hierarchial structures can exist among clinic staff and between staff and patients.

Presently the Clinic functions as an out patient service and can diagnose and treat many illnesses as well as educate people on what they can do to stay healthy. The lab can do blood and urine tests for such things as mono, hepatitis, pregnancy, VD, and other conditions and infections; the pharmacy carries antibiotics and other medicines to help make sick bodies well; and there is information and counseling for VD problems, sex education, abortion referral, and nutrition. The Clinic hopes to be able to expand its services in the future, but as more and more peoplecameto the clinic many people began to realize that the the Clinic was becoming just as bad as the honk institutions. Not only was it not acting as a model, but it took the responsibility from those who should have been d doing it. It became clear that the answer to the community's health needs did not lie only in the existence of a free clinic, but the existing institutions had to be forced to become responsive to the people of the community.

The Free Clinic knows that it alone will not be able to provide adequate health care to the people of this community so in addition to providing the services that it presently provides, the Clinic will be struggling to force the present medical institutions to use their vast facilities, which are said to be the best in the world, to the use of all the people. The Free Clinic calls for neighborhood clinics throughout the city which are controlled by the community and the staff of the clinics.

The Clinic is open Monday thru Thursday from 7 pm until all the patients have been seen. When you go you should go early to insure thay you are seen as early as possible. If you have some questions or just need some advice, you can call the Clinic at 761-8952 or stop by upstairs at the Community Center. What we demand is free, complete health care for everyone. Power to the People.

"The Free People's Clinic," *Ann Arbor Sun*, September 1, 1972, http://oldnews.aadl.org/node/195097.

introduction of a common medical application form that could be used to apply to many medical schools at once (the American Medical College Application Service, or AMCAS), applications for a 225-seat entering class skyrocketed from 1,728 in 1970 to 3,096 in 1971. A variety of federal and local programs contributed to increasing gender, racial, and socioeconomic diversity in the student body during the early 1970s.[108] The first-year cohort for the 1972–1973 academic year included a total of 247 students, of whom 21 percent were women and 13.7 percent were identified as "black, oriental, [or] chicano [*sic*]."[109] In the same year, the Robert Wood Johnson Foundation Student Aid Program provided funds to encourage applicants from "rural and inner-city areas" to study medicine at Michigan.[110] Student-led groups encouraged diversity. Women were finally allowed to join the Galens Honorary Medical Society in the early 1970s (although they had participated in Smoker performances before then), and newer student organizations such as the Black Medical Association (BMA) published newsletters and organized events to raise awareness of issues that affected students from minority groups. In 1973 the BMA planned a national symposium on "Community Health and the Emerging Black Physician" to be held in Ann Arbor and hosted annual health-care programs to commemorate Martin Luther King, Jr., Day.[111] The student Committee on Ethics, Humanism, and Medicine was formed in 1978 and organized conferences to address ethical issues in modern medicine over the next decade, with such panel titles as "Physicians: The Regulated or the Regulators?"[112] Clearly, medical students arrived at Michigan with progressive political ideals that would strongly affect their experience and the environment of the school in the late twentieth century.[113]

Over the course of the 1970s, more Michigan graduates chose to enter primary care as a professional field, a trend encouraged by the state and federal governments. Some 5,419 American medical school graduates sought research positions in 1968, but that number dropped to 1,883 only eleven years later.[114] At Michigan, the medical school established a Department of Family Practice as well as a preceptorship program to expose students to clinical practice in community health-care systems (and, not coincidentally, to provide an adequate patient base for the student population). By 1981, Dean John Gronvall estimated that about 60 percent of the medical school's graduates chose to become primary carc physicians, and the state had recommended incentives to "lure" those new doctors to practice in rural or poverty-stricken areas. The Robert Wood Johnson Foundation Student Aid Program, for example, directly encouraged its recipients to return to and practice medicine in their home communities after graduating from

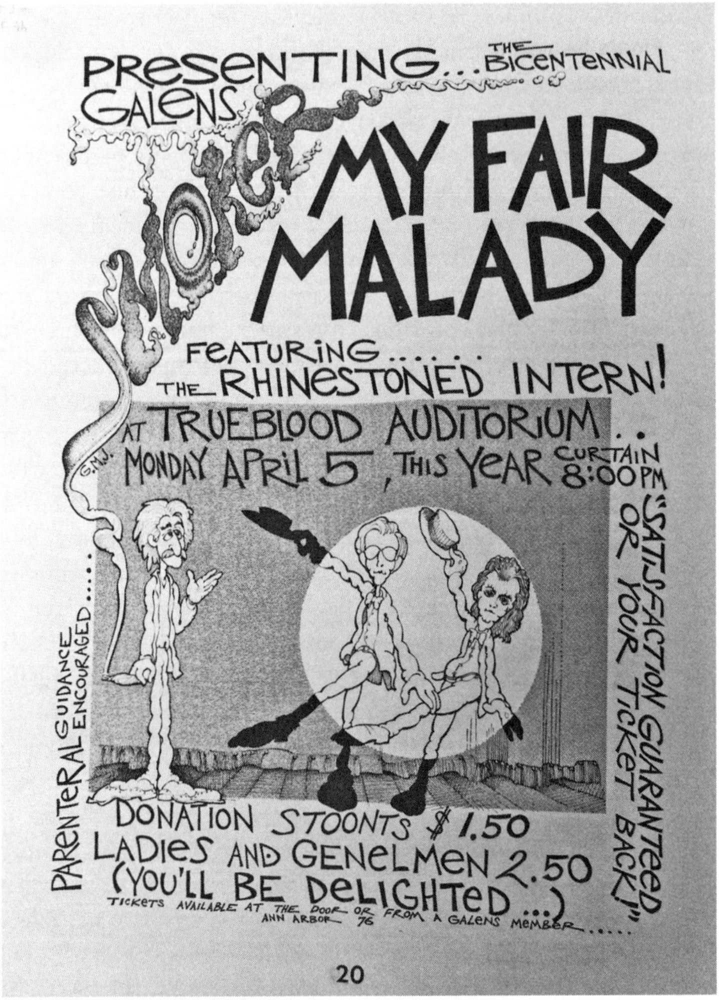

Advertisement for *My Fair Malady*, *The Paeon*, January–February 1976, p. 20. Box 5, Medical School (University of Michigan) Publications, Bentley Historical Library, University of Michigan, Ann Arbor.

the university.[115] By the mid-1990s, however, the trend toward primary care lagged at Michigan compared with the national average, although about half of the school's graduates still chose to enter the field. At the school's Match Day ceremony in 1994, Dean Giles Bole remarked, "'I love all this primary-care stuff'" and reportedly was "greeted with a handful of hisses from his audience of more than 200 graduating medical students. 'No, I'm serious about it,' he countered."[116]

Despite changes in medical student personal and professional identities, there were difficulties in realizing the progressive ideals of the medical profession in the late twentieth century. In particular, although the medical school "had one of the most diverse student bodies on campus as well as in comparison with medical schools across the country," too many reports of discrimination received significant attention within the school and in the local media.[117] Kenneth M. Ludmerer has noted that many medical schools in the United States were concerned about the performance of students from minority and underprivileged backgrounds in the era of affirmative action.[118] So, too, at Michigan in the 1990s, a considerable number of white faculty members (about 60 percent) believed that their academic standards had "been lowered to attract a more diverse student body—an assertion rejected by 91 percent of the black, 86 percent of the Hispanic and 85 percent of the Asian faculty."[119] Furthermore, far too many of Michigan's students complained that they continued to face indirect and direct discrimination and hostility in the program. In 1973 the BMA reported a lack of support from various departments in the school and even "threats of academic and/or professional reprisal."[120]

By the end of the 1970s, as medical school enrollments declined, student groups voiced concerns about disproportionate declines for minority groups. According to the BMA representative in 1979, "There is a growing hostility within the Medical School to a fair and equitable Black admissions policy," and the organization had "been receiving complaints from Black students at the undergraduate level of a rigid and unreceptive posture here at Michigan."[121] A university Senate Advisory Committee on University Affairs investigated all of the health sciences departments in 1987 and described the environment they observed as "a climate of coldness and disrespect" toward students of color—one that led many to forgo application to Michigan altogether.[122] The 1990 accreditation site visit to the school found it "apparent that the attrition rate of [underrepresented minority] students is approaching an unacceptable level" and claimed that "minority students do not feel welcome" in the program.[123] According to one Ann Arbor journalist in 1996, "The University of Michigan Medical School is such an inhospitable place for blacks that 19 out of the 20 African-American graduate students, medical students and house officers surveyed said they would not stay there if offered a position."[124] Women, too, continued to face limitations at Michigan, despite the growing proportion of female medical students (and, subsequently,

U.S. doctors) after 1980. Despite the gains, in 1994 women students said "they wish[ed] for more female role models in the classroom and in the hospital. At the highest ranks, doctoring is still dominated by men."[125] As the 1990s progressed, the percentage of women in incoming classes continued to increase, as did the numbers of female faculty.

Even so, the medical school maintained its strong national reputation, and its students took numerous opportunities to celebrate their successes. This was particularly true of rite-of-passage events. In recent years, the alumni society has sponsored a White Coat Ceremony for incoming students, in which they receive a ceremonial white coat to mark their entrance into the school. About four years later students celebrate Match Day, the national matching program through which graduating medical students are matched with postgraduate training programs. This is a rite of passage shared on the same day by students around the country as they learn where they will be spending the next few years—which could be on either side of the country. These graduating doctors cheer, laugh, and cry as they receive the results of the National Resident Matching Program and put pins on a

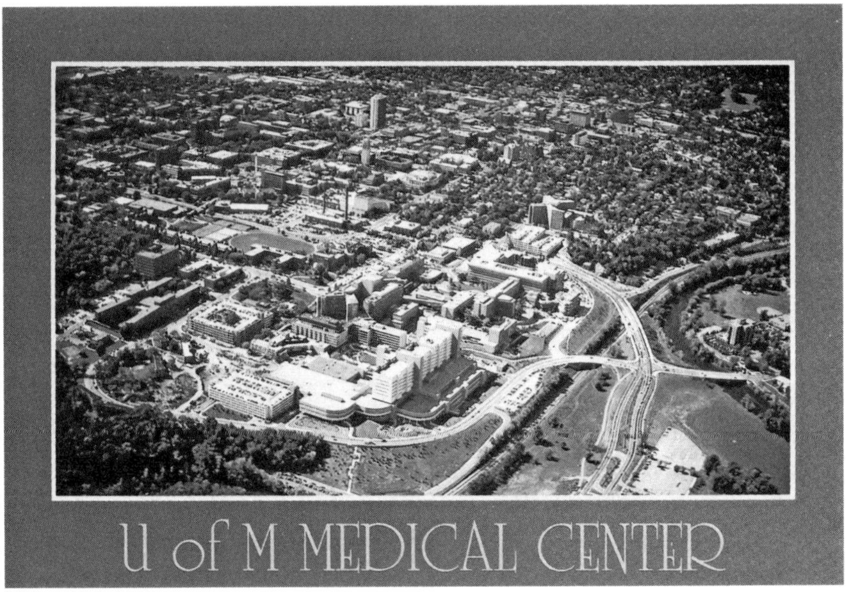

University of Michigan Medical Center (postcard), ca. 1986. Photograph by John Penrod. Penrod/Hiawatha Company Postcard Collection, Bentley Historical Library, University of Michigan, Ann Arbor.

map to indicate where they will be going.[126] Even with evidence of frustration and hostility, Michigan students clearly take pride in their school and accomplishments.

Conclusion

Like the medical profession generally, Michigan's medical school weathered significant changes during the final decades of the twentieth century. On the one hand, the school remained on the cutting edge of medical innovation, developing and introducing revolutionary techniques and treatments in a variety of fields. The size, diversity, and professional scope of the faculty; the expansion of the school's physical plant; and the quality of the student body continued to impress observers and helped maintain the University of Michigan Medical School as one of the top programs in the country. However, within the medical center, the program and administrative structure that seemed so strong, prosperous, and promising in 1969 had begun to implode. The center was reorganized in 1974 and again in the mid-1990s when both medical school dean Giles Bole and University of Michigan Health System CEO John D. Forsyth resigned from their positions after significant disagreements about budgeting and the relationship between the hospital and university. This move was designed to allow the Board of Regents to reorganize the varied missions of the school and clinical facilities into a single, consolidated unit under the executive vice provost for medical affairs.[127]

At the same time, public expectations for medical care and professionalism, political and economic pressures, and disillusionment with the "establishment" had in many ways dismantled older traditions in medical education and clinical practice, traditions that Michigan's physicians had a significant role in implementing. When, as Kenneth Ludmerer has argued, "the social contract between society and medical education had been unilaterally broken,"[128] the University of Michigan found itself in the precarious position of maintaining its distinctive reputation in the face of funding declines; tensions between research, clinical, and instructional priorities; demands for inclusion and diversity; and the effectiveness of clinical instruction at Ann Arbor's University Hospital. All of these issues included echoes of many of the school's earlier controversies and decisions. In many ways, the school's history of the late twentieth century contains reflections of its past, though not always clear ones.

Epilogue

Looking Back from the Twenty-First Century

In 2017 the University of Michigan celebrated the bicentennial of its 1817 founding as the Catholepistemiad. In 1837, two decades after the university's modest beginning as a single building in Detroit, the legislature of the newly formed state of Michigan decided to establish a university on forty acres of land in the village of Ann Arbor. The legislature specified that as an integral part of the institution there should be established a medical school, and in 1850 the doors opened for the first University of Michigan medical students. The medical school of today is obviously quite different from the school that greeted those first students. As of 2017, it is part of Michigan Medicine, a new name that encompasses the entire medical system. Despite what has happened during the intervening 167 years, the school's mission today remains in some fundamental ways similar to that envisioned by its original founders. Examining the institution's history not only gives us insight into how the choices were made that have shaped the institution of today but also highlights the possibilities for continual change through the choices that we continue to make.

Clearly, much has changed since 1850. The very idea of what it means to be a physician is quite different, in terms of both the types of knowledge necessary to practice medicine and how the profession is organized. Not only is the medical school curriculum longer (four years instead of two), but the curricular content now progresses from one year to the next. The emphasis today on the natural sciences, the idea that knowledge changes, and the linkage of classroom instruction with bedside learning are all fundamentally different concepts from those that students found in the medical school's original program. The larger system of medical education and practice today is much more structured. We now have standardized national exams to assess overall knowledge and national private specialty boards to label physicians as experts in specific areas; these systems of formal licensure and specialization simply did not exist in 1850.

And what is the best way to organize the time in medical school? One model for the structure of medical education was defined in part during the late nineteenth and early twentieth centuries at the University of Michigan and a handful of other pathbreaking schools after the standard curriculum was lengthened to four years: two years of basic science followed by two years of clinical instruction. This curricular model marked a distinct break with what had come before, and it soon became the standard for almost all U.S. medical schools throughout most of the twentieth century. While Michigan and other schools did implement some innovations from time to time, they were modifications that did not change in broad strokes the essential structure and assumptions of medical education, being what sociologist Samuel W. Bloom has aptly referred to as "reform without change."[1] However, that static model does now appear to be changing. Michigan's medical school curriculum currently is in the midst of a radical restructuring unlike any that the school has attempted since the introduction of scientific ideology as central to the curriculum more than a century ago. That transformation is taking place even as new curricular ideas, such as the flipped classroom, and new electronic technologies, such as innumerable smart-phone applications, hold the potential to change the ways that medical students learn and are taught. Precisely how this change in the curriculum will work out remains to be seen, but one can be certain that it will reflect larger social norms and the expectations of what it means to become an excellent physician, just as earlier changes also had done.

Another major change involves the geographical sweep of the school. Some early medical school faculty traveled to Europe and brought new insights, such as the ideas and technology for the germ theory of disease, back to the small Midwestern town of Ann Arbor. Some students came to attend school at Michigan from overseas, but not many, and not as part of any systematic program. Today's faculty and students span the globe in ways that may not have been imaginable during the early years of the school and in any event simply would not have been physically possible without the airline transportation of today. Students are increasingly interested in learning how to reduce the health-care disparities that result from differences in socioeconomic status, ethnicity, gender, or other factors and to do so not only in southeastern Michigan but also in faraway locales. Part of the new curriculum includes the opportunity for students to study in "Paths of Excellence," one of which, "Global Health and Disparities," emphasizes global medicine and gives it a formal place in the curricular structure. With the leadership of the Global REACH (Research, Education, and Collaboration in Health) program, founded in 2001, faculty members are working in seventy-four countries across six continents, and recent students have traveled to twenty countries, including Ghana, China, Brazil, Ethiopia, and India. Michigan's medical students today have opportunities to obtain a truly global education.

The medical students who make up that student body have also changed, in ways that reflect not only changes in social context but also changes in ideas about who ought to become a physician. While the original class of 1850 was all male, in 1870 Michigan became one of the first major American medical schools to admit women. Those early women paved the way for many others to follow. In 2016, the entering medical school class of 172 students (selected from more than 6,000 applicants) was more than 56 percent women. Michigan has also led the way toward training a racially and ethnically diverse group of students; in 2016 about 16 percent of the entering students were members of groups underrepresented in medicine. Residencies and fellowships were nonexistent when the medical school started. Today they are an essential part of learning to be a physician, and Michigan now hosts around twelve hundred residents and fellows in twenty-five accredited residency programs and seventy-eight accredited fellowship programs. Not all students in the medical school are training to become physicians. While the original medical school did not offer a Ph.D. degree, many students now come to the medical school to learn how to pursue basic research; today 588 students are pursuing graduate degrees, along with 604 postdoctoral fellows.

The physical plant has both expanded and fundamentally changed since the school's early days. The library is a prime example of this transformation. During the late nineteenth century the medical school made a prescient decision to subscribe to every major medical journal in the world, which reflected a radical shift in ideas about medical education and changing medical knowledge. Today, the school continues that philosophy of valuing new knowledge, but journals (and books) are far more often consulted in their electronic form. As a result, the medical library, once a monument to learning and education characterized by seemingly endless rows and rows of bookshelves, is now almost totally devoid of books and journals in their physical form. In 2015 the circa 1980 medical library was reopened after a two-year renovation that provides space explicitly designed not to house printed material but to support the needs of the new curriculum in other, electronic, ways.

From a single building, the medical school has come to include 2.3 million square feet of space spread over seventeen buildings, with 3,514 faculty and 3,825 staff members in 2016. In 2006, the Biomedical Science Research and Rachel Upjohn Buildings were opened. Significant additional space came from the Parke-Davis pharmaceutical company. Parke-Davis had started to construct research space in the area north of campus in the 1960s, a process that continued after the company's acquisition by Pfizer. When Pfizer decided to leave Ann Arbor, the university, led by the medical school, purchased the 174-acre campus and its twenty-eight buildings in 2009. It has since become the North Campus Research Complex (NCRC), home to a variety of research enterprises, partnerships with industry and government, and educational programs. While quite a reach from the central campus location of the original medical school, NCRC is consistent with the outward-looking scope of the changing medical school mission and provides much-needed space for research. Research was important from the early years of the medical school, but it was not until after World War II and the explosion in federal funds available for extramural research that the scale of the research enterprise grew to the proportions it now enjoys throughout the school. In 2016 the school spent more than $440 million on sponsored projects, of which almost $290 million came from the National Institutes of Health.

Starting in 1860 the medical school decided to move clinical instruction away from loose, unstructured, and relatively unsupervised associations with various health-care locations in the area and instead to own and operate its own twenty-bed facility on North University Street. Michigan's University Hospital, the first of its kind in the country, has served as a model for many others throughout the United States. In its various incarnations the hospital has remained in Ann Arbor, despite serious debates for a time over whether it would be better situated in Detroit. The number of beds has grown from about twenty to more than one thousand. The University Hospital now has more than two million clinic visits each year and discharges almost fifty thousand people yearly; doctors there deliver more than four thousand babies and perform more than fifty thousand surgeries each year. In 2007 the university's Cardiovascular Center—the largest in the United States—was dedicated, and in 2011 the departments of pediatrics and of obstetrics and gynecology relocated to the Von Voigtlander Women's Hospital, with fifty single maternity rooms. The models of care have transformed in ways that reflect a dynamically changing model of specialization, most recently marked by the creation of a new division (within the Department of Internal Medicine) of "hospitalist" medicine, in which physicians do not divide their time between seeing patients in the clinic and seeing them on the inpatient wards but specialize in the care of hospitalized patients. Since 1953 the VA Ann Arbor Healthcare System has been a major partner with the medical school for education, research, and patient care. Affiliations and associations with other health-care delivery sites continue to be implemented.

The 2017 bicentennial event has inspired another generation of commemoration and celebrations. But in many ways, the medical school and larger university have always been very close to their history. Many university buildings already bear the names of venerable leaders, and countless campus hallways are decorated with portraits and plaques dedicated to notable presidents, deans, professors, benefactors, and alumni. After the new hospital was constructed and occupied in 1986, the Department of Internal Medicine chose to name its inpatient services for historical figures at the University of Michigan, including earlier faculty members, department heads, and other notables.[2] Street and facility names on the Health System campus acknowledge the influence of trendsetters and significant figures in the school's past, such as Zina Pitcher and Victor Vaughan. Many endowed chairs carry the names and memories of former faculty and students, such as Alice Hamilton and Hugh Cabot.

As we look to the future from 2017, many of the same questions that have been present from the early years of the medical school still exist. At the onset it was not clear that the University of Michigan Medical School should be engaged in patient care. Michigan decided to do so in 1869 and in so doing established a model that many other universities have followed. But for many decades thereafter, the clinical system was relatively small. Money did not play much of a role. Patient care was paid for by the state. The system ran with very little administrative staff. And it was explicitly clear that the medical school was delivering patient care directly in pursuit of the goals of academic medicine, to help train the university's medical students (and later house officers). As the clinical care system continues to expand, the historical tensions between clinical care and the academic missions of teaching and research will require continued attention.

While much has changed since the school's early years, much remains the same. Medical students still come to Ann Arbor wanting to learn how to be skilled doctors. To do this they must acquire knowledge and the capacity for clinical reasoning. The mechanisms for doing so may change—from large lectures to small groups, from heavy physical textbooks to multimedia electronic documents—but the essential need to learn about medicine persists.

Students do not go to medical school only to learn facts and to learn how to think. They also go to learn how to take care of patients—to talk to patients, to examine them, to break bad news, to impart good news. And learning how to do this requires direct contact with patients. Despite all of the changes in content and context, the central goal of the nearly fifteen thousand students who have come though the University of Michigan Medical School since 1850 remains the same: to learn how best to care for other human beings. And to do this requires both intellectual knowledge and clinical expertise.

Why is it important to understand the history of this, or any, medical school? For one thing, it reminds us that the world changes: institutions change, leaders change, ideologies change, science changes, and knowledge changes. Especially for students, it is important always to realize that the facts being authoritatively presented one year may have changed dramatically by the next year. Much of the material that students hear their professors present will certainly change during the course of those students' professional careers. The same lesson is also valuable for the general public: medicine is not static.

But some things do not change. People want to stay healthy. People fall ill. People go to someone for help, for guidance on how to relieve their pain, for advice on how to get better. Often the person they go to is a physician. People enter the medical school hoping to become superb physicians and, in so doing, to follow in the footsteps of thousands of people before them.

The history of medicine can also be a poignant source of pride. Michigan's medical school has been a leader in many aspects of medical education and medical science in ways that have reached around the world. Some of that history has been recorded here. Unfortunately, there was not room in this book for much of it, including many interesting and important episodes from the past. We can learn both from past decisions we choose to praise and from past behaviors that we may now regret. Finally, learning about the history of the medical school may be most important because it is liberating. Reading the history, we learn about how those before us made consequential choices about what to teach, whom to teach, and how to teach. They made choices about whom to care for, what institutions to create, and what institutions to change. We, too, make choices. Realizing that we are not forced to follow past decisions can help us to celebrate the opportunity to shape the future.

Notes

INTRODUCTION

1. Harlan Hatcher, "Guest Editorial: The University and the Medical School," *University of Michigan Medical Center Journal* 33 (July–August 1967): 151.

2. Kenneth M. Ludmerer, *Learning to Heal: The Development of American Medical Education* (New York: Basic Books, 1985), 5.

3. For example, see Robert Oliver, *Making the Modern Medical School: The Wisconsin Stories* (Nantucket, MA: Science History, 2002); Constance E. Putnam, *The Science We Have Loved and Taught: Dartmouth Medical School's First Two Centuries* (Hanover, NH: University Press of New England, 2004); Leonard G. Wilson, *Medical Revolution in Minnesota: A History of the University of Minnesota Medical School* (St. Paul, MN: Midewiwin, 1989); Harry K. Beecher and Mark D. Altschule, *Medicine at Harvard: The First Three Hundred Years* (Hanover, NH: University Press of New England, 1977); Horace W. Davenport, *Not Just Any Medical School: The Science, Practice, and Teaching of Medicine at the University of Michigan, 1850–1941* (Ann Arbor: University of Michigan Press, 1999); and Joel D. Howell, "Introduction," in *Medical Lives and Scientific Medicine at Michigan, 1891–1969*, ed. Joel D. Howell (Ann Arbor: University of Michigan Press, 1993), 1–11.

4. See A. McGhee Harvey, *Science at the Bedside: Clinical Research in American Medicine, 1905–1945* (Baltimore: Johns Hopkins University Press, 1981), xvii; and Kenneth M. Ludmerer, *Time to Heal: American Medical Education from the Turn of the Century to the Era of Managed Care* (Oxford: Oxford University Press, 1999), xii. For more specific work on modern doctor-patient relations, see Christopher Crenner, *Private Practice: In the Early Twentieth-Century Medical Office of Dr. Richard Cabot* (Baltimore: Johns Hopkins University Press, 2005).

5. Reuben Peterson, "Landmarks in the Medical School: A Survey of the History of the University of Michigan Medical School and Its Hospital," *Michigan Alumnus Quarterly Review* 45 (April 1939): [1]. See also Howell, "Introduction," 2.

6. Davenport, *Not Just Any Medical School,* ix–xi; Kenneth M. Ludmerer, "The University of Michigan Medical School: A Tradition of Leadership," in *Medical Lives and Scientific Medicine at Michigan, 1891–1969*, ed. Joel D. Howell (Ann Arbor: University of Michigan Press, 1993), 14–15; Howell, "Introduction," 3, 6; Thomas Neville Bonner, *To the Ends of the Earth: Women's Search for Education in Medicine* (Cambridge,

MA: Harvard University Press, 1992), 141; Harvey, *Science at the Bedside*, 329. Historian Susan Lawrence notes that women were admitted to the first medical school class at the University of Iowa in 1870 and received a fully coeducational experience there. Susan C. Lawrence, "Iowa Physicians: Legitimacy, Institutions, and the Practice of Medicine, Part One: Establishing a Professional Identity, 1833–1886," *Annals of Iowa* 62 (Spring 2003): 174–175.

7. Howell, "Introduction," 3; Charles E. Rosenberg, "Martin Arrowsmith: The Scientist as Hero," in *No Other Gods: On Science and American Social Thought*, rev. ed., ed. Charles E. Rosenberg (Baltimore: Johns Hopkins University Press, 1997), 124, 128. *Arrowsmith* was awarded the Pulitzer Prize in 1926, but Lewis declined to accept.

8. John A. Woods, "Dr. Kevorkian's U-M Connection," *Ann Arbor News*, December 9, 1993.

9. Stephen Lurie, "Innovation and Service Traditional at University of Michigan Medical School," *Journal of the American Medical Association* 283, no. 7 (2000): 855.

10. Howard Markel, "The University of Michigan Medical School, 1850–2000: 'An Example Worthy of Imitation,'" *Journal of the American Medical Association* 283, no. 7 (2000): 915; Davenport, *Not Just Any Medical School*, ix.

11. See Joel D. Howell, "Telling Michigan's Story," *Medicine at Michigan* 18, no. 1 (2016), http://www.medicineatmichigan.org/history/2016/spring/telling-michigans-story.

12. January 1915 meeting, in *Proceedings of the Board of Regents* (Ann Arbor: University of Michigan, 2000), 93–96.

13. Constance E. Putnam makes a similar point in her history of Dartmouth Medical School. See Putnam, *The Science We Have Loved and Taught*, xx.

CHAPTER 1

1. Fanny J. Anderson, "The Role of the Physician in the History of the State of Michigan before the Civil War, 1837–1861," 1972, p. 30, Bentley Historical Library, University of Michigan, Ann Arbor; Howard H. Peckham, *The Making of the University of Michigan, 1817–1992*, ed. Margaret L. Steneck and Nicholas H. Steneck (Ann Arbor: University of Michigan Bentley Historical Library, 1994), 6–7, 17; William N. Hubbard, Jr., and Nicholas H. Steneck, *The Origins of Michigan's Leadership in the Health Sciences* (Ann Arbor: University of Michigan Historical Center for the Health Sciences, 1995), 44.

2. Horace H. Davenport, *University of Michigan Surgeons, 1850–1970* (Ann Arbor: University of Michigan Historical Center for the Health Sciences, 1993), 7; "Niagara Falls Route," *Ann Arbor Headlight*, 2, no. 15 (ca. 1896): 10, Box 1, Washtenaw County Historical Records, 1827–2013, Bentley Historical Library, University of Michigan, Ann Arbor; Wilfred B. Shaw, ed., *The University of Michigan: An Encyclopedic Survey*, vol. 1 (Ann Arbor: University of Michigan Press, 1942), 177–180; Orlando W. Stephenson, *Ann Arbor: The First Hundred Years* (Ann Arbor: Ann Arbor Chamber of Commerce, 1927), 335. The census does not include Native American inhabitants of the region. By 1850 Washtenaw County supported a total population of only 28,567. See Peckham, *Making of the University of Michigan*, 18.

3. Horace W. Davenport, *Not Just Any Medical School: The Science, Practice, and Teaching of Medicine at the University of Michigan, 1850–1941* (Ann Arbor: University of Michigan Press, 1999), 1; Frederick W. Mayer, *A Setting for Excellence: The Story of the Planning and Development of the Ann Arbor Campus of the University of Michigan* (Ann Arbor: University of Michigan Press, 2015), 51.

4. Martin Kaufman, "American Medical Education," in *The Education of American Physicians: Historical Essays*, ed. Ronald L. Numbers (Berkeley: University of California Press, 1980), 7–28.

5. J. H. Beech, "An Address to the Graduating Class of the Medical Department of the University of Michigan," *Peninsular and Independent Medical Journal* 1 (May 1858): 73.

6. Paul Starr, *The Social Transformation of American Medicine* (New York: Basic Books, 1982), 88, 93.

7. Davenport, *Not Just Any Medical School*, 2.

8. Anderson, "Role of the Physician," 30.

9. John Harley Warner, "Ideals of Science and Their Discontents in Late Nineteenth-Century American Medicine," *Isis* 82 (September 1991): 465. See also *To Spread the Light of Knowledge: 250 Years of the Nation's First Medical School* (Philadelphia: Perelman School of Medicine of the University of Pennsylvania, 2015), 39.

10. Anderson, "Role of the Physician," 30; Peckham, *Making of the University of Michigan*, 6–7, 17.

11. In some records, his surname is spelled "Douglass."

12. Davenport, *Not Just Any Medical School*, 2. For example, the chair of physiology was largely vacant for nearly two decades after Allen left the medical school, and the subject was for a time tied to anatomical instruction, but in 1872 physiology instruction was combined with materia medica and therapeutics. Several years later, the physiology chair was once more combined with anatomy when Ford was charged with taking over the topic, but the two fields were permanently separated when Johns Hopkins graduate and physician Henry Sewall was appointed to run the new Physiological Laboratory in the early 1880s. See Wilfred B. Shaw, ed., *The University of Michigan: An Encyclopedic Survey*, vol. 2 (Ann Arbor: University of Michigan Press, 1951), 811; and W. Bruce Fye, *The Development of American Physiology: Scientific Medicine in the Nineteenth Century* (Baltimore: Johns Hopkins University Press, 1987), 157–158.

13. "Report of the Committee on Medical Education," *Transactions of the American Medical Association* 6 (1853): 83–96, cited in Anderson, "Role of the Physician," 32. See also Davenport, *University of Michigan Surgeons*, 5; Thomas Neville Bonner, *Becoming a Physician: Medical Education in Britain, France, Germany, and the United States, 1750–1945* (Baltimore: Johns Hopkins University Press, 1995), 199; and Hubbard and Steneck, *Origins of Michigan's Leadership*, 36–37, 42.

14. Quoted in Anderson, "Role of the Physician," 34n158.

15. Ibid.

16. Ibid. See also Donald F. Huelke, "The History of the Department of Anatomy, the University of Michigan: Part I, 1850 to 1894," *University of Michigan Medical Bulletin* 27 (1961): 8–9; Shaw, *Encyclopedic Survey*, 2:939; and September 1858 meeting, in *Proceedings of the Board of Regents* (Ann Arbor: University of Michigan, 2000), 775.

17. Huelke, "History of the Department of Anatomy," 3, 13.

18. Theodore A. McGraw, "The Medical Schools of the Last Half-Century," *Journal of the Michigan State Medical Society* 14 (1915): 516.

19. Faculty meeting minutes, March 18, 1872, Faculty Meetings, 1850–1875, Box 127, Medical School (University of Michigan) Records, 1850–2010, Bentley Historical Library, Ann Arbor, MI. Lyster's appointment was reconsidered in 1879 and 1888, each time made conditional on his relocation to Ann Arbor. See Davenport, *University of Michigan Surgeons*, 18; faculty meeting minutes, February 16, 1888, Faculty Meetings, 1878–1891, Box 128, Medical School (University of Michigan) Records, 1850–2010, Bentley Historical Library.

20. Shaw, *Encyclopedic Survey*, 2:835–836, 939.

21. Shaw, *Encyclopedic Survey*, 1:177–180; Peckham, *Making of the University of Michigan*, 18; Stephenson, *Ann Arbor*, 335.

22. Huelke, "History of the Department of Anatomy," 3.

23. Beech, "Address," 70.

24. A. B. Palmer, "Report to the State Society on the Diseases of Children," *Peninsular and Independent Medical Journal* 1 (May 1858): 92. See also Stephenson, *Ann Arbor*, 360, 365.

25. Reynolds Farley, Sheldon Danziger, and Harry J. Holzer, *Detroit Divided* (New York: Russell Sage Foundation, 2000), 16; Davenport, *University of Michigan Surgeons*, 7.

26. Editorial, *Peninsular Journal of Medicine* 3 (1857): 163–166, cited in Anderson, "Role of the Physician," 33. According to Anderson, the author was Louis Robinson, but the cited editorial was printed anonymously.

27. Faculty meeting minutes, December 29, 1856, Faculty Meetings, 1850–1875, Box 127, Medical School (University of Michigan) Records, 1850–2010, Bentley Historical Library.

28. Faculty meeting minutes, March 25, 1857, Faculty Meetings, 1850–1875, Box 127, Medical School (University of Michigan) Records, 1850–2010, Bentley Historical Library.

29. Bonner, *Becoming a Physician*, 221; Anderson, "Role of the Physician," 34; Silas Farmer, *History of Detroit and Wayne County and Early Michigan: A Chronological Cyclopedia of the Past and Present*, 3rd ed. (Detroit: Silas Farmer, 1890), http://www.maritimehistoryofthegreatlakes.ca/documents/farmer/default.asp?ID=s015. Farmer refers to St. Mary's House of Invalids as "St. Mary's Hospital."

30. Meeting of September 28, 1958, in *Proceedings of the Board of Regents*, 764–781; Davenport, *University of Michigan Surgeons*, 8; Shaw, *Encyclopedic Survey*, 2:959; Anderson, "Role of the Physician," 35–36.

31. Cited in Davenport, *University of Michigan Surgeons*, 7. Other histories of the medical school suggest that many early faculty members, perhaps even a majority, favored a move to Detroit and/or opposed the construction of a teaching hospital in Ann Arbor. See also Reuben Peterson, "University Hospital Manuscript" (39), pp. 4–5, Box 2, Reuben Peterson Papers, Bentley Historical Library, University of Michigan, Ann Arbor.

32. [Moses Gunn], "Removal of the Medical Department," *Peninsular and Independent Medical Journal* 1 (May 1858): 106–109.

33. Ibid., 109 (emphasis in original).

34. Ibid. (emphasis in original).

35. Ibid., 110 (emphasis in original).

36. Anderson, "Role of the Physician," 36; faculty meeting minutes, March 22, 1867, Faculty Meetings, 1850–1875, Box 127, Medical School (University of Michigan) Records, 1850–2010, Bentley Historical Library. Huelke suggests that Gunn's failed cause may have contributed to his decision to leave the University of Michigan in 1867, but that decision was more likely motivated by the death of his son Glyndon, who drowned in the Detroit River in 1866. Huelke, "History of Anatomy," 9.

37. Zina Pitcher, *A Memoir Embracing an Epitome of the Transactions of the Regents of the University, with Some Reasons for the Adoption of Their More Important Measures, from 1837 to June 30, 1851* (Lansing, MI: Ingals, Hedges, 1852), cited in Anderson, "Role of the Physician," 30.

38. *Ohio Medical and Surgical Journal* 1 (1848): 185–187, cited in Anderson, "Role of the Physician," 32.

39. "University of Michigan, Department of Medicine and Surgery, Order of Exercises, Second Semester, 1889–1890," Miscellaneous, 1894–1903, Box 135, Medical School (University of Michigan) Records, 1850–2010, Bentley Historical Library.

40. The Bentley Historical Library contains a collection of 1,449 medical student theses from this period at Michigan's medical school. To request theses, see http://quod.lib.umich.edu/b/bhlead/umich-bhl-87223?rgn=Entire+Finding+Aid;view=text;q1=thesis.

41. J. Adams Allen, *Introductory Address to the Third Session of the College of Medicine and Surgery of the University of Michigan* (Detroit: George E. Pomeroy, 1852); "Third Annual Commencement of the Medical Department of the University of Michigan, Wednesday, March 30, 1853," Faculty Meetings, 1850–1875, Box 127, Medical School (University of Michigan) Records, 1850–2010, Bentley Historical Library.

42. Shaw, *Encyclopedic Survey*, 2:846.

43. Faculty meeting minutes, August 25, 1851, Faculty Meetings, 1850–1875, Box 127, Medical School (University of Michigan) Records, 1850–2010, Bentley Historical Library. For anatomical museum organization and budgetary considerations, see also the minutes from August 20, 1852, July 22, 1855, October 16, 1855, and December 13, 1855.

44. Rollo McCotter, "A History of the Anatomy Department of the University of Michigan," address given at honorary dinner, February 7, 1947, p. 3, Bentley Historical Library; Shaw, *Encyclopedic Survey*, 2:810.

45. For example, it decided at an 1856 meeting that the AMA's "proposed modification of the Course of Instruction in [the] Medical College . . . [was] upon the whole quite impracticable in the present state of the profession." The specific proposed reform was not described in detail. Faculty meeting minutes, February 8, 1856, Faculty Meetings, 1850–1875, Box 127, Medical School (University of Michigan) Records, 1850–2010, Bentley Historical Library.

46. Michael Sappol, *A Traffic of Dead Bodies: Anatomy and Embodied Social Identity in Nineteenth-Century America* (Princeton, NJ: Princeton University Press, 2002), 78.

47. Huelke, "History of the Department of Anatomy," 7. This account suggests that Gunn's dissection took place in his private office or in the basement of the old Ann Arbor courthouse, "which may have been one and the same place." Ibid.

48. Zina Pitcher, "Notice of the Territorial and State Medical Societies of Michigan," *Peninsular Medical Journal* 1 (1854): 500–506, cited in Anderson, "Role of the Physician," 32–33n152.

49. Robert C. Kedzie, "The Early Days of the Medical Department," *Michigan Alumnus* 8 (1902): 207, cited in Shaw, *Encyclopedic Survey*, 2:809.

50. Thomas V. Abowd, Tom R. De Meester, and Donald Lucas, "Our Heritage: A History of the Medical School," *University of Michigan Medical Center Journal* 33 (1967): 176.

51. Faculty meeting minutes, February 29, 1860, Faculty Meetings, 1850–1875, Box 127, Medical School (University of Michigan) Records, 1850–2010, Bentley Historical Library.

52. Davenport, *Not Just Any Medical School*, 10.

53. Quoted in Davenport, *Not Just Any Medical School*, 10. Sappol has highlighted the social class dimensions of nineteenth-century anatomical instruction, indicating that dissecting the bodies of deceased members of racial minorities and members of the working class contributed to the professional and class identity of American physicians. Sappol, *A Traffic of Dead Bodies*, 82–83. See also Theodore Russell Chase, class book of 1849, Class of 1849 (University of Michigan) Records, 1889 and 1899, Bentley Historical Library.

54. Huelke, "History of the Department of Anatomy," 9.

55. Davenport, *Not Just Any Medical School*, 10; McCotter, "History of the Anatomy Department," 3; "Body Snatching Was Once Lucrative Profession," *Ann Arbor News*, July 4, 1969; Bonner, *Becoming a Physician*, 225.

56. W. Herdman to the Honorable Board of Regents, June 28, 1880, Box 135, Medical School (University of Michigan) Records, 1850–2010, Bentley Historical Library.

57. *Medical Independent* 3 (1857): 422–432, cited in Anderson, "Role of the Physician," 34.

58. Shaw, *Encyclopedic Survey*, 2:939–941.

59. See Lawrence D. Longo, "Obstetrics and Gynecology," in *The Education of American Physicians: Historical Essays*, ed. Ronald L. Numbers (Berkeley: University of California Press, 1980), 205–225.

60. Judith Walzer Leavitt, *Brought to Bed: Childbearing in America, 1750–1950* (New York: Oxford University Press, 1986), 4–5; Bonner, *Becoming a Physician*, 224; Richard W. Stander and Warren H. Pearse, *Obstetrics, Gynecology and the University of Michigan* (Ann Arbor: n.p., 1968), 7; Shaw, *Encyclopedic Survey*, 2:859, 872.

61. Elizabeth M. Farrand, *History of the University of Michigan* (Ann Arbor: Register, 1885), 87, cited in Anderson, "Role of the Physician," 31; Shaw, *Encyclopedic Survey*, 2:780. The adjective "respectable" implied that the preceptor should be an allopath, not a sectarian or alternative practitioner.

62. Cited in Shaw, *Encyclopedic Survey*, 2:959. See also Anderson, "Role of the Physician," 36.

63. Shaw, *Encyclopedic Survey*, 2:780.

64. A. McGhee Harvey, *Science at the Bedside: Clinical Research in American Medicine, 1905–1945* (Baltimore: Johns Hopkins University Press, 1981), xv; Fye, *Development of American Physiology*, 2.

65. Horace W. Davenport, *Doctor Dock: Teaching and Learning Medicine at the Turn of the Century* (New Brunswick, NJ: Rutgers University Press, 1987), 5. See also Davenport, *Not Just Any Medical School*, 4.

66. Fye, *Development of American Physiology*, 119–120.

67. The Board of Regents accepted Allen's forced resignation after receiving a resolution from university president Henry Philip Tappan and twelve of Allen's colleagues stating that "the prosperity of the Medical College and the general welfare and harmony of the University are seriously affected by the connection of Dr. J. Adams Allen with the institution as a Professor." Davenport, acknowledging that little documentary evidence of this event exists, argues that Allen's political stance as a northern Democrat in 1854, the year of the inflammatory Kansas-Nebraska Act, was probably the main contributing factor to his ouster. Allen became president of the Michigan State Medical Society and, later, professor and president of Rush Medical College in Chicago. Shaw, *Encyclopedic Survey*, 2:911–912; Davenport, *Not Just Any Medical School*, 14.

68. Abowd et al., "Our Heritage," 181.

69. McGraw, "Medical Schools," 516; Bonner, *Becoming a Physician*, 248, 265; Davenport, *Doctor Dock*, 5; Davenport, *Not Just Any Medical School*, 6; Allan M. Brandt and Martha Gardner, "Antagonism and Accommodation: Interpreting the Relationship between Public Health and Medicine in the United States during the 20th Century," *American Journal of Public Health* 90 (May 2000): 707–709.

70. Margaret Humphreys, *Marrow of Tragedy: The Health Crisis of the American Civil War* (Baltimore: Johns Hopkins University Press, 2013), 1, see also 6–8.

71. Florence Nightingale, *Notes on Hospitals*, 3rd ed. (London: Longman, Green, Longman, Roberts, and Green, 1863), 7, 13–20.

72. Richard M. Doolen, "The Founding of the University of Michigan Hospital: An Innovation in Medical Education," *Journal of Medical Education* 39 (January 1964): 50–57; Edward G. Voss, "Founding of the First University Hospital," *Journal of Medical Education* 39 (August 1964): 797–798.

73. Ida C. Brown, "Introduction," in *Michigan Men in the Civil War: A Guide to the Resources in the Bentley Historical Library (1959–1977)* (Ann Arbor: University of Michigan), http://bentley.umich.edu/legacy-support/civilwar/introduction.php (accessed February 24, 2017).

74. Peckham, *Making of the University of Michigan*, 63.

75. *The President's Report to the Board of Regents for the Year Ending June 30, 1879* (Ann Arbor: University of Michigan, 1879), 12.

76. *The President's Report to the Board of Regents for the Year Ending June 30, 1875* (Ann Arbor: University of Michigan, 1875), 9.

77. Davenport, *Not Just Any Medical School*, 1; Bonner, *Becoming a Physician*, 214. Davenport assumes that the "respectable" description of a physician preceptor meant "regular," or allopathic, but provides no other evidence to indicate that apprentices with irregular or eclectic physicians were rejected by the medical school.

78. "Medical College of the University of Michigan, Session of 1855–6: Weekly Schedule," pasted in faculty meeting minutes, September 25, 1855, Faculty Meetings, 1850–1875, Box 127, Medical School (University of Michigan) Records, 1850–2010, Bentley Historical Library. See also Bonner, *Becoming a Physician*, 215.

79. Faculty meeting minutes, November 7 and 26, 1878, Faculty Meetings, 1878–1891, Box 128, Medical School (University of Michigan) Records, 1850–2010, Bentley Historical Library.

80. Bonner, *Becoming a Physician*, 217; *The President's Report to the Board of Regents for the Year Ending June 30, 1873* (Ann Arbor: University of Michigan, 1873), 9;

Henry B. Baker, "Notes Relative to the Benefits of Vaccination," supplement, *Proceedings, Addresses, and Discussions at the Second Annual Conference of the Health Officers in Michigan, at Ann Arbor, Mich., June 14 and 15, 1894: Report of the Michigan State Board of Health*, no. 417 (1894): 50.

81. Shaw, *Encyclopedic Survey*, 2:793. During the school's first twenty-five years, only eleven medical students from nine other countries (England, Ireland, Scotland, France, Germany, Russia, Jamaica, Hawaii, and Liberia) were enrolled, and it is likely that several of those were the children of American missionaries living abroad.

82. Albert B. Prescott, "Silas Hamilton Douglas: Founder of the Chemical Laboratory," Faculty History Project, http://www.lib.umich.edu/faculty-history/faculty/silas-hamilton-douglas/founder-chemical-laboratory (accessed February 24, 2017).

83. Cheney J. Schopieray, "'Col[ore]d Men Are Not Admitted Here,'" *The Quarto* 46 (Fall–Winter 2016): 6–7.

84. Dorothy Gies McGuigan, *A Dangerous Experiment: 100 Years of Women at the University of Michigan* (Benton Harbor, MI: R. W. Patterson for the University of Michigan Center for Continuing Education of Women, 1970), 2, 35–36; M.F., "Building the Next Generation of African-American Physicians," *Medicine at Michigan* 4, no. 3 (2002): 34–35; Georgia A. Lewis Johnson, *Black Graduates of the University of Michigan (1872–1960 Inclusive) and Selected Black Michigan Physicians* (Lansing, MI: Georgia A. Johnson, 1994), 55. Discussions of African Americans and other racial minority representatives in the medical student body are largely anecdotal and are found in secondary sources. For instance, McGuigan notes that Virginia Watts was the first African American woman to graduate from the University of Michigan, and she received that degree from the medical school in 1885; but the article in *Medicine at Michigan* claims that honor belongs to Sarah Bethena Jones, and Johnson claims it was Sophia R. or B. Jones.

85. Shaw, *Encyclopedic Survey*, 2:426.

86. Faculty meeting minutes, March 28, 1871, Faculty Meetings, 1850–1875, Box 127, Medical School (University of Michigan) Records, 1850–2010, Bentley Historical Library; Anderson, "Role of the Physician," 31; McGuigan, *Dangerous Experiment*, 1–2; Stephen Lurie, "Innovation and Service Traditional at University of Michigan Medical School," *Journal of the American Medical Association* 283, no. 7 (2000): 855; Janet Tarolli, "Five Women Determined to Be Doctors and the Role Michigan Played in Helping Them Achieve Their Dream," *Medicine at Michigan* 2, no. 3 (2000): 32; Shaw, *Encyclopedic Survey*, 2:794, 811. Shaw points out that Sanford's graduation "was followed, within a half hour, by Miss Sarah Kilgore, who received the degree of bachelor of laws." Shaw, *Encyclopedic Survey*, 2:794.

87. McGuigan, *Dangerous Experiment*, 38; Thomas Neville Bonner, *To the Ends of the Earth: Women's Search for Education in Medicine* (Cambridge, MA: Harvard University Press, 1992), 141–142; "University of Michigan. 22nd Annual Commencement of the Medical Department, Wednesday, March 27th, 1872, at Ten O'Clock A.M.," Faculty Meetings, 1850–1875, Box 127, Medical School (University of Michigan) Records, 1850–2010, Bentley Historical Library. See also Carol Marinch, "A Fair Chance for the Girls: Medical Education for Women at the University of Michigan, 1870–1890" (Senior Resident Research Project, Department of Internal Medicine, University of Michigan, 1986).

88. Bonner, *To the Ends of the Earth*, 141n12; Bonner, *Becoming a Physician*, 313.

89. "Memorial on Female Medical Education," March 25, 1870, in *Proceedings of the Board of Regents*, 35–37, cited in Shaw, *Encyclopedic Survey*, 2:794. See also McGuigan, *Dangerous Experiment*, 35; Sappol, *Traffic of Dead Bodies*, 88–90; Susan Wells, *Out of the Dead House: Nineteenth-Century Women Physicians and the Writing of Medicine* (Madison: University of Wisconsin Press, 2001), 200.

90. "Memorial on Female Medical Education," 36. See also McGuigan, *Dangerous Experiment*, 36.

91. July 1870 meeting, in *Proceedings of the Board of Regents*, 51–52, cited in Shaw, *Encyclopedic Survey*, 2:794. See also McCotter, "History of the Anatomy Department," 3; and McGuigan, *Dangerous Experiment*, 37n4.

92. Faculty meeting minutes, October 1, 1870, Faculty Meetings, 1850–1875, Box 127, Medical School (University of Michigan) Records, 1850–2010, Bentley Historical Library; McGuigan, *Dangerous Experiment*, 36–37; Shaw, *Encyclopedic Survey*, 2:794, 811. The faculty had also proposed establishing a Female Medical College in Ann Arbor or Detroit to accommodate women, but the Board of Regents rejected the idea.

93. Shaw, *Encyclopedic Survey*, 2:794.

94. Sappol, *Traffic of Dead Bodies*, 80–81.

95. Doris E. Attaway and Marjorie Rabe Barritt, eds., *Women's Voices: Early Years at the University of Michigan* (Ann Arbor: Bentley Historical Library, 2000), 26; Shaw, *Encyclopedic Survey*, 2:811; Bonner, *To the Ends of the Earth*, 141–142; Wells, *Out of the Dead House*, 200.

96. Faculty meeting minutes, January 14 and 25, 1873, Faculty Meetings, 1850–1875, Box 127, Medical School (University of Michigan) Records, 1850–2010, Bentley Historical Library. Originally, the faculty voted to expel the student from the school, but on a motion from Alonzo Palmer, decided on temporary suspension. See also faculty meeting minutes, March 20, 1872, Faculty Meetings, 1850–1875, Box 127, Medical School (University of Michigan) Records, 1850–2010, Bentley Historical Library.

97. McGuigan, *Dangerous Experiment*, 38; "22nd Annual Commencement of the Medical Department, Wednesday, March 27th, 1872," Photographs, Classes by Year (1872), Box 136, Medical School (University of Michigan) Records, 1850–2010, Bentley Historical Library.

98. Portions of this section were previously published in Dea Boster, "War of the Pathies: The Conflict around Homeopathic Medicine at Michigan in the Mid-19th Century," *Medicine at Michigan* 17 (Summer 2015): 12–13.

99. See Starr, *Social Transformation*, 80, 90–91, 95; Warner, "Ideals of Science," 465; Jacalyn Duffin, *History of Medicine: A Scandalously Short Introduction* (Toronto: University of Toronto Press, 2001), 92; and John Burnham, *What Is Medical History?* (Cambridge, UK: Polity, 2005), 24–25, 107.

100. For more information on sectarian conflicts in medicine, see Starr, *Social Transformation*, 97, 100; Erwin H. Ackerknecht, *A Short History of Medicine* (Baltimore: Johns Hopkins University Press, 1982), 144; Anderson, "Role of the Physician," 16; and Leonard G. Wilson, *Medical Revolution in Minnesota: A History of the University of Minnesota Medical School* (St. Paul, MN: Midewiwin, 1989), 44–45.

101. Duffin, *History of Medicine*, 92. See also Burnham, *What Is Medical History?*, 24–25, 107; Ackerknecht, *Short History of Medicine*, 144.

102. I. N. Eldridge, "Some Fragmentary Reminiscences of the Early History of Homeopathy in Michigan," *Journal of the American Institute of Homeopathy* 39, no. 3 (1946): 71–73; and *Journal of the American Institute of Homeopathy* 39, no. 4 (1946): 112.

103. "Eclecticism," *Michigan Homoeopathic Journal* 2, no. 9 (1854): 163.

104. Eldridge, "Some Fragmentary Reminiscences," *Journal of the American Institute of Homeopathy* 39, no. 3 (1946): 71; Shaw, *Encyclopedic Survey*, 2:1003–1005; Peterson, "University Hospital Manuscript," 39; Anderson, "Role of the Physician," 18.

105. Beech, "Address," 75–76 (emphasis in original).

106. Shaw, *Encyclopedic Survey*, 2:1003; Anderson, "Role of the Physician," 17–19.

107. Shaw, *Encyclopedic Survey*, 2:1003–1004.

108. Peterson, "University Hospital Manuscript," 30.

109. "Eclecticism," 165.

110. Eldridge, "Some Fragmentary Reminiscences," *Journal of the American Institute of Homeopathy* 39, no. 4 (1946): 116; Shaw, *Encyclopedic Survey*, 2:1004–1005; Anderson, "Role of the Physician," 20.

111. Shaw, *Encyclopedic Survey*, 2:1004–1005.

112. Royal S. Copeland to M. L. Burton, December 15, 1921, Correspondence, 1920–1922, Box 24, Royal S. Copeland Papers, Bentley Historical Library.

113. "THE UNIVERSITY: Protest of the Medical Faculty against the Action of the Regents" [March 1867?], in Faculty Minutes Book, 1867–1868, Faculty Meetings, 1850–1875, Box 127, Medical School (University of Michigan) Records, 1850–2010, Bentley Historical Library.

114. See "Last Day's [?] Proceedings of the Annual Meeting: Interesting Reports and Papers Presented; The Homeopathic Question in the University," [June 1868?], in Faculty Minutes Book, 1867–1868, Faculty Meetings, 1850–1875, Box 127, Medical School (University of Michigan) Records, 1850–2010, Bentley Historical Library; and Shaw, *Encyclopedic Survey*, 2:1006.

115. Shaw, *Encyclopedic Survey*, 2:1007. The *Encyclopedic Survey* notes that students in the new dentistry school also completed coursework in the Department of Medicine and Surgery in the 1870s, which added to the increased teaching burden. Ibid., 812–813.

116. Huelke, "History of the Department of Anatomy," 14.

117. "Statement of the Medical Faculty of the University of Michigan, Relative to Their Controversy with Their State Society," 1876, p. 2, Box 2, University of Michigan (Medical School) Publications, Bentley Historical Library. See also Shaw, *Encyclopedic Survey*, 2:860.

118. "Statement of the Medical Faculty," 8.

119. John J. Mulheron, "Addresses: I," in *Memorial Addresses and Resolutions on George E. Frothingham, M.D.* (Detroit: Wayne County Medical Society, [1900?]), 2–3, http://catalog.hathitrust.org/Record/003200539. After resigning from the medical school in 1889, Frothingham rejoined the Michigan State Medical Society and ultimately became its president. Ibid., 4.

120. "To the Honorable the [*sic*] Board of Regents of the University of Michigan," Homeopathic Hospital Student Petition, [1878], Box 135, Medical School (University of Michigan) Records, 1850–2010, Bentley Historical Library; meeting of April 11, 1878, in *Proceedings of the Board of Regents*, 220–221, cited in Casey B. White, "The

Role of Homeopathic Medicine in U.S. Medical Practice and Its Influence on Medical Education at the University of Michigan" (unpublished student paper, n.d.), 24. The Bentley's records erroneously date the petition to 1872.

121. "Medical Quackery. An Argument for the Protection of the People Therefrom," *Detroit Free Press*, March 11, 1879, p. 3.

122. Untitled news item, *True Northerner*, April 11, 1879, p. 3.

123. [Jonathan Adams Allen, Jr.], "President's Address," 7th Report of the State Medical Association (1859), 31, cited in Shaw, *Encyclopedic Survey*, 2:911.

124. Davenport, *Not Just Any Medical School*, 18.

125. March 1860 meeting, in *Proceedings of the Board of Regents*, 901.

126. Shaw, *Encyclopedic Survey*, 2:953–954, 959; Davenport, *Doctor Dock*, 13; Peterson, "University Hospital Manuscript," 13.

127. Elizabeth Gaspar Brown, "Notes on the University Hospital: The Early Decades," *Michigan Quarterly Review* 3 (1964): 10.

128. Davenport, *Doctor Dock*, 13; Davenport, *Not Just Any Medical School*, 18.

129. Shaw, *Encyclopedic Survey*, 9:953–954; "Dr. Sager's Report: On the Organization of the Hospital," [1869], Faculty Meetings, 1850–1875, Box 127, Medical School (University of Michigan) Records, 1850–2010, Bentley Historical Library; faculty meeting minutes, September 14, 1869, Faculty Meetings, 1850–1875, Box 127, Medical School (University of Michigan) Records, 1850–2010, Bentley Historical Library; "Contract: The Board of Regents of the University of Michigan and John Carrington of Ann Arbor Mich.," [September 23, 1869], Faculty Meetings, 1850–1875, Box 127, Medical School (University of Michigan) Records, 1850–2010, Bentley Historical Library.

130. A. Sager, "Case of Delivery by Caesarian Section," *Michigan University Medical Journal* 2 (September 1871): 385–393, cited in Shaw, *Encyclopedic Survey*, 2:859; Peterson, "University Hospital Manuscript," 35–36.

131. McGraw, "Medical Schools," 516; Davenport, *University of Michigan Surgeons*, 26.

132. Maintenance charges were estimated at about four dollars per week in 1869, which was "about the maximum at present in our western institutions." "Dr. Sager's Report."

133. McGraw, "Medical Schools," 516. See also Shaw, *Encyclopedic Survey*, 2:859, 975.

134. Nightingale, *Notes on Hospitals*, 56–57.

135. Shaw, *Encyclopedic Survey*, 2:1011.

136. George Dock, "The University Hospital: Its Past, Present, and Future," *Michigan Alumnus* 9 (1903): 186; Shaw, *Encyclopedic Survey*, 2:954, 959; Davenport, *Doctor Dock*, 13.

137. June 1879 meeting, in *Proceedings of the Board of Regents*, 391; Shaw, *Encyclopedic Survey*, 2:861–862.

138. "Dr. Sager's Report." See also Longo, "Obstetrics and Gynecology."

139. "Dr. Sager's Report"; September 1869 meeting, in *Proceedings of the Board of Regents*, 366, cited in Shaw, *Encyclopedic Survey*, 2:975; Shaw, *Encyclopedic Survey*, 1:182.

140. June 1872 meeting, in *Proceedings of the Board of Regents*, 189–191, cited in Shaw, *Encyclopedic Survey*, 2:976.

141. Shaw, *Encyclopedic Survey*, 2:954. The *Encyclopedic Survey* also suggests that controversies over the proposed Homeopathic Hospital at the University of Michigan in the mid-1870s may have contributed to the regents' disinclination to request appropriations for a large state hospital in Ann Arbor. Ibid., 2:976–977.

142. Kenneth M. Ludmerer, "The University of Michigan Medical School: A Tradition of Leadership," in *Medical Lives and Scientific Medicine at Michigan, 1891–1969*, ed. Joel D. Howell (Ann Arbor: University of Michigan Press, 1993), 15.

143. See Warner, "Ideals of Science," 456; Kenneth M. Ludmerer, *Learning to Heal: The Development of American Medical Education* (New York: Basic Books, 1985), 56–57; Ludmerer, "University of Michigan Medical School," 16; Huelke, "History of the Department of Anatomy," 5; and Shaw, *Encyclopedic Survey*, 2:811.

CHAPTER 2

1. Victor N. Kobayashi, "From 'Germ Theory' to Bacteriology: A Case in Academic Freedom at the University of Michigan" (unpublished paper, 1962), 6; Wilfred B. Shaw, ed., *The University of Michigan: An Encyclopedic Survey*, vol. 2 (Ann Arbor: University of Michigan Press, 1951), 824, http://quod.lib.umich.edu/u/umsurvey/AAS3302.0002.001/1:1?rgn=div1;view=fulltext; Powel H. Kazanjian, "The Beginnings of Bacteriology in American Medicine: Works of Frederick Novy, 1888–1933" (Ph.D. diss., University of Michigan, 2012), 42–43. Kobayashi notes that Vaughan and Novy were "moderate" in their perspective on germ theory, adopting the view that "the presence of bacilli was not conclusive evidence of infection and that other factors such as climate and heredity were important in the causation of diseases." Kobayashi, "From 'Germ Theory' to Bacteriology," 9–10.

2. Nancy Tomes, *The Gospel of Germs: Men, Women, and the Microbe in American Life* (Cambridge, MA: Harvard University Press, 1998), 6–8; Kobayashi, "From 'Germ Theory' to Bacteriology," 5; Shaw, *Encyclopedic Survey*, 2:821–822.

3. Kenneth M. Ludmerer, *Learning to Heal: The Development of American Medical Education* (New York: Basic Books, 1985), 47.

4. Ibid., 76. See also Naomi Rogers, "Thomas Francis, Jr.: From the Bench to the Field," in *Medical Lives and Scientific Medicine at Michigan, 1891–1969*, ed. Joel D. Howell (Ann Arbor: University of Michigan Press, 1993), 163–164.

5. Ludmerer, *Learning to Heal*, 20–21, 72–74; W. Bruce Fye, "Albion Walter Hewlett: Teacher, Clinician, Scientist, and Missionary for 'Pathologic Physiology,'" in *Medical Lives and Scientific Medicine at Michigan, 1891–1969*, ed. Joel D. Howell (Ann Arbor: University of Michigan Press, 1993), 52; Shaw, *Encyclopedic Survey*, 2:811; Regina Morantz-Sanchez, *Sympathy and Science: Women Physicians in American Medicine* (Chapel Hill: University of North Carolina Press, 1985), 75. Regina Morantz-Sanchez identifies what was likely Rush Medical College as "Chicago Medical College."

6. Morantz-Sanchez, *Sympathy and Science*, 75; Ludmerer, *Learning to Heal*, 86, 141.

7. Ludmerer, *Learning to Heal*, 43–44.

8. John J. Mulheron, "Addresses: I," in *Memorial Addresses and Resolutions on George E. Frothingham, M.D.* (Detroit: Wayne County Medical Society, [1900?]), 4.

9. Quoted in Charles H. McIntyre, "Victor C. Vaughan," in *Builders of American Medicine: Being a Collection of Original Papers Read before the Victor C. Vaughan Society of the University of Michigan Medical School* (Ann Arbor, MI: George Wahr, 1932), 224–225.

10. Ibid. See also Horace W. Davenport, *Not Just Any Medical School: The Science, Practice, and Teaching of Medicine at the University of Michigan, 1850–1941* (Ann Arbor: University of Michigan Press, 1999), 22.

11. Kobayashi, "From 'Germ Theory' to Bacteriology," 6–9; Ludmerer, *Learning to Heal*, 52.

12. Orlando W. Stephenson, *Ann Arbor: The First Hundred Years* (Ann Arbor, MI: Ann Arbor Chamber of Commerce, 1927), 332–342, 346, 361.

13. "Michigan's Pride: The Great University of the Northwest," *Ann Arbor Register*, September 24, 1891, p. 7.

14. Horace W. Davenport, *Doctor Dock: Teaching and Learning Medicine at the Turn of the Century* (New Brunswick, NJ: Rutgers University Press, 1987), 125, 187, 237, 242.

15. Howard H. Peckham, *The Making of the University of Michigan, 1817–1992*, ed. Margaret L. Steneck and Nicholas H. Steneck (Ann Arbor: University of Michigan Bentley Historical Library, 1994), 94–95.

16. Jonathan Marwil, *A History of Ann Arbor* (Ann Arbor: University of Michigan Press, 1990), 77–78, 85. Regarding hospital funding, Ann Arbor voters approved $25,000 for the University Hospital in 1889 (with an additional $17,500 the following decade) and in 1913 approved $25,000 to erect a contagious disease facility. Wilfred B. Shaw, ed., *The University of Michigan: An Encyclopedic Survey*, vol. 1 (Ann Arbor: University of Michigan Press, 1942), 182.

17. Ann Arbor District Library, "Ann Arbor: Population and Size," http://www.aadl.org/research/a2populationandsize (accessed February 27, 2017); "Detroit Population History, 1900–2000," *Somacon*, September 7, 2015, http://www.somacon.com/p469.php. See also Abraham Flexner, *Medical Education in the United States and Canada: A Report to the Carnegie Foundation for the Advancement of Teaching* (New York: Carnegie Foundation for the Advancement of Teaching, 1910), 245, http://www.carnegiefoundation.org/sites/default/files/elibrary/Carnegie_Flexner_Report.pdf.

18. Marwil, *History of Ann Arbor*, 58.

19. *Ann Arbor Democrat*, April 10, 1879, cited in Marwil, *History of Ann Arbor*, 58; see also 77.

20. Davenport, *Not Just Any Medical School*, 16. See also Shaw, *Encyclopedic Survey*, 2:811–813. Johns Hopkins Medical School is often credited as the model for modern scientific medical instruction, but Harvard, Pennsylvania, and Michigan had already implemented such changes before Johns Hopkins opened. See Kenneth M. Ludmerer, *Time to Heal: American Medical Education from the Turn of the Century to the Era of Managed Care* (Oxford: Oxford University Press, 1999), 4–5.

21. "University of Michigan, Department of Medicine and Surgery, Order of Exercises, Second Semester, 1889–1890," Miscellaneous, 1894–1903, Box 135, Medical School (University of Michigan) Records, 1850–2010, Bentley Historical Library, University of Michigan, Ann Arbor.

22. Faculty meeting minutes, October 8, 1887, Faculty Meetings, 1878–1891, Box 128, Medical School (University of Michigan) Records, Bentley Historical Library.

23. Shaw, *Encyclopedic Survey*, 2:825; faculty meeting minutes, February 14, 1898, p. 25, Faculty Meetings, 1897–1903, Box 128, Medical School (University of Michigan) Records, 1850–2010, Bentley Historical Library; Morantz-Sanchez, *Sympathy and Science*, 77; Kenneth M. Ludmerer, "The University of Michigan Medical School: A Tradition of Leadership," in *Medical Lives and Scientific Medicine at Michigan, 1891–1969*, ed. Joel D. Howell (Ann Arbor: University of Michigan Press, 1993), 15–16.

24. Shaw, *Encyclopedic Survey*, 2:802, 807, 822; Davenport, *Not Just Any Medical School*, 15–16; Ludmerer, *Learning to Heal*, 96–98; John Parascandola, *The Development of American Pharmacology: John J. Abel and the Shaping of a Discipline* (Baltimore: Johns Hopkins University Press, 1992), 62–63; Kazanjian, "Beginnings of Bacteriology," 53. Sewall left Michigan in 1889 for health reasons; he had tuberculosis and relocated to a western climate.

25. Rollo McCotter, "A History of the Anatomy Department of the University of Michigan," address given at honorary dinner, February 7, 1947, pp. 4–8, Bentley Historical Library. Between 1881 and 1940, more than ten thousand cadavers had been received at the medical school (four hundred to five hundred per year by 1940). Shaw, *Encyclopedic Survey*, 2:820.

26. Fye, "Albion Walter Hewlett," 58; Ludmerer, *Learning to Heal*, 33; McIntyre, "Victor C. Vaughan," 224; Parascandola, *Development of American Pharmacology*, 40–42. Abel had earned his medical degree at Michigan in 1883 but had traveled to Leipzig to continue his studies before accepting the faculty job; he left for Johns Hopkins in 1893. Parascandola, *Development of American Pharmacology*, 47.

27. Albion Walter Hewlett, "Eight Years in the Department of Internal Medicine," *Transactions of the Clinical Society of the University of Michigan* 7 (June 1916), cited in Fye, "Albion Walter Hewlett," 68–69.

28. McIntyre, "Victor C. Vaughan," 224.

29. JoAnne Yates, *Control through Communication: The Rise of System in American Management* (Baltimore: Johns Hopkins University Press, 1993), xvii.

30. "Niagara Falls Route," *Ann Arbor Headlight*, souvenir edition 2, no. 15 [1896?]: 21, Box 1, Washtenaw County Historical Society Records, 1827–2013, Bentley Historical Library.

31. Ludmerer, *Time to Heal*, 23.

32. Portions of this section were previously published in Dea Boster, "Finding the 'Sick' in Cheese: Victor Vaughan and Michigan Public Health in the Late 19th Century," *Medicine at Michigan* 17 (Winter 2015): 14–15.

33. Davenport, *Not Just Any Medical School*, ix, 6; McIntyre, "Victor C. Vaughan," 221. It is likely that the Board of Regents in the mid-1870s would have been more concerned about the religion of faculty members than they were in later decades. In his discussion of the acceptance of the germ theory at the medical school, Kobayashi notes, "Towards the end of the nineteenth century, the University of Michigan had become more secular. School officials had to put more effort into proving to its major critics that the University policy was non-sectarian, rather than into proving that the school was not irreligious." Kobayashi, "From 'Germ Theory' to Bacteriology," 12.

34. Shaw, *Encyclopedic Survey*, 2:797, 821, 824; McIntyre, "Victor C. Vaughan," 222; Davenport, *Doctor Dock*, 5; Davenport, *Not Just Any Medical School*, 8, 44.

35. McIntyre, "Victor C. Vaughan," 230.

36. H. B. Baker, "Poisonous Cheese," in *Twelfth Annual Report of the Secretary of the State Board of Health of the State of Michigan for the Fiscal Year Ending September 30, 1884* (Lansing, MI: W. S. George, 1885), 123; Edward Geist, "When Ice Cream Was Poisonous: Adulteration, Ptomaines, and Bacteriology in the United States, 1850–1910," *Bulletin of the History of Medicine* 86 (Fall 2012): 345.

37. V. C. Vaughan, "Poisonous Cheese," in *Thirteenth Annual Report of the Secretary of the State Board of Health of the State of Michigan for the Fiscal Year Ending September 30, 1885* (Lansing, MI: W. S. George, 1886), 224. See also "Tyrotoxicon—Cheese Poison," *Ann Arbor Courier*, July 22, 1885; "Milk and Its Relation to the Public Health," special issue, *Hygienic Laboratory Bulletin*, no. 56 (1909): 375; Geist, "When Ice Cream Was Poisonous," 335, 345; and Davenport, *Not Just Any Medical School*, 7.

38. Vaughan, "Poisonous Cheese," 224–225; Victor C. Vaughan and Frederick G. Novy, *Ptomaines and Leucomaines, or the Putrefactive and Physiological Alkaloids* (Philadelphia: Lea Brothers, 1888), 56; Geist, "When Ice Cream Was Poisonous," 346.

39. Vaughan, "Poisonous Cheese," 221–222; Davenport, *Not Just Any Medical School*, 7.

40. "Tyrotoxicon—Cheese Poison."

41. Ibid.; Vaughan, "Poisonous Cheese," 223–224.

42. Geist, "When Ice Cream Was Poisonous," 336.

43. "Adrian Press Washtenawisms," *Ann Arbor Argus*, August 18, 1893.

44. Victor Vaughan, "Appendix 3: The Michigan State Board of Health," in *A Doctor's Memories* (Indianapolis, IN: Bobbs-Merrill, 1926), http://vaughan.org/bios/vcv/aDoctorsMemories/Text/vcvmemAp3.html. See also Geist, "When Ice Cream Was Poisonous," 348–349; Davenport, *Doctor Dock*, 187; Davenport, *Not Just Any Medical School*, 7–8; Shaw, *Encyclopedic Survey*, 2:824; McIntyre, "Victor C. Vaughan," 231; and Kazanjian, "Beginnings of Bacteriology," 47–52. The Hygienic Laboratory was moved to the West Medical Building in 1903.

45. Kobayashi, "From 'Germ Theory' to Bacteriology," 13; Tomes, *Gospel of Germs*, 18.

46. Geist, "When Ice Cream Was Poisonous," 347–348, 351.

47. "Milk and Its Relation to the Public Health," 377.

48. Vaughan, *A Doctor's Memories*. See also Geist, "When Ice Cream Was Poisonous," 353.

49. See Powel Kazanjian, *Frederick Novy and the Development of Bacteriology in Medicine* (New Brunswick, NJ: Rutgers University Press, 2017).

50. Shaw, *Encyclopedic Survey*, 2:822–825; Davenport, *Not Just Any Medical School*, 16, 45–46; Kazanijian, "Beginnings of Bacteriology," 34–38; Henry Sewall, "Experiments on the Preventive Inoculation of Rattlesnake Venom," *Journal of Physiology* 8 (August 1887): 203–210.

51. Parascandola, *Development of American Pharmacology*, 105–106; George Dock, "Mosquitoes and Malaria: The Present Knowledge of Their Relations, with Some Observations in Ann Arbor and Vicinity," *Journal of the Michigan State Medical Society* 2 (February 1903): 37–45; Davenport, *Doctor Dock*, 125.

52. Ludmerer, *Time to Heal*, 13.

53. John Abel to Mary Hinman, March 11 and April 1, 1883, cited in Parascandola, *Development of American Pharmacology*, 24.

54. "The Etiology of Cholera," *Nature* 33 (December 1885): 97; Kobayashi, "From 'Germ Theory' to Bacteriology," 9. See also Shaw, *Encyclopedic Survey*, 2:824–825, 887–888.

55. Vaughan, *A Doctor's Memories*, 147, cited in Kobayashi, "From 'Germ Theory' to Bacteriology," 6.

56. Davenport, *Doctor Dock*, 11–12; Kobayashi, "From 'Germ Theory' to Bacteriology," 11n35, 14. Kobayashi notes that the regents did not notify Gibbes of the reason for his dismissal (at least not in the records of their proceedings) and warns that the situation had more to do with academic freedom than the triumph of science, particularly at a time when the "germ theory" was in favor but not universally accepted: "It is unfair to explain away the attitudes and contributions of such pioneers as Novy or Vaughan as a reflection of the new scientific orthodoxy, but certainly, it would not be fair either, to label Gibbes as merely a reactionary conservative who acted as a barrier to scientific progress." Kobayashi, "From 'Germ Theory' to Bacteriology," 13.

57. McCotter, "History of the Anatomy Department," 7–8; Davenport, *Not Just Any Medical School*, 26. The original medical building was declared unsafe in 1906, was abandoned altogether after a fire five years later, and ultimately was demolished.

58. Zina Pitcher, *An Address to the First Graduates of the Medical Department of the University of Michigan* (Detroit: William Harsha, 1851).

59. Cited in McIntyre, "Victor C. Vaughan," 225; see also Davenport, *Doctor Dock*, 12.

60. Davenport, *Doctor Dock*, 13. See also Ludmerer, *Learning to Heal*, 65; and George Weisz, *Divide and Conquer: A Comparative History of Medical Specialization* (Oxford: Oxford University Press, 2006), xxii.

61. Shaw, *Encyclopedic Survey*, 2:923.

62. Ferol B. Brinkman, ed., *The University of Michigan: An Encyclopedic Survey*, vol. 5, *The University of Michigan, 1940–75* (Ann Arbor: University of Michigan Bentley Historical Library, 1977), 193. For more on medical specialization during this time period more generally, see Weisz, *Divide and Conquer*; and Rosemary Stevens, *American Medicine and the Public Interest* (Berkeley: University of California Press, 1998).

63. Shaw, *Encyclopedic Survey*, 1:326; June 1893 meeting, in *Proceedings of the Board of Regents* (Ann Arbor: University of Michigan, 2000), 160.

64. Shaw, *Encyclopedic Survey*, 2:928.

65. Shaw, *Encyclopedic Survey*, 2:807, 927. The Homeopathic College also appointed a lecturer on mental diseases in 1894.

66. Shaw, *Encyclopedic Survey*, 2:927–929; faculty meeting minutes, January 23, 1902, p. 143, Faculty Meetings, 1897–1903, Box 128, Medical School (University of Michigan) Records, 1850–2010, Bentley Historical Library.

67. Shaw, *Encyclopedic Survey*, 2:899–900; Davenport, *Not Just Any Medical School*, 23. Davenport notes that "in a contest for a professorship at Michigan there is usually an insider versus an outsider" and that Dock's exemplary training "overwhelmed" the insider candidate, Osbourne F. Chadbourne. Davenport, *Not Just Any Medical School*, 23.

68. Shaw, *Encyclopedic Survey*, 2:807, 931. The school's official program in roentgenology was not established until 1907, with the hiring of Dr. James G. Van Zwaluwenberg; before that point, Herdman offered instruction in the new technology.

69. Davenport, *Not Just Any Medical School*, 29–31; Davenport, *Doctor Dock*, 18–20.

70. Davenport, *Doctor Dock*, 31.

71. Ludmerer, *Learning to Heal*, 64.

72. Ludmerer, "University of Michigan Medical School," 18, 24, 26.

73. Davenport, *Doctor Dock*, 39; Joel D. Howell, *Technology in the Hospital: Transforming Patient Care in the Early Twentieth Century* (Baltimore: Johns Hopkins University Press, 1995), 16–18; Christopher Crenner, *Private Practice: In the Early Twentieth-Century Medical Office of Dr. Richard Cabot* (Baltimore: Johns Hopkins University Press, 2005), 3, 5.

74. "Dr. Maclean Downed," *Ann Arbor Register*, May 2, 1889, James H. Wade Scrapbook (February 1897), "Detroit, Newspaper Clippings regarding Relocation of Clinical Work, 1889" folder, Box 135, Medical School (University of Michigan) Records, 1850–2010, Bentley Historical Library. The newspaper titles were handwritten on the clippings, without reference to their cities.

75. "Dr. Lyster on the Clinic," *Detroit Evening News*, April 26, 1889, James H. Wade Scrapbook (February 1897), "Detroit, Newspaper Clippings regarding Relocation of Clinical Work, 1889" folder, Box 135, Medical School (University of Michigan) Records, 1850–2010, Bentley Historical Library. See also "Doctors Wax Warm," *Detroit Evening News*, April 25, 1889, James H. Wade Scrapbook (February 1897), "Detroit, Newspaper Clippings regarding Relocation of Clinical Work, 1889" folder, Box 135, Medical School (University of Michigan) Records, 1850–2010, Bentley Historical Library; and "Dr. Maclean Downed."

76. Faculty meeting minutes, February 10 and May 2, 1887, Faculty Meetings, 1878–1891, Box 128, Medical School (University of Michigan) Records, 1850–2010, Bentley Historical Library. See also Shaw, *Encyclopedic Survey*, 2:861–862.

77. Grace Shackman, "The Private Hospital Era," *Ann Arbor Observer*, March 1994.

78. October 1889 meeting, in *Proceedings of the Board of Regents*, 375–376; Shaw, *Encyclopedic Survey*, 2:955.

79. Faculty meeting minutes, October 11, 1889, Faculty Meetings, 1878–1891, Box 128, Medical School (University of Michigan) Records, 1850–2010, Bentley Historical Library. See also Davenport, *Doctor Dock*, 13; and Davenport, *Not Just Any Medical School*, 20.

80. Reuben Peterson to Dr. Amos Wheelock, May 14, 1927, Correspondence, 1890–1927, Box 1, Reuben Peterson Papers, Bentley Historical Library; Shaw, *Encyclopedic Survey*, 2:873. Howell identified a clear shift in accounting and budget practices during the life of the Catherine Street hospital and noted that the role of superintendent, initially a general manager, ultimately was taken over by a group of administrators. Howell, *Technology in the Hospital*, 36–37. See also David Rosner, *A Once Charitable Enterprise: Hospitals and Health Care in Brooklyn and New York, 1885–1915* (Cambridge: Cambridge University Press, 1982).

81. Peckham, *Making of the University of Michigan*, 102. See also Barbara Melosh, *"The Physician's Hand": Work Culture and Conflict in American Nursing* (Philadelphia: Temple University Press, 1982); and Susan M. Reverby, *Ordered to Care: The Dilemma of American Nursing, 1850–1945* (Cambridge: Cambridge University Press, 1987).

82. Paul Starr, *The Social Transformation of American Medicine* (New York: Basic Books, 1982), 123. Davenport notes that although the formal preceptorship requirement was eliminated in 1877, students continued to apprentice until the 1920s. Davenport, *Not Just Any Medical School*, 34.

83. Reuben Peterson, "University Hospital Manuscript" (39), p. 3, Box 2, Reuben Peterson Papers, Bentley Historical Library. See also Davenport, *Doctor Dock*, 17; and Fye, "Albion Walter Hewlett," 64–65.

84. A. W. Hewlett to Shirley W. Smith (secretary to regent Walter Sawyer), December 16, 1908, Correspondence, December 1908, Box 1, Walter H. Sawyer Papers, Bentley Historical Library. See also Hewlett, "Eight Years," 148; and Fye, "Albion Walter Hewlett," 64.

85. Shaw, *Encyclopedic Survey*, 2:872, 879, 882. See also Ludmerer, *Time to Heal*.

86. Faculty meeting minutes, April 13, 1903, p. 187, Faculty Meetings, 1897–1903, Box 128, Medical School (University of Michigan) Records, 1850–2010, Bentley Historical Library; Davenport, *Not Just Any Medical School*, 11; Shaw, *Encyclopedic Survey*, 2:901.

87. Shaw, *Encyclopedic Survey*, 1:326; Shaw, *Encyclopedic Survey*, 2:931; Davenport, *Doctor Dock*, 9–10.

88. Shaw, *Encyclopedic Survey*, 2:867–872.

89. George Dock, "Some Reasons Why There Should Be a Hospital for Consumptives in Connection with the University Hospital," *Physician and Surgeon* 24 (1902): 61, 64.

90. Shaw, *Encyclopedic Survey*, 2:903; see also 2:839, 842; and Davenport, *Doctor Dock*, 237–239, 242.

91. Reuben Peterson, "The New Contagious Hospital at the University of Michigan and Its Proposed Plan of Operation," *Journal of the Michigan State Medical Society*, May 1914, p. 10.

92. Davenport, *Doctor Dock*, 239, 244, 255–259; Shaw, *Encyclopedic Survey*, 2:903.

93. Sinclair Lewis, *Arrowsmith* (New York: Signet, 1998); Howard Markel, "Prescribing *Arrowsmith*," *New York Times*, September 24, 2000, http://www.nytimes.com/2000/09/24/books/bookend-prescribing-arrowsmith.html. See also Charles E. Rosenberg, "Martin Arrowsmith: The Scientist as Hero," in *No Other Gods: On Science and American Social Thought*, rev. ed., ed. Charles E. Rosenberg (Baltimore: Johns Hopkins University Press, 1997), 123–131; and Kazanjian, "Beginnings of Bacteriology."

94. George Dock and T. L. Chadbourne, "An Etiologic Study of Tuberculosis in Country-People," *Philadelphia Medical Journal* 2 (1898): 966; Davenport, *Doctor Dock*, 21, 132–133, 208, 225.

95. Fye, "Albion Walter Hewlett," 57.

96. Peterson, "University Hospital Manuscript," 4. See also "Niagara Falls Route," 11.

97. "Michigan's Pride," 7; Aldred Scott Warthin, "The University Medical School and the State," in *Indiana University, 1820–1920: Centennial Memorial Volume* (Bloomington: Indiana University, 1921): 161–162.

98. Hewlett, "Eight Years," 146; Fye, "Albion Walter Hewlett," 57; Shaw, *Encyclopedic Survey*, 2:977.

99. Horace W. Davenport, "George Dock at Michigan, 1891–1908," in *Medical Lives and Scientific Medicine at Michigan, 1891–1969*, ed. Joel D. Howell (Ann Arbor: University of Michigan Press, 1993), 35; Shaw, *Encyclopedic Survey*, 2:807; Fye, "Albion Walter Hewlett," 46; Hewlett, "Eight Years," 148.

100. Reuben Peterson to Victor Vaughan, February 25, 1889, and Reuben Peterson to medical faculty, January 8, 1908, Correspondence, 1890–1927, Box 1, Reuben Peterson Papers, Bentley Historical Library.

101. Shaw, *Encyclopedic Survey*, 2:872.

102. Ibid., 2:873.

103. Hewlett, "Eight Years," 148.

104. Ibid., 147. See also Howell, *Technology in the Hospital*, 269n16.

105. Dock, "Some Reasons," 60.

106. Emil Amberg to Loyal E. Knappen (regent), November 25 or 28, 1904, Detroit, 1904–10, Box 125, Medical School (University of Michigan) Records, 1850–2010, Bentley Historical Library.

107. "Statement of the Delta County Medical Society, Escanaba, Michigan," Correspondence, 1890–1927, Box 1, Reuben Peterson Papers, Bentley Historical Library. See also Dock, "Some Reasons," 64–65. The Marquette County Medical Society made a similar resolution around the same time, sending it to Regent Henry W. Carey. See secretary of Marquette County Medical Society to Henry W. Carey, December 19, 1904, Detroit, 1904–10, Box 135, Medical School (University of Michigan) Records, 1850–2010, Bentley Historical Library.

108. Charles E. Rosenberg, *The Care of Strangers: The Rise of America's Hospital System* (New York: Basic Books, 1987), 21.

109. Shaw, *Encyclopedic Survey*, 2:871–872, 901, 975; Peterson, "University Hospital Manuscript," 7; Warthin, "University Medical School," 161.

110. Davenport, *Doctor Dock*, 31.

111. Hewlett, "Eight Years," 147.

112. "Requirements for Admission to the Department of Medicine and Surgery, University of Michigan, 1909 and Thereafter," *University Bulletin* 10 (March 1909): 1–2, Box 1, University of Michigan (Medical School) Publications, Bentley Historical Library. See also Davenport, *Not Just Any Medical School*, 24–25, 33.

113. Faculty meeting minutes, June 8, 1903, pp. 203, 205, Faculty Meetings, 1897–1903, Box 128, Medical School (University of Michigan) Records, 1850–2010, Bentley Historical Library. Letter grades were not introduced in the medical school until 1915. Davenport, *Not Just Any Medical School*, 34.

114. "To the Faculty of the Med. Dept. of the Univ. of Michigan," ca. 1898, Miscellaneous, 1894–1903, Box 135, Medical School (University of Michigan) Records, 1850–2010, Bentley Historical Library.

115. Faculty meeting minutes, February 23, 1903, p. 177, Faculty Meetings, 1897–1903, Box 128, Medical School (University of Michigan) Records, 1850–2010, Bentley Historical Library. See also Davenport, *Not Just Any Medical School*, 35.

116. For example, see faculty meeting minutes, February 25 and June 17, 1902, and June 19, 1908, pp. 147–149, 161, 221–225, Faculty Meetings, 1897–1903, Box 128, Medical School (University of Michigan) Records, 1850–2010, Bentley Historical Library.

117. Faculty meeting minutes, November 22, 1889, Faculty Meetings, 1878–1891, Box 128, Medical School (University of Michigan) Records, 1850–2010, Bentley Historical Library; faculty meeting minutes, May 26, 1900, p. 97, Faculty Meetings, 1897–1903, Box 128, Medical School (University of Michigan) Records, 1850–2010, Bentley Historical Library.

118. Faculty meeting minutes, May 23, 1889, Faculty Meetings, 1878–1891, Box 128, Medical School (University of Michigan) Records, 1850–2010, Bentley Historical Library; faculty meeting minutes, September 28, 1901, p. 131, Faculty Meetings, 1897–1903, Box 128, Medical School (University of Michigan) Records, 1850–2010, Bentley Historical Library.

119. Faculty meeting minutes, June 8, 1903, p. 207, Faculty Meetings, 1897–1903, Box 128, Medical School (University of Michigan) Records, 1850–2010, Bentley Historical Library.

120. Howard H. Cummings, "The Early History of Psi Chapter of Phi Chi," *Phi Chi Quarterly* 25, no. 4 (1928): 612, 615.

121. Walter A. Donnelly, Wilfred B. Shaw, and Ruth W. Gjelsness, eds., *The University of Michigan: An Encyclopedic Survey*, vol. 4 (Ann Arbor: University of Michigan Press, 1958), 1927; Marvin J. Lubeck, "History of the Galens Honorary Medical Society," *Medical Bulletin* 21 (February 1955): 41–42.

122. Lubeck, "History of the Galens," 42. Women were admitted to Galens starting in 1971, according to Bentley Historical Library, "Galens Medical Society Records: 1914–2001," http://quod.lib.umich.edu/b/bhlead/umich-bhl-9859?rgn=Entire+Finding+Aid;view=text;q1=galens (accessed February 27, 2017).

123. Lubeck, "History of the Galens," 44–45. Lubeck claims the idea of the Smoker had been discussed in 1914, but 1918 was the first known event to take place.

124. Davenport, *Not Just Any Medical School*, x–xi.

125. Morantz-Sanchez, *Sympathy and Science*, 232; Office of Medical School Education, "The University of Michigan Medical School Male-Female Graduates," in the author's possession.

126. "Michigan's Pride," 7. Morantz-Sanchez notes that by 1893, only 37 of 105 "orthodox" medical schools in the United States admitted women. Morantz-Sanchez, *Sympathy and Science*, 65.

127. Faculty meeting minutes, September 29, 1887, Faculty Meetings, 1891–1897, Box 128, Medical School (University of Michigan) Records, 1850–2010, Bentley Historical Library. See also Davenport, *Not Just Any Medical School*, 9–10, 24–25; McCotter "History of the Anatomy Department," 4–8; and Shaw, *Encyclopedic Survey*, 2:792.

128. Davenport, *Doctor Dock*, 17.

129. Davenport, *Not Just Any Medical School*, 16, 31.

130. Ibid., 31.

131. Flexner, *Medical Education*, 178–179. See also Morantz-Sanchez, *Sympathy and Science*, 67, 71, 128.

132. Survey and Mosher quoted in Morantz-Sanchez, *Sympathy and Science*, 55, 60.

133. Shaw, *Encyclopedic Survey*, 2:867–868. When the Bates estate first envisioned the endowment in 1890, obstetrics/gynecology and pediatrics were not distinct fields; even after the professional division was made, the name of the professorship at Michigan remained the same until the 1920s.

134. See Flexner, *Medical Education*, 179; Starr, *Social Transformation*, 124; and Morantz-Sanchez, *Sympathy and Science*, 4–6.

135. Barbara Sicherman, *Alice Hamilton: A Life in Letters* (Urbana: University of Illinois Press, 2003), 1–2, 34–35.

136. Ann Arbor's African American population grew by more than 50 percent during the first decade of the twentieth century. Marwil, *History of Ann Arbor*, 79.

137. James Tobin, "Doc Susie," *Medicine at Michigan* 16 (Spring–Summer 2014): 14–15; Virginia Cornell, *Doc Susie: The True Story of a Country Physician in the Colorado Rockies* (New York: Ballantine, 1991).

138. S. R. Beckwith, "What I Saw in Ann Arbor," 1880, pp. 2–3, Homeopathic Medical School Reports, Box 1, Homeopathic Medical School (University of Michigan) Records, Bentley Historical Library.

139. Royal Samuel Copeland, "The New Homoeopathic Hospital Nurses' Home," *Michigan Alumnus* 7 (November 1900): 56. See also Flexner, *Medical Education*, 159n1, 244; Shaw, *Encyclopedic Survey*, 2:782, 1011–1012.

140. Copeland, "New Homoeopathic Hospital," 54.

141. Flexner, *Medical Education*, 244.

142. Faculty meeting minutes, March 25, 1886, and June 23, 1890, Faculty Meetings, 1878–1891, Box 128, Medical School (University of Michigan) Records, 1850–2010, Bentley Historical Library. In 1894, however, the faculty did vote to accept two homeopathic students as transfers to the regular program, in the junior class. Faculty meeting minutes, February 23, 1894, Faculty Meetings, 1878–1891, Box 128, Medical School (University of Michigan) Records, 1850–2010, Bentley Historical Library.

143. Reuben Peterson to Victor Vaughan, February 14, 1895, Correspondence, 1890–1927, Box 1, Reuben Peterson Papers, Bentley Historical Library. See also McIntyre, "Victor C. Vaughan," 220–221; Mulheron, "Addresses: I," 3; and Shaw, *Encyclopedic Survey*, 2:877.

144. "A Very Hot Time: State Homeopathic Society Forces a Resignation," *Weekly Expositor* (Brockway Centre, MI), May 12, 1893, p. 2. Dean Obetz was cleared of the charges and not forced to resign at that point, as the article's title implies, but he did leave the university the following year; his successor, Wilbert Hinsdale, served as homeopathic dean until the school closed in 1922. Shaw, *Encyclopedic Survey*, 2:1009.

145. Faculty meeting minutes, February 11, 1895, Faculty Meetings, 1891–1897, Box 128, Medical School (University of Michigan) Records, 1850–2010, Bentley Historical Library; "Doings at Lansing. Work of the State Legislature," *True Northerner* (Paw Paw, MI), March 15, 1895, p. 3; "Record Is Broken: Bills and Resolutions Introduced at Lansing," *Copper County Evening News* (Calumet, MI), March 3, 1897, p. 5; Shaw, *Encyclopedic Survey*, 2:1008.

146. Royal S. Copeland to M. L. Burton, December 15, 1921, p. 6, "Correspondence, 1920–1922, concerning the Reorganization of the Medical School of the University of Michigan" folder, Box 24, Royal S. Copeland Papers, Bentley Historical Library.

147. "Michigan's Pride," 7; "Feel Proud! Homeopath Students at the U. of M.," *Detroit Free Press*, November 24, 1895, p. 10; "Niagara Falls Route," 24.

148. Copeland to Burton, 11; Ann Arbor District Library, "Ann Arbor City Council Minutes, July 03, 1899," p. 205, http://councilminutes.aadl.org/councilminutes/18990703.

149. Arthur Dean Bevan and N. P. Colwell to Victor Vaughan, September 17, 1920, and Victor Vaughan to N. P. Colwell, September 20, 1920, in "N. P. Colwell, AMA" folder, Box 33, Medical School (University of Michigan) Records, 1850–2010, Bentley Historical Library.

150. Portions of this section were included in Dea Boster and Joel Howell, "'Raising Oranges in Canada': Education, Locality, and Conflict at the University of Michigan Medical School in the Late Nineteenth Century," paper presented at the American Association for the History of Medicine Annual Meeting, New Haven, CT, May 2015.

151. "University Items," *Ann Arbor Courier*, March 4, 1885; faculty meeting minutes, October 8, 1887, Faculty Meetings, 1878–1891, Box 128, Medical School (University of Michigan) Records, 1850–2010, Bentley Historical Library; Davenport, *Doctor Dock*, 11; Davenport, *Not Just Any Medical School*, 20; "Ann Arbor or Detroit," *Ann Arbor Courier*, July 11, 1888.

152. "A Professor's Defiance," *Ann Arbor Argus*, April 26, 1889, and "On the Warpath Again," *Detroit Evening Journal*, April 20, 1889, James H. Wade Scrapbook (February 1897), "Detroit, Newspaper Clippings regarding Relocation of Clinical Work, 1889" folder, Box 135, Medical School (University of Michigan) Records, 1850–2010, Bentley Historical Library. See also Davenport, *Doctor Dock*, 11; and Davenport, *Not Just Any Medical School*, 20.

153. "Doctors Wax Warm."

154. "Dr. Lyster on the Clinic"; "Dr. Maclean Downed." For more on Lyster's appointment to the university, see faculty meeting minutes, February 16, 1888, Faculty Meetings, 1878–1891, Box 128, Medical School (University of Michigan) Records, 1850–2010, Bentley Historical Library.

155. "A Professor's Defiance."

156. Frothingham had been the proprietor and editor of the *Ann Arbor Register* several years before, a role that the rival *Ann Arbor Courier* claimed was retaliation against the *Courier* for publishing something unfavorable about one of Frothingham's colleagues. In an 1883 editorial, the *Courier* observed, "Dr. Frothingham has probably learned by this time that the editor of a paper has the same right to make his own editorials to suit himself as a doctor has to treat one of his patients, as he chooses." "Prof. Frothingham," *Ann Arbor Courier*, August 24, 1883. See also Edgar B. Smith, "Addresses: II," in *Memorial Addresses and Resolutions on George E. Frothingham, M.D.* (Detroit: Wayne County Medical Society, [1900?]), 7–8, http://catalog.hathitrust.org/Record/003200539.

157. "Dr. Maclean Downed."

158. McIntyre, "Victor C. Vaughan," 217.

159. "Doctors Wax Warm." See also Howell, *Technology in the Hospital*, 3.

160. "Dr. Maclean Downed." Reuben Peterson, in his amateur history of the University Hospital, noted that "this idea was so thoroughly drilled into the people of Michigan that clinical professors received letters into the early nineteen hundreds from people amply able to pay for medical services, saying they were willing to go 'before the class.'" Peterson, "University Hospital Manuscript," 4.

161. *The Leucocyte* 6 (1899): 17, cited in Thomas Neville Bonner, *Becoming a Physician: Medical Education in Britain, France, Germany, and the United States, 1750–1945* (Baltimore: Johns Hopkins University Press, 1995), 318.

162. "Doctors Wax Warm." See also Peterson, "University Hospital Manuscript," 13.

163. Reprinted in *Ann Arbor Argus*, May 3, 1889, James H. Wade Scrapbook (February 1897), "Detroit, Newspaper Clippings regarding Relocation of Clinical Work, 1889" folder, Box 135, Medical School (University of Michigan) Records, 1850–2010, Bentley Historical Library. See also Davenport, *Not Just Any Medical School*, 27.

164. "Dr. Maclean Downed."

165. For cxample, see Davenport, *Doctor Dock*, 32.

166. "On the Warpath Again." See also "A Professor's Defiance."

167. Davenport, *Not Just Any Medical School*, 20.

168. "Dr. Maclean Downed." For another example of mistrust aimed at Detroit personnel, see "Ann Arbor or Detroit."

169. "Frothingham's Scalp," *Detroit Tribune*, April 22, 1889, James H. Wade Scrapbook (February 1897), "Detroit, Newspaper Clippings regarding Relocation of Clinical Work, 1889" folder, Box 135, Medical School (University of Michigan) Records, 1850–2010, Bentley Historical Library.

170. "A Professor's Defiance." See also "Ann Arbor Shaken Up," *Detroit Evening News*, April 20, 1889, James H. Wade Scrapbook (February 1897), "Detroit, Newspaper Clippings regarding Relocation of Clinical Work, 1889" folder, Box 135, Medical School (University of Michigan) Records, 1850–2010, Bentley Historical Library; and "State News."

171. "Ann Arbor Shaken Up."

172. "The Moderator," *Ann Arbor Courier*, May 8, 1889. For a reprinted letter to the editor of the *Ithaca (NY) Journal* indicating how widespread this controversy became, see also "Bounce Them!," *Ann Arbor Courier*, May 2, 1889, James H. Wade Scrapbook (February 1897), "Detroit, Newspaper Clippings regarding Relocation of Clinical Work, 1889" folder, Box 135, Medical School (University of Michigan) Records, 1850–2010, Bentley Historical Library.

173. June 1889 meeting, in *Proceedings of the Board of Regents*, 325. See also Davenport, *Not Just Any Medical School*, 20–21; Parascandola, *Development of American Pharmacology*, 38; Mulheron, "Addresses: I," 4. Despite the controversy, official records from the dean's office and faculty in 1889 are largely silent on the Detroit issue; indeed, the collection of faculty meeting minutes contain no entries at all for that spring, a rather conspicuous omission. Records of the Board of Regents' proceedings during that period are terse, with brief mentions of Frothingham's and Maclean's misconduct and subsequent resignations, but little otherwise. When Frothingham died in 1900, memorials specifically noted that he took the initiative to resign from his position at the University of Michigan, having "realized that he owed something to himself, his family, and the dignity of the profession," rather than being "dismissed" (as Davenport described the situation), although the distinction seems to be a fine one in the circumstances. Smith, "Addresses: II," 8.

174. Ann Arbor District Library, "Ann Arbor City Council Minutes, December 19, 1904," p. 133, http://councilminutes.aadl.org/councilminutes/19041219.

175. Victor Vaughan to Walter Sawyer, March 8, 1906, "Correspondence, January–June 1906" folder, Box 1, Walter H. Sawyer Papers, Bentley Historical Library.

176. See Dock, "Some Reasons," 64; Reuben Peterson to Walter Sawyer, April 1, 1908, "Correspondence, April 1908" folder, Box 1, Walter H. Sawyer Papers, Bentley Historical Library; and Davenport, *Doctor Dock*, 22–23.

177. "Merger Question," *Detroit Free Press,* [December 5, 1906?], "Miscellaneous" folder, Box 22, Ann Arbor Private Hospitals Records, Bentley Historical Library.

178. Davenport, *Doctor Dock,* 11, 317.

179. Starr, *Social Transformation,* 117–118, 120; Ludmerer, *Time to Heal,* xxii; Thomas Neville Bonner, "Searching for Abraham Flexner," *Academic Medicine* 73 (February 1998): 162; Flexner, *Medical Education,* viii.

180. Flexner, *Medical Education,* x.

181. Ibid., xii; Starr, *Social Transformation,* 119, 121, 230; Erwin H. Ackerknecht, *A Short History of Medicine* (Baltimore: Johns Hopkins University Press, 1982), 226; Ronald L. Numbers, "The Fall and Rise of the American Medical Profession," in *The Professions in American History,* ed. Nathan O. Hatch (Notre Dame, IN: University of Notre Dame Press, 1985). In some secondary sources, Flexner's report is cited as an example of Progressive-era "muckraking."

182. Flexner, *Medical Education,* 56.

183. Ibid., xi, xvi, 103.

184. Ibid., 73.

185. Ibid., 157; Starr, *Social Transformation,* 117–118, 120; Ludmerer, *Learning to Heal,* 96–99. Flexner did not mention Michigan in his chapter titled "Historical and General"; instead, he identified Johns Hopkins, Harvard, and Penn as the important trendsetters of American medical education.

186. Flexner, *Medical Education,* 243, 247. See also Davenport, *Not Just Any Medical School,* 27.

187. Flexner, *Medical Education,* 29, 32, 37, 171, 246.

188. Ibid., 28n1, 72n1.

189. Ibid., 29, 43.

190. Ibid., 135; see also 134, 143, 247.

191. Ibid., 144, 148, 246. See also Fye, "Albion Walter Hewlett," 58–59.

192. Fye, "Albion Walter Hewlett," 60.

193. Flexner, *Medical Education,* 144; see also 109, 111n2.

194. Victor Vaughan, "Report from the Dean of the Medical School," September 1915, Box 32, Medical School (University of Michigan) Records, 1850–2010, Bentley Historical Library, cited in Fye, "Albion Walter Hewlett," 62–63.

195. Flexner, *Medical Education,* 119, 244, 247.

196. Ludmerer, *Learning to Heal,* 158. See also Ludmerer, *Time to Heal,* 19.

CHAPTER 3

1. Portions of this section were previously published in Dea Boster, "Founding the Simpson Memorial," *Medicine at Michigan* 17 (Fall–Winter 2015): 12–13.

2. Horace W. Davenport, *Not Just Any Medical School: The Science, Practice, and Teaching of Medicine at the University of Michigan, 1850–1941* (Ann Arbor: University of Michigan Press, 1999), 168; Steven C. Martin, "Cyrus Cressey Sturgis and American Internal Medicine, 1913–1957," in *Medical Lives and Scientific Medicine at Michigan, 1891–1969,* ed. Joel D. Howell (Ann Arbor: University of Michigan Press, 1993), 88; Cyrus C. Sturgis, "The Thomas Henry Simpson Memorial Institute for Medical Re-

search," *Phi Chi Quarterly* 25 (May 1928): 602–603. In various secondary sources and memorials at the University of Michigan, Christine McDonald Simpson is referred to as "Catherine," but primary records from Detroit before her husband's death identify her as "Christine." For example, see *The Social Secretary of Detroit*, 1922 ed. (Detroit: Social Secretary, 1922), 128.

3. Henry A. Christian, "The Significance and Relationships of the Thomas Henry Simpson Memorial Institute for Medical Research," *Science* 65 (April 1927): 360. See also Martin, "Cyrus Cressey Sturgis," 88–89; and Davenport, *Not Just Any Medical School*, 169.

4. Martin, "Cyrus Cressey Sturgis," 84; Kenneth M. Ludmerer, *Time to Heal: American Medical Education from the Turn of the Century to the Era of Managed Care* (Oxford: Oxford University Press, 1999), xxii. As mentioned chapter 2, Flexner's study did not initiate the revolution in medical science and education, but it certainly is remembered as the frontrunner of the ideal. See Robert H. Ebert, "Medical Education at the Peak of the Era of Experimental Medicine," *Daedalus* 115, no. 2 (1986): 63.

5. Naomi Rogers, "Thomas Francis, Jr.: From the Bench to the Field," in *Medical Lives and Scientific Medicine at Michigan, 1891–1969*, ed. Joel D. Howell (Ann Arbor: University of Michigan Press, 1993), 164. See also Martin, "Cyrus Cressey Sturgis," 75–78; and Joel D. Howell, *Technology in the Hospital: Transforming Patient Care in the Early Twentieth Century* (Baltimore: Johns Hopkins University Press, 1995), 3.

6. Wilfred B. Shaw, ed., *The University of Michigan: An Encyclopedic Survey*, vol. 2 (Ann Arbor: University of Michigan Press, 1951), 891–892; Kenneth M. Ludmerer, *Learning to Heal: The Development of American Medical Education* (New York: Basic Books, 1985), 227; Davenport, *Not Just Any Medical School*, 105.

7. Davenport, *Not Just Any Medical School*, 145.

8. University of Michigan Medical School secretary to N. P. Colwell, July 26, 1917, "N. P. Colwell, AMA" folder, Box 33, Medical School (University of Michigan) Records, 1850–2010, Bentley Historical Library, University of Michigan, Ann Arbor.

9. Marvin J. Lubeck, "History of the Galens Honorary Medical Society," *Medical Bulletin* 21 (February 1955): 43.

10. Davenport, *Not Just Any Medical School*, 35.

11. Martin, "Cyrus Cressey Sturgis," 83; Ferol B. Brinkman, ed., *The University of Michigan: An Encyclopedic Survey*, vol. 5, *The University of Michigan, 1940–75* (Ann Arbor: University of Michigan Bentley Historical Library, 1977), 194; Davenport, *Not Just Any Medical School*, 317.

12. Davenport, *Not Just Any Medical School*, 164–166.

13. Shaw, *Encyclopedic Survey*, 2:945–946.

14. Ludmerer, *Learning to Heal*, 104; Shaw, *Encyclopedic Survey*, 2:945, 949; Steven J. Peitzman, "Louis Harry Newburgh and Metabolism at Michigan," in *Medical Lives and Scientific Medicine at Michigan, 1891–1969*, ed. Joel D. Howell (Ann Arbor: University of Michigan Press, 1993), 148.

15. Martin, "Cyrus Cressey Sturgis," 91–92.

16. Sturgis, "Thomas Henry Simpson Memorial Institute," 609. See also "Section II: Development of the Institute's Research Activities," *Research News* 16, no. 4 (1965): 12–14.

17. Department of Cardiac Surgery, "The Department of Cardiac Surgery at the University of Michigan," Department of Anesthesiology, "A History of the Department of Anesthesiology, University of Michigan Medical School," and Department of Internal Medicine, "Recent History of the Michigan Department of Internal Medicine," in *University of Michigan: An Encyclopedic Survey, Bicentennial Edition* (Ann Arbor: Michigan Publishing, forthcoming), https://quod.lib.umich.edu/b/bicentennial.

18. Cited in Wilfred B. Shaw, ed., *The University of Michigan: An Encyclopedic Survey*, vol. 1 (Ann Arbor: University of Michigan Press, 1942), 302–304.

19. "Schools Not All of High Grade," *Yale (MI) Expositor*, July 1, 1910, p. 6; Shaw, *Encyclopedic Survey*, 2:1010; M. L. Burton to Royal S. Copeland, July 22, 1920, Box 24, Correspondence, 1920–1922, Concerning the Reorganization of the Medical School of the University of Michigan, Royal S. Copeland Papers, Bentley Historical Library.

20. D. A. MacLachlan, MD, to Royal Copeland, November 11, 1921, and D. A. MacLachlan to M. L. Burton, December 2, 1921, Box 24, Correspondence, 1920–1922, Concerning the Reorganization of the Medical School of the University of Michigan, Royal S. Copeland Papers, Bentley Historical Library.

21. James C. Wood to Royal Copeland, November 29, 1921, Box 24, Correspondence, 1920–1922, Concerning the Reorganization of the Medical School of the University of Michigan, Royal S. Copeland Papers, Bentley Historical Library.

22. Royal Copeland to M. L. Burton, December 15, 1921, Royal Copeland to Arthur Brisbane, December 5, 1921, and Royal Copeland to Milton A. Darling, January 19, 1922, Correspondence, 1920–1922, concerning the Reorganization of the Medical School of the University of Michigan, Box 24, Royal S. Copeland Papers, Bentley Historical Library. Reuben Peterson saw echoes of this conflict in later discussions of "socialized" medicine in the United States, claiming that opposition to state-regulated medical care inspired the same threats as those aimed at sectarians in Michigan during the late nineteenth century. Reuben Peterson, "University Hospital Manuscript" (39), p. 38, Box 2, Reuben Peterson Papers, Bentley Historical Library.

23. Harley A. Haynes, "The University Hospital: University of Michigan," *Methods and Problems of Medical Education* 18 (1930): 59; Howell, *Technology in the Hospital*, 4–5, 17.

24. Peterson, "University Hospital Manuscript," 7; Charles H. McIntyre, "Victor C. Vaughan," in *Builders of American Medicine: Being a Collection of Original Papers Read before the Victor C. Vaughan Society of the University of Michigan Medical School* (Ann Arbor, MI: George Wahr, 1932), 225.

25. "'U' Hospital Building 40 Years Old Today," *Ann Arbor News*, August 12, 1965.

26. Shaw, *Encyclopedic Survey*, 2:807, 895–897. See also Haynes, "University Hospital," 60; and Nitin K. Ahuja, "Fordism in the Hospital: Albert Kahn and the Design of Old Main, 1917–25," *Journal of the History of Medicine and Allied Sciences* 67 (2011): 398–427.

27. Haynes, "University Hospital," 71.

28. Ibid., 60, 71, 74.

29. Haynes, "University Hospital," 74; see also 71, 73. The volume of patients and expansion of hospital services, however, made Dock's earlier model for clinical clerkships impractical. Ibid., 73.

30. Shaw, *Encyclopedic Survey*, 2:904–905.

31. Rogers, "Thomas Francis, Jr.," 165.

32. [John C. Burgher?], "Interview with Dr. N. F. Miller," January 2, 1936, p. 1, in "1935 Curriculum Revision Committee" folder, Box 40, Medical School (University of Michigan) Records, 1850–2010, Bentley Historical Library.

33. Shaw, *Encyclopedic Survey*, 2:873. See also Christine Kae Bass, "'It Did Not Seem like a Hospital, It Seemed like Home': Women's Experiences as Patients at Peterson's Hospital, Ann Arbor, Michigan, 1902–1933" (Ph.D. diss., Program in American Culture, University of Michigan, 1999).

34. Shaw, *Encyclopedic Survey*, 1:327.

35. Haynes, "University Hospital," 60; Shaw, *Encyclopedic Survey*, 2:901.

36. Aldred Scott Warthin, "The University Medical School and the State," in *Indiana University, 1820–1920: Centennial Memorial Volume* (Bloomington: Indiana University, 1921), 157, 160.

37. "Hospital One of University's Great Agencies of Service," *Ann Arbor Daily News*, [1935?], p. 76. See also Shaw, *Encyclopedic Survey*, 2:975.

38. Haynes, "University Hospital," 60–61.

39. Warthin, "University Medical School and the State," 162.

40. Shaw, *Encyclopedic Survey*, 2:905.

41. "Report of the Medical School 1939–40," p. 5, Box 1, University of Michigan (Medical School) Publications, Bentley Historical Library.

42. "Report of the Medical School 1939–40," 11; Davenport, *Not Just Any Medical School*, 36.

43. C. S. Yoakum to Dean Hugh Cabot, February 3, 1928, "1928, A, including Admission Standards and AAMC" folder, Box 37, Medical School (University of Michigan) Records, 1850–2010, Bentley Historical Library.

44. Howard B. Lewis to C. S. Yoakum, January 27, 1928, "1928, A, including Admission Standards and AAMC" folder, Box 37, Medical School (University of Michigan) Records, 1850–2010, Bentley Historical Library. See also Davenport, *Not Just Any Medical School*, 30.

45. A. C. Curtis (medical school secretary) to A. C. Furstenberg, March 28, 1935, and "University of Michigan Medical School Report," p. 2, "1935 Curriculum Revision Committee" folder, Box 40, Medical School (University of Michigan) Records, 1850–2010, Bentley Historical Library.

46. Raphael Isaacs to A. C. Furstenberg, August 21, 1936, and U. J. Wile to A. C. Furstenberg, August 14, 1936, "1936 Medical School Report, Replies To" folder, Box 40, Medical School (University of Michigan) Records, 1850–2010, Bentley Historical Library.

47. Paul Starr, *The Social Transformation of American Medicine* (New York: Basic Books, 1982), 124–126.

48. Abraham Flexner to Victor Vaughan, July 9, 1919, and Victor Vaughan to Abraham Flexner, July 14, 1919, "Flexner, Abraham, Gen Ed Board, 1917–21" folder, Box 33, Medical School (University of Michigan) Records, 1850–2010, Bentley Historical Library.

49. Abraham Flexner to Victor Vaughan, July 7, 1919, and Victor Vaughan to Abraham Flexner, July 11, 1919, "Flexner, Abraham, Gen Ed Board, 1917–21" folder, Box 33, Medical School (University of Michigan) Records, 1850–2010, Bentley Historical Library.

50. C. W. Edmunds to N. P. Colwell, July 21, 1920, "N. P. Colwell, AMA" folder, Box 33, Medical School (University of Michigan) Records, 1850–2010, Bentley Historical Library. See also Thomas Neville Bonner, "Searching for Abraham Flexner," *Academic Medicine* 73 (February 1998): 164.

51. Davenport, *Not Just Any Medical School*, 31–32. See also Ludmerer, *Time to Heal*, 63.

52. Davenport, *Not Just Any Medical School*, x–xi, 29; Hugh Cabot to University of Michigan president Little, June 22, 1927, "Correspondence (Regents' Communications) Regarding Admission Requirements and Salaries, 1925–27" folder, Box 135, Medical School (University of Michigan) Records, 1850–2010, Bentley Historical Library. In 1935, medical school secretary A. C. Curtis informed Dean Furstenberg that "in the past five years, but two students have been accepted for advanced standing and in both cases . . . these students were Jews," implying that the department was setting an undesirable precedent for admitting Jewish students. A. C. Curtis to A. C. Furstenberg, March 28, 1935, "1935 E-G" folder, Box 40, Medical School (University of Michigan) Records, 1850–2010, Bentley Historical Library.

53. Regina Markell Morantz, Cynthia Stodola Pomerleau, and Carol Hansen Fenichel, eds., *In Her Own Words: Oral Histories of Women Physicians* (New Haven, CT: Yale University Press, 1982), 111. See also Ludmerer, *Time to Heal*, 63; "Report of the Medical School 1939–40," 5; and Starr, *Social Transformation*, 124.

54. Shaw, *Encyclopedic Survey*, 2:793–794; minutes of Barbour Scholarship Committee, March 16, 1928, p. 2, and "Suggested Outline. Barbour Scholarship Committee," March 16, 1928, "1928, B, includes Barbour Scholarship Committee" folder, Box 37, Medical School (University of Michigan) Records, 1850–2010, Bentley Historical Library.

55. "University of Michigan Medical School Report," 1, 4, "1935 Curriculum Committee Revision" folder, Box 40, Medical School (University of Michigan) Records, 1850–2010, Bentley Historical Library; "Report of the Medical School 1939–40," 4; Davenport, *Not Just Any Medical School*, 31.

56. Shaw, *Encyclopedic Survey*, 2:1927–1928; Lubeck, "History of the Galens," 44–48; John A. D. Cooper et al., "Survey Report, University of Michigan School of Medicine, Ann Arbor, Michigan, 1958," p. 9, Box 2, University of Michigan (Medical School) Publications, Bentley Historical Library. Lubeck claims that Galens was responsible for Michigan's first "official" honor system, which contradicts evidence of the honor system in place at the turn of the century. However, Galens was instrumental in revising later versions of the school's honor system policy, particularly in the mid-1920s, "when there were reports of instances of dishonesty occurring during examinations." Lubeck, "History of the Galens," 43.

57. See Ebert, "Medical Education," 60.

58. Faculty meeting minutes, October 19, 1933, p. 146, Box 128, Faculty Meetings, Sept. 1930–February 1935, Medical School (University of Michigan) Records, 1850–2010, Bentley Historical Library; faculty meeting minutes, November 1, 1938, p. 135, Box 128, Faculty Meetings, March 1935–June 1939, Medical School (University of Michigan) Records, 1850–2010, Bentley Historical Library; "Report of the Medical School 1939–40," 12; Davenport, *Not Just Any Medical* School, 247; Shaw, *Encyclopedic Survey*, 2:946.

59. "Report of the Medical School 1939–40," 4.

60. Valerie P. Castle, Dick MacDonald, and Faye Silverstein, "Department of Pediatrics and Communicable Diseases," in *University of Michigan: An Encyclopedic Survey, Bicentennial Edition* (Ann Arbor: Michigan Publishing, forthcoming), https://quod.lib.umich.edu/b/bicentennial; Howard Markel, "When It Rains It Pours: Endemic Goiter, Iodized Salt, and David Murray Cowie," *American Journal of Public Health* 77 (1987): 219–229.

61. Peitzman, "Louis Harry Newburgh," 150.

62. Shaw, *Encyclopedic Survey*, 2:891.

63. Brinkman, *Encyclopedic Survey* 5:196; Shaw, *Encyclopedic Survey*, 2:899; Castle, MacDonald, and Silverstein, "Department of Pediatrics"; Davenport, *Not Just Any Medical School*, 247.

64. Cyrus C. Sturgis, *Hematology* (Springfield, IL: Charles C. Thomas, 1947), x, quoted in Martin, "Cyrus Cressey Sturgis," 99.

65. Martin, "Cyrus Cressey Sturgis," 93; Brinkman, *Encyclopedic Survey*, 5:194.

66. Davenport, *Not Just Any Medical School*, 189.

67. Shaw, *Encyclopedic Survey*, 2:945–946; Martin, "Cyrus Cressey Sturgis," 94–95; John W. Henderson, *The University of Michigan Department of Ophthalmology: A Proud Heritage* (Ann Arbor: Department of Ophthalmology, University of Michigan, 1986), 111; Davenport, *Not Just Any Medical School*, 189.

68. Hugh Cabot and Harley Haynes to regents, November 4, 1926, "Correspondence (Regents Communications) regarding Admission Requirements and Salaries, 1925–27" folder, Box 135, Medical School (University of Michigan) Records, 1850–2010, Bentley Historical Library.

69. *Washtenaw Tribune*, February 7, 1930, cited in Davenport, *Not Just Any Medical School*, 191–192.

70. Copeland to Burton, December 15, 1921.

71. Davenport, *Not Just Any Medical School*, 191. Frederick Novy served as an interim dean from 1933 to 1935.

72. See "University of Michigan Department of Medicine and Surgery: Schedule of Work, First Semester, 1910–11," "University of Michigan Department of Medicine and Surgery: Schedule of Work, Second Semester, 1911," "University of Michigan Department of Medicine and Surgery: Schedule, First Semester, 1921–1922," and "University of Michigan Department of Medicine and Surgery: Schedule, Second Semester, 1921–1922," Box 2, University of Michigan (Medical School) Publications, Bentley Historical Library; and Davenport, *Not Just Any Medical School*, 37.

73. "Report of the Medical School 1939–40," 3. See also Davenport, *Not Just Any Medical School*, 34.

74. Davenport, *Not Just Any Medical School*, 35.

75. Executive Committee of the Medical School to the Executive Faculty of the Medical School, October 23, 1935, "1935 E-G" folder, Box 40, Medical School (University of Michigan) Records, 1850–2010, Bentley Historical Library.

76. "Medical School, Summer Session, 1934, June 25 to August 3 and 17," Box 2, University of Michigan (Medical School) Publications, Bentley Historical Library; "University of Michigan Medical School Report," pp. 2, 4, "1935 Curriculum Revision Committee" folder, Box 40, Medical School (University of Michigan) Records, 1850–2010, Bentley Historical Library. See also Davenport, *Not Just Any Medical School*, 30–31, 36–37.

77. A. C. Curtis to A. C. Furstenberg, March 28, 1935, "1935 Curriculum Revision Committee" folder, Box 40, Medical School (University of Michigan) Records, 1850–2010, Bentley Historical Library.

78. Executive Committee to Executive Faculty, October 23, 1935. See also "Summary of Discussion with Dr. Max Peet concerning Changes in the Curriculum," January 17, 1936, and [John C. Burgher?], "Interview with Dr. Newburgh," n.d., "1935 Curriculum Revision Committee" folder, Box 40, Medical School (University of Michigan) Records, 1850–2010, Bentley Historical Library.

79. [John C. Burgher?], "Interview with Dr. N. F. Miller," 2. See also [John C. Burgher?], "Interview with Dr. Newburgh."

80. [John C. Burgher?], "Interview with Dr. F. J. Hodges," December 19, 1935, p. 1, "1935 Curriculum Revision Committee" folder, Box 40, Medical School (University of Michigan) Records, 1850–2010, Bentley Historical Library.

81. Executive Committee to Executive Faculty, October 23, 1935, and Vocational Education Department to A. C. Furstenberg, July 15, 1935, "1935 E-G" folder, Box 40, Medical School (University of Michigan) Records, 1850–2010, Bentley Historical Library.

82. Executive Committee to Executive Faculty, October 23, 1935.

83. "University of Michigan Medical School Report," 7; see also 5, 8; and Davenport, *Not Just Any Medical School*, 30–31.

84. [John C. Burgher?], "Interview with Dr. Newburgh," 1; "University of Michigan Medical School Report," 7. See also [Cyrus C. Sturgis?], "Revision of the Curriculum based on Conversation with Dr. Barrett," December 23, 1935, 1, and [John C. Burgher?], "Interview with Dr. Frank Wilson," January 16, 1936, p. 1, "1935 Curriculum Revision Committee" folder, Box 40, Medical School (University of Michigan) Records, 1850–2010, Bentley Historical Library.

85. [John C. Burgher?], "Interview with Dr. Newburgh," 2; [John C. Burgher?], "Interview with Dr. Frank Wilson," 2; "[Interview with] Dr. Camp," n.d., pp. 1–2, "1935 Curriculum Revision Committee" folder, Box 40, Medical School (University of Michigan) Records, 1850–2010, Bentley Historical Library; [John C. Burgher?], "Interview with Dr. F. J. Hodges," 1.

86. "I: The Selection of Students," pp. 1–2, "1936 Med School Reports, Replies To" folder, Box 40, Medical School (University of Michigan) Records, 1850–2010, Bentley Historical Library.

87. "II: The Training of the Students," p. 4, "1936 Med School Reports, Replies To" folder, Box 40, Medical School (University of Michigan) Records, 1850–2010, Bentley Historical Library. See also [John C. Burgher?], "Interview with Dr. Newburgh," 2.

88. Anonymous to A. C. Furstenberg, September 18, 1936, "1936 Med School Reports, Replies To" folder, Box 40, Medical School (University of Michigan) Records, 1850–2010, Bentley Historical Library.

89. Elizabeth Crosby to A. C. Furstenberg, November 11, 1936, "1936 Med School Reports, Replies To" folder, Box 40, Medical School (University of Michigan) Records, 1850–2010, Bentley Historical Library.

90. L. H. Newburgh to A. C. Furstenberg, August 11, 1936, "1936 Med School Reports, Replies To" folder, Box 40, Medical School (University of Michigan) Records, 1850–2010, Bentley Historical Library.

91. Howard B. Lewis to A. C. Furstenberg, November 17, 1936, p. 2, "1936 Med School Reports, Replies To" folder, Box 40, Medical School (University of Michigan)

Records, 1850–2010, Bentley Historical Library. See also Crosby to Furstenberg, November 11, 1936.

92. Newburgh to Furstenberg, August 11, 1936.

93. Lewis to Furstenberg, November 17, 1936.

94. Newburgh to Furstenberg, August 11, 1936.

95. N. P. Colwell (AMA medical education council secretary) to Charles W. Edmunds (assistant dean), September 16, 1919, and Charles W. Edmunds to N. P. Colwell, November 4, 1919, "N. P. Colwell, AMA" folder, Box 33, Medical School (University of Michigan) Records, 1850–2010, Bentley Historical Library. See also Davenport, *Not Just Any Medical School*, xi.

96. Victor Vaughan to N. P. Colwell, April 15, 1919, "N. P. Colwell, AMA" folder, Box 33, Medical School (University of Michigan) Records, 1850–2010, Bentley Historical Library.

97. Hugh Cabot to Aaron Brown, September 22, 1928, "1928, B, Includes Barbour Scholarship Committee" folder, Box 37, Medical School (University of Michigan) Records, 1850–2010, Bentley Historical Library.

98. Shaw, *Encyclopedic Survey*, 2:949–950; Brinkman, *Encyclopedic Survey*, 5:196; "IV: Employment of the Young Graduate," "1936 Med School Reports, Replies To" folder, Box 40, Medical School (University of Michigan) Records, 1850–2010, Bentley Historical Library; Ludmerer, *Time to Heal*, 186.

99. Martin, "Cyrus Cressey Sturgis," 80, 86.

100. Walter Donnelly, Wilfred B. Shaw, and Ruth W. Gjelsness, eds., *The University of Michigan: An Encyclopedic Survey*, vol. 4 (Ann Arbor: University of Michigan Press, 1958), 1661–1662. For more on the reputed decadence of interns, see Ludmerer, *Time to Heal*, 82–83.

101. Ludmerer, *Time to Heal*, 116; McIntyre, "Victor C. Vaughan," 225; Larry D. Gruppen, R. Van Harrison, and Roland G. Hiss, "Department of Medical Education at the University of Michigan," in *University of Michigan: An Encyclopedic Survey, Bicentennial Edition* (Ann Arbor: Michigan Publishing, forthcoming), https://quod.lib.umich.edu/b/bicentennial.

102. Shaw, *Encyclopedic Survey*, 2:923–925; Gruppen, Van Harrison, and Hiss, "Department of Medical Education."

CHAPTER 4

1. "University of Michigan Medical School Ninety-Seventh Annual Opening Exercises: Program for October 5, 1942," Box 5, University of Michigan (Medical School) Publications, Bentley Historical Library, University of Michigan, Ann Arbor.

2. Janet Tarolli, "Epilogue: Building the Modern Medical Center, 1941 to Present," in *Not Just Any Medical School: The Science, Practice, and Teaching of Medicine at the University of Michigan 1850–1941*, by Horace W. Davenport (Ann Arbor: University of Michigan Press, 1999), 297.

3. Steven C. Martin, "Cyrus Cressey Sturgis and American Internal Medicine, 1913–1957," in *Medical Lives and Scientific Medicine at Michigan, 1891–1969*, ed. Joel D. Howell (Ann Arbor: University of Michigan Press, 1993), 97; Tarolli, "Epilogue," 298.

4. University of Michigan, *President's Report for 1943–44*, 97, cited in Tarolli, "Epilogue," 298. See also Ferol B. Brinkman, ed., *The University of Michigan: An Encyclopedic Survey*, vol. 5, *The University of Michigan, 1940–75* (Ann Arbor: University of Michigan Bentley Historical Library, 1977), 186; and Kenneth M. Ludmerer, *Time to Heal: American Medical Education from the Turn of the Century to the Era of Managed Care* (Oxford: Oxford University Press, 1999), 127. Support for a three-year curriculum continued well after the war ended and was proposed at Michigan's 1958 teaching institute as a possibility to improve the curriculum. See Robert Lovell's remarks in "Summary of Activities of the Discussion Panels," *University of Michigan Medical Bulletin* 24 (August 1958): 326.

5. Tarolli, "Epilogue," 297, 299.

6. Ludmerer, *Time to Heal*, xix–xxii; Robert H. Ebert, "Medical Education at the Peak of the Era of Experimental Medicine," *Daedalus* 115, no. 2 (1986): 58; Howard Markel, "Foreword," in *Not Just Any Medical School: The Science, Practice, and Teaching of Medicine at the University of Michigan, 1850–1941*, by Horace W. Davenport (Ann Arbor: University of Michigan Press, 1999), v–vi; Department of Internal Medicine, "Recent History of the Michigan Department of Internal Medicine," in *University of Michigan: An Encyclopedic Survey, Bicentennial Edition* (Ann Arbor: Michigan Publishing, forthcoming), https://quod.lib.umich.edu/b/bicentennial; Brinkman, *Encyclopedic Survey*, 5:182–184, 195; Joel D. Howell, "Introduction," in *Medical Lives and Scientific Medicine at Michigan, 1891–1969*, ed. Joel D. Howell (Ann Arbor: University of Michigan Press, 1993), 9; Naomi Rogers, "Thomas Francis, Jr.: From the Bench to the Field," in *Medical Lives and Scientific Medicine at Michigan, 1891–1969*, ed. Joel D. Howell (Ann Arbor: University of Michigan Press, 1993), 183.

7. Brinkman, *Encyclopedic Survey*, 5:184.

8. Reuben Peterson, "University Hospital Manuscript" (39), p. 7, Box 2, Reuben Peterson Papers, Bentley Historical Library.

9. Tarolli, "Epilogue," 298–299; Brinkman, *Encyclopedic Survey*, 5:185, 190, 200. For an example of the "sprawling" adjective, see Elizabeth Gaspar Brown, "Notes on the University Hospital: The Early Decades," *Michigan Quarterly Review* 3 (1964): 8.

10. Ebert, "Medical Education," 64–65. Ebert also notes that doctors continued to be drafted into the military after the war had ended, which interrupted some residencies or placed a break between internships and subspecialty fellowships. Ibid., 66.

11. "Medical School Takes Too Long, Dean Says," *Ann Arbor News*, June 7, 1958.

12. Larry D. Gruppen, R. Van Harrison, and Roland G. Hiss, "The Department of Medical Education at the University of Michigan," in *University of Michigan: An Encyclopedic Survey, Bicentennial Edition* (Ann Arbor: Michigan Publishing, forthcoming), https://quod.lib.umich.edu/b/bicentennial; Ebert, "Medical Education," 66. Ebert notes that the growth of specialization had more to do with advances in medical science than postwar NIH funding, but the influx of government money did have a strong impact on clinical departments and curricula, since "the organization of the NIH is categorical, meaning oriented to diseases and to organs. . . . Monies came directly to subspecialty divisions and to individuals in those divisions so that the schism of loyalty between the NIH and the university or hospital or even clinical department was inevitably accentuated." Ebert, "Medical Education," 61–62.

13. Brinkman, *Encyclopedic Survey*, 5:188–189; Valerie P. Castle, Dick MacDonald, and Faye Silverstein, "Department of Pediatrics and Communicable Diseases," in *Uni-*

versity of Michigan: An Encyclopedic Survey, Bicentennial Edition (Ann Arbor: Michigan Publishing, forthcoming), https://quod.lib.umich.edu/b/bicentennial.

14. Brinkman, *Encyclopedic Survey*, 5:203–204; Department of Anesthesiology, "A History of the Department of Anesthesiology, University of Michigan Medical School," in *University of Michigan: An Encyclopedic Survey, Bicentennial Edition* (Ann Arbor: Michigan Publishing, forthcoming), https://quod.lib.umich.edu/b/bicentennial.

15. See John A. D. Cooper et al., "Survey Report, University of Michigan School of Medicine, Ann Arbor, Michigan, 1958," pp. 22, 72, Box 2, Medical School (University of Michigan) Publications, Bentley Historical Library.

16. "University of Michigan Medical School: Medicine, September 1955," pp. i–iii, and "University of Michigan Medical School: Medicine, September 1958," p. iii, "Medical School Printed Brochures, Medicine, 1955–1994" folder, Box 1, Medical School (University of Michigan) Publications, Bentley Historical Library.

17. Ebert, "Medical Education," 59.

18. Ibid., 65. See also Martin, "Cyrus Cressey Sturgis," 74, 98.

19. Lowell T. Coggeshall, *Planning for Medical Progress through Education* (Evanston, IL: Association of American Medical Colleges, 1975); Joel D. Howell, "Lowell T. Coggeshall and American Medical Education: 1901–1987," *Academic Medicine* 67 (1992): 711–718.

20. E. H. Watson, "By Precept: A Critical Appraisal of Medical Teaching," *Medical Education* 28 (May 1953): 12.

21. July 1969 meeting, in *Proceedings of the Board of Regents* (Ann Arbor: University of Michigan, 2000), 18–19.

22. "Report of the Medical School 1939–40," pp. 4–5, 11, Box 1, University of Michigan (Medical School) Publications, Bentley Historical Library; Howell, "Introduction," 8–9.

23. Howell, "Introduction," 10–11; Rogers, "Thomas Francis, Jr.," 174, 183; University of Michigan School of Public Health, "1955 Polio Vaccine Trial Announcement," https://sph.umich.edu/polio/ (accessed February 27, 2017).

24. Brinkman, *Encyclopedic Survey*, 5:206; "One Hundredth Annual Opening Exercises: Program for September 30, 1950," Box 5, Medical School (University of Michigan) Publications, Bentley Historical Library; "'U' to Get New Charge of Cobalt," *Ann Arbor News*, November 19, 1958.

25. Howell, "Introduction," 9; Brinkman, *Encyclopedic Survey*, 5:191–192, 197; Department of Anesthesiology, "A History of the Department"; Castle, MacDonald, and Silverstein, "Department of Pediatrics."

26. Tarolli, "Epilogue," 298–299; Brinkman, *Encyclopedic Survey*, 5:199, 210; Howard Markel, "The University of Michigan Medical School, 1850–2000: 'An Example Worthy of Imitation,'" *Journal of the American Medical Association* 283, no. 7 (2000): 919.

27. Cooper et al., "Survey Report," 72.

28. Brinkman, *Encyclopedic Survey*, 5:184–185. See also Ebert, "Medical Education," 63; and Martin, "Cyrus Cressey Sturgis," 97. Although the school received a significant amount of federal money, compared with other major medical schools—including Yale, Columbia, Johns Hopkins, and Harvard—Michigan had the smallest number of NIH research fellowships in the 1950s. This was most likely due to the availability of funding from university and private sources. Martin, "Cyrus Cressey Sturgis," 98.

29. Brinkman, *Encyclopedic Survey*, 5:191, 195, 203.

30. John W. Konnak and Dev S. Pardanani, *A History of Urology at the University of Michigan 1920–2001* (University of Michigan Historical Center for the Health Sciences, 2002), 88–90.

31. Brinkman, *Encyclopedic Survey*, 5:181, 195–196, 207–209.

32. Ibid., 5:193–194, 201–202; Tarolli, "Epilogue," 299–300; Department of Emergency Medicine, "The History of the Department of Emergency Medicine at Michigan," in *University of Michigan: An Encyclopedic Survey, Bicentennial Edition* (Ann Arbor: Michigan Publishing, forthcoming), https://quod.lib.umich.edu/b/bicentennial.

33. University of Michigan, *President's Report for 1959–60*, 79, cited in Tarolli, "Epilogue," 299.

34. Cooper et al., "Survey Report," 5–6, 72. See also Brinkman, *Encyclopedic Survey*, 5:189–190.

35. "Report of the Medical School 1939–40," 18.

36. Watson, "By Precept," 11.

37. Rollo McCotter, "A History of the Anatomy Department of the University of Michigan," address given at honorary dinner, February 7, 1947, p. 8, Bentley Historical Library.

38. Fred Jenner Hodges, "Origin and Growth of Michigan's Medical Center," *University of Michigan Medical Bulletin* 16 (September 1950): 242; Tarolli, "Epilogue," 299.

39. Cooper et al., "Survey Report," 12; Brinkman, *Encyclopedic Survey*, 5:186–187.

40. A. C. Furstenberg, "History and Purpose of the Teaching Institute," *University of Michigan Medical Bulletin* 24 (August 1958): 295. See also Cooper et al., "Survey Report," 73.

41. Cooper et al., "Survey Report," 9, 24–25.

42. Watson, "By Precept," 11, 13.

43. George E. Miller, "What Are We Trying to Do?" *University of Michigan Medical Bulletin* 24 (August 1958): 301; "Some Observations on Activities of the Institute Panels," *University of Michigan Medical Bulletin* 24 (August 1958): 314.

44. Cooper et al., "Survey Report," 10.

45. Ibid., 2, 9.

46. Ibid., 25–26. See also Miller, "What Are We Trying to Do?," 300–301; and John A. Cooper, "Educational Patterns in Medicine," *University of Michigan Medical Bulletin* 24 (August 1958): 316, 321.

47. Cooper et al., "Survey Report," 24, 73.

48. D. L. Hinerman, "Introduction: Our Challenge for the Future of Medical Education," *University of Michigan Medical Bulletin* 24 (August 1958): 291 292.

49. Furstenberg, "History and Purpose," 296. See also Harlan Hatcher, "Address of Welcome," *University of Michigan Medical Bulletin* 24 (August 1958): 295; and Hinerman, "Introduction," 291.

50. Hatcher, "Address of Welcome," 293.

51. See Robert S. Harnack, "How Do We Go about Doing It?," *University of Michigan Medical Bulletin* 24 (August 1958): 309; "Some Observations," 312; and "Summary of Activities," 329–330.

52. Miller, "What Are We Trying to Do?," 298–299.

53. Harnack, "How Do We Go about Doing It?," 306; "Summary of Activities," 331; "Some Observations," 313.

54. "Doctors Seek Curriculum Improvement," *Ann Arbor News*, June 3, 1958.

55. Brinkman, *Encyclopedic Survey*, 5:189; Harry A. Towsley, "Introduction: The Goals of Medical Television," *University of Michigan Medical Bulletin* 28 (November 1962): 303–304.

56. Brinkman, *Encyclopedic Survey*, 5:186.

57. Cooper et al., "Survey Report," 23, 73.

58. Letter to the editor, *The Paeon*, November 1966, p. 6 (emphasis in original).

59. Miller, "What Are We Trying to Do?," 302.

60. "Medical School—Office of the Dean—Memo of Record, Week of January 2–5, 1968," pp. 3–5, "Enrollment Expansion 1965–72" folder, Box 78, Medical School (University of Michigan) Records, Bentley Historical Library.

61. Cooper et al., "Survey Report," 8–9. The MCAT originated with aptitude tests that spread in popularity between the 1930s and 1940s and became more standardized by 1948.

62. A. C. Furstenberg to A. M. Chickening, November 17, 1942, in "1942-D" folder, Box 45, Medical School (University of Michigan) Records, Bentley Historical Library; executive faculty meeting minutes, December 1, 1938, Box 128, Executive Faculty Minutes, 1935–1939, Medical School (University of Michigan) Records, 1850–2010, Bentley Historical Library; Ludmerer, *Time to Heal*, 61.

63. Brinkman, *Encyclopedic Survey*, 5:187. See also Cooper et al., "Survey Report," 8.

64. Cooper et al., "Survey Report," 10.

65. "Third of Medical Students Are from Low-Income Families," *Ann Arbor News*, June 28, 1956.

66. "Summary of Activities," 328.

67. "Medical School Takes Too Long."

68. "Report of the Medical School 1939–40," 1–3. The house was built with funding from the Public Works Administration during the New Deal and was constructed on the site of a ward building that had been destroyed by fire in 1927. During World War II, the house was requisitioned for use by the U.S. Navy. See Horace W. Davenport, *Not Just Any Medical School: The Science, Practice, and Teaching of Medicine at the University of Michigan 1850–1941* (Ann Arbor: University of Michigan Press, 1999), 36.

69. "Intramurals," *The Paeon*, November 1966, p. 7; Davenport, *Not Just Any Medical School*, 37; Cooper et al., "Survey Report," 10; "Student Health Organization," *Paeon*, February 1967, pp. 1–8, and September 1967, pp. 2–3.

70. Eleanor Goldberg, "Galens Provide Service to City," *Michigan Daily*, April 19, 1957.

71. Lee R. Britton to William N. Hubbard, Jr., January 10, 1968, Charles Newton to William N. Hubbard, Jr., May 8, 1967, Todd Grant to William N. Hubbard, Jr., April 30, 1966, University of Michigan News Service, "Press Release," January 22, 1968, Robert H. Hartlett to William N. Hubbard, Jr., March 15, 1963, and Terry J. Bergstrom to William N. Hubbard, Jr., April 30, 1965, "Student Organizations—Galens Medical Society 1963–79" folder, Box 235, Medical School (University of Michigan) Records, 1850–2010, Bentley Historical Library. See also Marvin J. Lubeck, "History of the Galens Honorary Medical Society," *Medical Bulletin* 21 (February 1955): 48.

72. William N. Hubbard, Jr., to Charles Robinson, February 22, 1968, "Student Organizations—Galens Medical Society 1963–79" folder, Box 235, Medical School (University of Michigan) Records, Box 235, Bentley Historical Library; Bergstrom to Hubbard, April 30, 1965; Britton to Hubbard, January 10, 1968.

73. Cooper et al., "Survey Report," 10; "U-M Medical School Applications Dropping, Says Dean Furstenberg," *Ann Arbor News*, April 12, 1956; Furstenberg, "History and Purpose," 295–296.

74. "The University of Michigan Medical School: Initial Enrollment of Student Totals at the Beginning of Each Academic Year and Percent Attrition during Progression in Medical School," and Harlan Hatcher to George Romney, March 11, 1966, "Enrollment Expansion 1965–72" folder, Box 78, Medical School (University of Michigan) Records, 1850–2010, Bentley Historical Library.

75. Brinkman, *Encyclopedic Survey*, 5:186–187.

76. Watson, "By Precept," 15–16; "Some Observations," 313–314.

77. Glenn W. Geelhoed, letter to the editor, *The Paeon*, October 1, 1966, pp. 1, 4. By 1987, the paper had become more irreverent and farcical, akin to the *Harvard Lampoon*. A collection of issues is available in Box 5, Medical School (University of Michigan) Publications, Bentley Historical Library.

78. Bergstrom to Hubbard, April 30, 1965. See also Hartlett to Hubbard, March 15, 1963.

79. Davenport, *Not Just Any Medical School*, 37.

80. Tarolli, "Epilogue," 297–298.

81. Brinkman, *Encyclopedic Survey*, 5:186, 204–206; Department of Anesthesiology, "A History of the Department"; Castle, MacDonald, and Silverstein, "Department of Pediatrics"; Department of Cardiac Surgery, "The Department of Cardiac Surgery at the University of Michigan," in *University of Michigan: An Encyclopedic Survey, Bicentennial Edition* (Ann Arbor: Michigan Publishing, forthcoming), https://quod.lib.umich.edu/b/bicentennial. In 1962, the state legislature pulled its funding for the Veterans' Center and that facility became the North Outpatient Building.

82. A. C. Furstenberg, "Conclusion," *University of Michigan Medical Bulletin* 24 (August 1958): 337.

83. *President's Report for 1959–60*, 79, cited in Tarolli, "Epilogue," 299.

84. Cooper et al., "Survey Report," 21, 73. See also Tarolli, "Epilogue," 299.

85. "Big Changes Due in Hospital Area," *Ann Arbor News*, May 17, 1965.

86. Brinkman, *Encyclopedic Survey*, 5:196–197; Tarolli, "Epilogue," 298; "A Career Spent Turning Childbirth into a Family Affair," *Ann Arbor News*, June 3, 1973. In 1969, Avery became the first woman, and the first nonphysician, to join the school's Norman F. Miller Obstetrics and Gynecology Honor Society.

87. "Medical School—Office of the Dean—Memo of Record, Week of January 2–5, 1968," p. 4, "Enrollment Expansion 1965–72" folder, Box 78, Medical School (University of Michigan) Records, 1850–2010, Bentley Historical Library.

88. Castle, MacDonald, and Silverstein, "Department of Pediatrics"; Brinkman, *Encyclopedic Survey*, 5:201.

89. Brinkman, *Encyclopedic Survey*, 5:201; Tarolli, "Epilogue," 299; Castle, MacDonald, and Silverstein, "Department of Pediatrics." Mott was a major shareholder of General Motors.

90. Charles F. Wilkinson, "Intern Training in the Hospital System," *Rhode Island Medical Journal* 31 (March 1947): 2, Box 2, Medical School (University of Michigan) Publications, Bentley Historical Library.

91. Ibid., 2, 3–5; Gruppen, Van Harrison, and Hiss, "Department of Medical Education."

92. Wilkinson, "Intern Training," 7–8. For more on pediatrics, see Wilfred B. Shaw, ed., *The University of Michigan: An Encyclopedic Survey*, vol. 2 (Ann Arbor: University of Michigan Press, 1951), 909; and Brinkman, *Encyclopedic Survey*, 5:200.

93. Furstenberg, "Conclusion," 338; Brinkman, *Encyclopedic Survey*, 5:188, 207, 210.

94. Harlan Hatcher, "Guest Editorial: The University and the Medical School," *University of Michigan Medical Center Journal* 33 (July–August 1967): 151.

95. Brinkman, *Encyclopedic Survey*, 5:190; Tarolli, "Epilogue," 300.

96. Ebert, "Medical Education," 63–64.

97. Ibid., 61; Kenneth M. Ludmerer, *Learning to Heal: The Development of American Medical Education* (New York: Basic Books, 1985), xix.

98. "University of Michigan Medical School: Medicine, September 1966," Medical School Printed Brochures, Medicine, 1965–1994, Box 1, Medical School (University of Michigan) Publications, Bentley Historical Library.

99. "UMMS 1964 Class Day Ceremony and Honors Convocation, Program for June 5, 1964," Box 5, Medical School (University of Michigan) Publications, Bentley Historical Library.

100. James Tobin, "JFK at the Union: The Unknown Story of the Peace Corps Speech," http://peacecorps.umich.edu/Tobin.html (accessed May 1, 2017).

101. James Tobin, "1964: Michigan, LBJ, and the Great Society," *Michigan Today*, May 23, 2012, http://michigantoday.umich.edu/a8273/.

CHAPTER 5

1. Ferol B. Brinkman, ed., *The University of Michigan: An Encyclopedic Survey*, vol. 5, *The University of Michigan, 1940–75* (Ann Arbor: University of Michigan Bentley Historical Library, 1977), 185, 190, 204, http://quod.lib.umich.edu/u/umsurvey/AAS3302.0005.001/1:1?rgn=div1;view=fulltext; R. W. Fleming to Frederick T. Cioffi, November 26, 1969, "Compliance, General 1969" folder, Box 77, Medical School (University of Michigan) Records, 1850–2010, Bentley Historical Library, University of Michigan, Ann Arbor.

2. Harlan Hatcher, "Guest Editorial: The University and the Medical School," *University of Michigan Medical Center Journal* 33 (July–August 1967): 151.

3. Alexandra Minna Stern, "Innovation, Expansion, and Specialization in Women's Health: The University of Michigan's Department of Obstetrics and Gynecology, 1964–2014," in *University of Michigan: An Encyclopedic Survey, Bicentennial Edition* (Ann Arbor: Michigan Publishing, forthcoming), https://quod.lib.umich.edu/b/bicentennial.

4. J. A. Gronvall, "President's Report for 1967–68: The Medical School," 1, cited in Janet Tarolli, "Epilogue: Building the Modern Medical Center, 1941 to Present," in *Not Just Any Medical School: The Science, Practice, and Teaching of Medicine at the*

University of Michigan, 1850–1941, by Horace W. Davenport (Ann Arbor: University of Michigan Press, 1999), 300, see also 301; Kenneth M. Ludmerer, *Time to Heal: American Medical Education from the Turn of the Century to the Era of Managed Care* (Oxford: Oxford University Press, 1999), 271; Robert H. Ebert, "Medical Education at the Peak of the Era of Experimental Medicine," *Daedalus* 115, no. 2 (1986): 55, 61, 69–70; "Warren Bicentennial Notes," in *University of Michigan: An Encyclopedic Survey, Bicentennial Edition* (Ann Arbor: Michigan Publishing, forthcoming), https://quod.lib.umich.edu/b/bicentennial; John C. Burnham, "American Medicine's Golden Age: What Happened to It?" *Science* 225 (March 1982): 1474, 1478; Charles G. Child to Allan F. Smith, February 10, 1971, "Af[firmative] Action, Women 1970–71" folder, Box 91, Medical School (University of Michigan) Records, 1850–2010, Bentley Historical Library.

5. W. N. Hubbard, Jr., to R. W. Fleming, January 14, 1969, "Compliance, General 1969" folder, Box 77, Medical School (University of Michigan) Records, 1850–2010, Bentley Historical Library.

6. Fleming to Cioffi, November 26, 1969.

7. Ibid. See also Frederick T. Cioffi to Dr. Robben [*sic*] Fleming, October 15, 1969, p. 4, "Compliance, General 1969" folder, Box 77, Medical School (University of Michigan) Records, 1850–2010, Bentley Historical Library.

8. Hubbard to Fleming, January 14, 1969. See also Ebert, "Medical Education," 71.

9. Stephen Selbst, "Black Conference Held," *Michigan Daily*, February 4, 1973, p. 1.

10. "Doctor Surplus Predicted," *Ann Arbor News*, September 30, 1980; Max Gates, "U-M Vows to Cut Medical School Enrollment 24% If State Maintains Aid Level," *Ann Arbor News*, December 17, 1982; Tarolli, "Epilogue," 301.

11. Ebert, "Medical Education," 69–71.

12. Jane Dorr, "Hospitals Fear Loss of U-M Medical Students," *Ann Arbor News*, June 7, 1982; Max Gates, "Regents OK Medical School Cut Despite Questions about Money," *Ann Arbor News*, February 26, 1983; Max Gates, "U-M Medical School Defers Enrollment Cut," *Ann Arbor News*, August 29, 1983.

13. Max Gates, "Medical Tuition to Reach $20,000 a Year?," *Ann Arbor News*, July 25, 1982.

14. "Appendix 2: Memorandum to Liaison Committee on Medical Education," May 14, 1982, p. 59, Box 2, University of Michigan (Medical School) Publications, Bentley Historical Library.

15. Ebert, "Medical Education," 78. See also Paul B. Beeson, "The Changing Role Model, and the Shift in Power," *Daedalus* 115, no. 2 (1986): 92.

16. "Report of the Survey of the University of Michigan Medical School, Ann Arbor, Michigan, May 14–17, 1990," p. 4, Box 2, University of Michigan (Medical School) Publications, Bentley Historical Library.

17. Horace W. Davenport, *Not Just Any Medical School: The Science, Practice, and Teaching of Medicine at the University of Michigan, 1850–1941* (Ann Arbor: University of Michigan Press, 1999), xi. See also Tarolli, "Epilogue," 301.

18. John W. Henderson, *The University of Michigan Department of Ophthalmology: A Proud Heritage.* (Ann Arbor: Department of Ophthalmology, University of Michigan, 1986), 162; "Historical Perspective—The Development of the Medical Service Plans at the University of Michigan," in *University of Michigan Medical Service Plans*

Annual Report, 1977, pp. A-1, A-2, Box 4, Medical School (University of Michigan) Publications, Bentley Historical Library.

19. Stern, "Innovation, Expansion, and Specialization"; see also Ludmerer, *Time to Heal*, 226.

20. Department of Radiology, "History of the Department of Radiology at the University of Michigan: From the Whitehouse Era to the Present Day," in *University of Michigan: An Encyclopedic Survey, Bicentennial Edition* (Ann Arbor: Michigan Publishing, forthcoming), https://quod.lib.umich.edu/b/bicentennial; "Impact of Medical Service Plans on Education, Research, Patient Care, Hospital Occupancy, and the Recruitment and Retention of Faculty," in *University of Michigan Medical Service Plans Annual Report*, 1977, p. C-3, Box 4, Medical School (University of Michigan) Publications, Bentley Historical Library.

21. Stern, "Innovation, Expansion, and Specialization"; Department of Obstetrics and Gynecology, "Annual Report," July 1, 1968–June 30, 1969, Box 3, Willson Papers, Bentley Historical Library, cited in ibid.

22. "Impact of Medical Service Plans," C-2.

23. Ibid., C-1–C-4; "Historical Perspective," A-3. See also Ludmerer, *Time to Heal*, 338.

24. "Impact of Medical Service Plans," C-3; Ebert, "Medical Education," 68; Child to Smith, February 10, 1971; "Historical Perspective" A-2, A-3.

25. "Warren Bicentennial Notes." See also Brinkman, *Encyclopedic Survey*, 5:185; Joel D. Howell, *Technology in the Hospital: Transforming Patient Care in the Early Twentieth Century* (Baltimore: Johns Hopkins University Press, 1995), 5–6; Beeson, "Changing Role Model," 93; Ludmerer, *Time to Heal*, xxiii, 269.

26. Department of Internal Medicine, "Recent History of the Michigan Department of Internal Medicine," in *University of Michigan: An Encyclopedic Survey, Bicentennial Edition* (Ann Arbor: Michigan Publishing, forthcoming), https://quod.lib.umich.edu/b/bicentennial.

27. "Impact of Medical Service Plans," C-3.

28. Ebert, "Medical Education," 58; see also "Memorandum to Liaison Committee," 59.

29. Department of Internal Medicine, "Recent History."

30. Ibid.; Stern, "Innovation, Expansion, and Specialization."

31. Brinkman, *Encyclopedic Survey*, 5:190–191; John A. D. Cooper et al., "Survey Report, University of Michigan School of Medicine, Ann Arbor, Michigan, 1958," p. 6, Box 2, Medical School (University of Michigan) Publications, Bentley Historical Library.

32. Department of Internal Medicine, "Recent History"; Stern, "Innovation, Expansion, and Specialization"; Department of Obstetrics and Gynecology, "The University of Michigan's Department of Obstetrics and Gynecology, 1964–2014: Milestones," Department of Neurosurgery, "History of Michigan Neurosurgery, 1967–2017," and Department of Biomedical Engineering, "Biomedical Engineering at Michigan: A Product of Vision and Persistence," in *University of Michigan: An Encyclopedic Survey, Bicentennial Edition* (Ann Arbor: Michigan Publishing, forthcoming), https://quod.lib.umich.edu/b/bicentennial. Before 2001, neurosurgery was a division within the Department of Surgery.

33. Department of Internal Medicine, "Recent History"; Department of Radiology, "History of the Department."

34. "Report of the Survey," 40.

35. Brinkman, *Encyclopedic Survey*, 5:211; Department of Internal Medicine, "Recent History."

36. Department of Internal Medicine, "Recent History."

37. Department of Pathology, "Overview of Research in the Department of Pathology: 1980–Present," in *University of Michigan: An Encyclopedic Survey, Bicentennial Edition* (Ann Arbor: Michigan Publishing, forthcoming), https://quod.lib.umich.edu/b/bicentennial. See also Department of Internal Medicine, "Recent History."

38. Department of Internal Medicine, "Recent History"; Department of Radiology, "History of the Department"; Department of Pathology, "Overview of Research."

39. Department of Internal Medicine, "Recent History."

40. Stern, "Innovation, Expansion, and Specialization."

41. "Report of the Survey," 40. See also Department of Internal Medicine, "Recent History."

42. Stern, "Innovation, Expansion, and Specialization."

43. Ludmerer, *Time to Heal*, 309, 331; "U-M College of Literature, Science and the Arts: Medical School; Task Force on Medical Education Report, July 30, 1984," pp. 21–22, Box 4, Medical School (University of Michigan) Publications, Bentley Historical Library.

44. Stephen Cain, "Changing Med School a Daunting Task," *Ann Arbor News*, March 14, 1996.

45. David Wahlberg, "Travel Necessary for Research, Education, Doctors at U-M Say," *Ann Arbor News*, September 14, 1997.

46. David Wahlberg, "U-M Faculty Worried about Tenured Jobs," *Ann Arbor News*, March 21, 1998.

47. "Table I: Active Instructional Staff by School or College, Title and Sex; The University of Michigan, Fall 1970," "Af[firmative] Action, Women 1970–71" folder, Box 91, Medical School (University of Michigan) Records, 1850–2010, Bentley Historical Library.

48. John M. Weller to Allan F. Smith, February 12, 1971, "Af[firmative] Action, Women 1970–71" folder, Box 91, Medical School (University of Michigan) Records, 1850–2010, Bentley Historical Library.

49. Child to Smith, February 10, 1971.

50. See Stern, "Innovation, Expansion, and Specialization."

51. "Report of the Survey," 63.

52. Stephen Cain, "Blacks See Med School as 'Cold,'" *Ann Arbor News*, March 13, 1996.

53. Cain, "Changing Med School a Daunting Task."

54. Hatcher, "Guest Editorial," 152. See also Ebert, "Medical Education," 56–57.

55. Department of Pathology, "Department of Pathology Teaching Programs," in *University of Michigan: An Encyclopedic Survey, Bicentennial Edition* (Ann Arbor: Michigan Publishing, forthcoming), https://quod.lib.umich.edu/b/bicentennial; Department of Radiology, "History of the Department." See also "Student Curriculum Evaluation: Part II," *Paeon*, January–February 1976, pp. 8–9, Box 5, Medical School (University of Michigan) Publications, Bentley Historical Library.

56. Dean's Committee on Curriculum Improvement, "Medical Education Retreat, May 17, 1991," p. 1, Box 4, Medical School (University of Michigan) Publications, Bentley Historical Library. See also Brinkman, *Encyclopedic Survey*, 5:188.

57. Integrated Premedical/Medical Program brochure, [1983?], "Brochures 1975–1997, undated" folder, p. 1, Box 1, U-M Integrated Premedical/Medical Program Publications, Bentley Historical Library.

58. "U-M College of Literature," 7, 12; Tarolli, "Epilogue," 300–301.

59. "Minority Students Can Explore Careers," *Ann Arbor News*, April 28, 1995.

60. Alphonse R. Burdi, "The University of Michigan's Alternative Pathway to Becoming a Successful Physician: Inteflex," [1988?], Box 1, U-M Integrated Premedical/Medical Program Publications, Bentley Historical Library. See also "U-M College of Literature," 1, 12; and Brinkman, *Encyclopedic Survey*, 5:188.

61. "Scott E. Ewing, Ex-Student, Appeals Dismissal," *Michigan Daily*, April 2, 1983; Stuart Taylor, Jr., "High Court Backs Dismissal of Michigan Medical Student," *New York Times*, December 13, 1985; "Student Loses Bid in High Court," *Chicago Tribune*, December 13, 1985.

62. "Appendix C: Problems Associated with the Current Medical School Environment," in *Report to the Dean from the Dean's Committee on Curriculum Improvement*, November 1991, Box 4, Medical School (University of Michigan) Publications, Bentley Historical Library. The previous year during its accreditation site visit the LCME recommended keeping the Inteflex program but suggested that its management not be separated from medical school administration, presumably for the same reason. "Report of the Survey," 6.

63. "U-M College of Literature," 12.

64. Ebert, "Medical Education," 56.

65. "Memorandum to Liaison Committee," 60.

66. Dean's Committee on Curriculum Improvement, "Medical Education Retreat," 14.

67. William Thompson, "U-Nevada Doctor Wants Stress on Patient Care," *Michigan Daily*, December 9, 1978, p. 2.

68. "U-M College of Literature," 6; Dean's Committee on Curriculum Improvement, "Medical Education Retreat," 5, 11–12, 14; "Appendix C"; "The University of Michigan Medical School: Curriculum for the 21st Century," [1993?], p. iv, Box 1, Medical School (University of Michigan) Publications, Bentley Historical Library. See also Ludmerer, *Time to Heal*, xxiv, 233.

69. "U-M College of Literature," 7–9; "Curriculum for the 21st Century," 23–24. See also "Report of the Survey," 73. According to Janet Tarolli, "More than 50 percent of the clinical education of medical students occurred at hospitals other than University Hospital," including Henry Ford Hospital, Wayne County General Hospital, St. Joseph Mercy Hospital, and the VA Hospital. Tarolli, "Epilogue," 301.

70. Department of Internal Medicine, "Recent History"; Mary Morgan, "High-Tech Teaching Tool," *Ann Arbor News*, June 9, 1999; Kim Clarke, "Anatomically Correct," *Ann Arbor News*, October 21, 1993; "Medical Donors: Gift Adds to Memory of Deceased," *Ann Arbor News*, September 15, 1996.

71. Max Gates, "Getting Doctors to Think about Prevention," *Ann Arbor News*, December 11, 1982.

72. "Curriculum for the 21st Century," 26.

73. "Report of the Survey," 2–5. See also "Curriculum for the 21st Century," 3–4, 6. The 1993 document is decidedly less critical than the accreditation reports on these issues.

74. "Curriculum for the 21st Century," i–ii, 2; Dean's Committee on Curriculum Improvement, "Medical Education Retreat," 1.

75. Dean's Committee on Curriculum Improvement, "Medical Education Retreat," 3–4; Department of Pathology, "Department of Pathology Teaching Programs." See also "Curriculum for the 21st Century," 4, 12–13, 19.

76. Julie Wiernik, "Med School Brings in Human Factor," *Ann Arbor News*, April 26, 1992.

77. David Wahlberg, "Alternative Medicine Gains Ground," *Ann Arbor News*, September 4, 1998. This article also notes that the medical school applied for an NIH grant to study Chinese *qi* and therapeutic touch healing to help patients recover from surgery.

78. "Curriculum for the 21st Century," iii, iv.

79. Ibid., iv, 6, 11.

80. Dean's Committee on Curriculum Improvement, "Medical Education Retreat," 13.

81. Ibid., 10 (emphasis in original).

82. Ludmerer, *Time to Heal*, xxiii. See also Ebert, "Medical Education," 74; and Department of Internal Medicine, "Recent History."

83. "Department of Internal Medicine Annual Report, University of Michigan," 1982, pp. 11, 16, in the author's possession; Department of Internal Medicine, "Recent History."

84. Department of Internal Medicine, "Recent History."

85. "Warren Bicentennial Notes"; Department of Pathology, "Anatomic Pathology, 1970–2014," in *University of Michigan: An Encyclopedic Survey, Bicentennial Edition* (Ann Arbor: Michigan Publishing, forthcoming), https://quod.lib.umich.edu/b/bicentennial.

86. Henderson, *Department of Ophthalmology*, 179–180, 186–187; Brinkman, *Encyclopedic Survey*, 5:197–198; Stern, "Innovation, Expansion, and Specialization."

87. Department of Radiology, "History of the Department."

88. Department of Internal Medicine, "Recent History"; Stern, "Innovation, Expansion, and Specialization."

89. Department of Radiology, "History of the Department."

90. "U-M Hails Hospital Verdict," *Ann Arbor News*, August 18, 1981; Larry Bush, "Hospital Helps Medical School," *Ann Arbor News*, October 16, 1981.

91. Stern, "Innovation, Expansion, and Specialization"; Department of Internal Medicine, "Recent History."

92. Department of Pathology, "Anatomic Pathology"; Liz Cobbs, "U-M M-Labs to Perform Autopsies," *Ann Arbor News*, June 5, 1993.

93. Department of Internal Medicine, "Recent History"; Department of Radiology, "History of the Department."

94. Department of Emergency Medicine, "The History of the Department of Emergency Medicine at Michigan," in *University of Michigan: An Encyclopedic Survey, Bicentennial Edition* (Ann Arbor: Michigan Publishing, forthcoming), https://quod.lib.umich.edu/b/bicentennial.

95. Stern, "Innovation, Expansion, and Specialization"; Brinkman, *Encyclopedic Survey*, 5:197.

96. "Abortion: U-M Ob-Gyn Chief Takes Bold Step," *Ann Arbor News*, July 21, 1993. See also Stern, "Innovation, Expansion, and Specialization."

97. Tarolli, "Epilogue," 299.

98. See "The University of Michigan Medical School Recognition Ceremony for Members of the AIMED Class of 1987, May 1, 1987," Box 2, University of Michigan (Medical School) Publications, Bentley Historical Library; and "Grant Will Aid Needy U-M Medical Students," *Ann Arbor News*, October 5, 1972. AIMED is an acronym for Assistance to Increase Matriculation and Earn Degrees and was adopted at Michigan as the result of a 1984 grant.

99. See examples from 1955, 1970, 1978, and 1982 in "Medical School Printed Brochures" folder, Box 1, Medicine, 1955–1994, Medical School (University of Michigan) Publications, Bentley Historical Library.

100. Gates, "Medical Tuition to Reach $20,000 a Year?" See also "25% Cutback Proposed for U-M Medical School," *Ann Arbor News*, November 4, 1981.

101. "Medical Students Fighting Tuition Hikes," *Ann Arbor News*, November 25, 1975; "Student Debt Worries Medical, Dental Units," *Ann Arbor News*, March 16, 1978; "Regents Hear Tuition Complaints," *Michigan Daily*, May 1978; "Report of the Survey," 29.

102. Max Gates, "Money Is Rx for Medical Students," *Ann Arbor News*, September 4, 1980.

103. "The Medical Students Guide to Life in Ann Arbor," 1974, p. 2, Box 5, Medical School (University of Michigan) Publications, Bentley Historical Library.

104. Ibid., 5–7. It is worth noting that community service opportunities were missing from later editions of the handbook, such as the 1977–1978 version.

105. Ibid., 19. The medical students of the 1970s were certainly not the first to indulge in recreational use of cannabis, but the forthright mention of it in the student handbook is telling of how common the practice had become at that time.

106. "U-M College of Literature," 14.

107. "Study Center to Hold Open House," *Ann Arbor News*, June 7, 1974. See also "Memorandum to Liaison Committee," 31, 60; "Report of the Survey," 30; and Julie Selbst, "Campus Buildings Honored with Architecture Awards," *Michigan Daily*, September 15, 1979, p. 3.

108. "U-M College of Literature," 6. See also Ebert, "Medical Education," 71.

109. Memorandum from Office of the Dean to Drs. Gronvall, Green, DeMuth, Campbell, and Votaw, September 7, 1972, "Enrollment Expansion, 1965–1972" folder, Box 78, Medical School (University of Michigan) Records, 1850–2010, Bentley Historical Library.

110. "Grant Will Aid Needy U-M Medical Students."

111. University of Michigan news release, January 22, 1973, "Student Organizations—Black Med Assoc, 1973–79" folder, Box 235, Medical School (University of Michigan) Records, 1850–2010, Bentley Historical Library. Examples of programs can be found in "Medical School Conferences/Symposia, Martin Luther King Day Commemorative Health Care Program" folder, Box 5, Medical School (University of Michigan) Publications, Bentley Historical Library.

112. "Thirteenth Conference on Ethics, Humanism, and Medicine," March 16, 1985, Box 5, Medical School (University of Michigan) Records, 1850–2010, Bentley Historical Library.

113. See Ebert, "Medical Education," 72.

114. Ibid., 67, 73.

115. "U-M Medical Dean Favors Plan to Freeze Enrollment," *Ann Arbor News*, April 3, 1981; "Grant Will Aid Needy U-M Medical Students."

116. Kim Clarke, "'Match Day' Shows the Way," *Ann Arbor News*, March 17, 1994. See also David Wahlberg, "Primary Choice: Primary Care," *Ann Arbor News*, March 19, 1998; and Ebert, "Medical Education," 73.

117. Cain, "Blacks See Med School as 'Cold.'"

118. Ludmerer, *Time to Heal*, 252, 300.

119. Cain, "Blacks See Med School as 'Cold.'"

120. Donald L. Rucknagel and David E. Schteingart to University Medical Center personnel, February 23, 1972, "Compliance, General" folder, Box 77, Medical School (University of Michigan) Records, 1850–2010, Bentley Historical Library; Bernard N. Stulberg to Executive Committee, February 16, 1973, and BMA to John Gronvall, December 14, 1976, "Student Organizations—Black Med Assoc, 1973–79" folder, Box 235, Medical School (University of Michigan) Records, 1850–2010, Bentley Historical Library. The 1976 letter was copied to a number of other recipients, including the National Association for the Advancement of Colored People, Urban League, and William L. Cash, Jr., assistant to the president for human relations.

121. Miguel West to John Gronvall, April 4, 1979, "Student Organizations—Black Med Assoc, 1973–79" folder, Box 235, Medical School (University of Michigan) Records, 1850–2010, Bentley Historical Library.

122. Cain, "Changing Med School a Daunting Task."

123. "Report of the Survey," 5. See also "Appendix C." Minority enrollments continued to decline during the late 1990s. See David Wahlberg, "Ethnic Diversity Enriches College, Former Students Say," *Ann Arbor News*, January 16, 1998.

124. Cain, "Blacks See Med School as 'Cold.'" This article was reporting on results of a cultural diversity assessment conducted at Michigan by Nichols and Associates, an outside firm.

125. Delia M. Rios and Reshma Kapadia, "A New Prescription," *Ann Arbor News*, November 20, 1994. See also Ebert, "Medical Education," 75.

126. Jennifer Bagwell, "New Medical Students Begin Their Climb," *Ann Arbor News*, August 18, 1997; William B. Treml, "Rarin' to Go: Match Day Party Is Good Medicine for U-M's Next Crop of Doctors," *Ann Arbor News*, March 21, 1996.

127. "Department of Medicine, University of Michigan, 1995–96 Annual Report," p. 1, Box 1, Department of Internal Medicine (University of Michigan) Publications, Bentley Historical Library; David Wahlberg and Stephen Cain, "U-M May Consolidate Hospitals, Med School," *Ann Arbor News*, July 3, 1996.

128. Ludmerer, *Time to Heal*, xxv.

EPILOGUE

1. Samuel W. Bloom, "Structure and Ideology in Medical Education: An Analysis of Resistance to Change," *Journal of Health and Social Behavior* 29 (1988): 294–306.

2. Joel D. Howell, "Introduction," in *Medical Lives and Scientific Medicine at Michigan, 1891–1969*, ed. Joel D. Howell (Ann Arbor: University of Michigan Press, 1993), 4–5.

Bibliography

DIGITIZED COLLECTIONS

Ann Arbor District Library. *Ann Arbor City Council Meeting Minutes*. http://councilminutes.aadl.org/.

Ann Arbor District Library. *Old News*. http://oldnews.aadl.org/.

Proceedings of the Board of Regents. Ann Arbor: University of Michigan, 2000. http://quod.lib.umich.edu/u/umregproc/.

University of Michigan. *University of Michigan: An Encyclopedic Survey, Bicentennial Edition*. Ann Arbor: Michigan Publishing, forthcoming. https://quod.lib.umich.edu/b/bicentennial.

MANUSCRIPT COLLECTIONS AT BENTLEY HISTORICAL LIBRARY, UNIVERSITY OF MICHIGAN, ANN ARBOR

Board of Regents (University of Michigan) Records, 1817–2011
Class of 1849 (University of Michigan) Records, 1889 and 1899
Department of Internal Medicine (University of Michigan) Publications
Homeopathic Medical School (University of Michigan) Records
Hospitals (University of Michigan) Records
Medical School (University of Michigan) Publications
Medical School (University of Michigan) Records, 1850–2010
Reuben Peterson Papers
Royal S. Copeland Papers
Walter H. Sawyer Papers
Washtenaw Country Historical Society Records

NEWSPAPERS

Alpena (MI) Weekly Argus
Ann Arbor Argus

Ann Arbor Courier
Ann Arbor Daily News
Ann Arbor News
Ann Arbor Observer
Ann Arbor Register
Chicago Tribune
Copper County Evening News (Calumet, MI)
Detroit Evening Journal
Detroit Evening News
Detroit Free Press
Detroit Tribune
Michigan Daily
New York Times
Toledo Blade
True Northerner (Paw Paw, MI)
Weekly Expositor (Brockway Centre, MI)
Yale (MI) Expositor

PUBLISHED PRIMARY SOURCES

Allen, J. Adams. *Introductory Address to the Third Session of the College of Medicine and Surgery of the University of Michigan.* Detroit: George E. Pomeroy, 1852.

Baker, Henry B. "Notes Relative to the Benefits of Vaccination." Supplement, *Proceedings, Addresses, and Discussions at the Second Annual Conference of the Health Officers in Michigan, at Ann Arbor, Mich., June 14 and 15, 1894: Report of the Michigan State Board of Health*, no. 417 (1894): 50–59.

Baker, Henry B. "Poisonous Cheese." In *Twelfth Annual Report of the Secretary of the State Board of Health of the State of Michigan for the Fiscal Year Ending September 30, 1884*, 122–128. Lansing, MI: W. S. George, 1885.

Beech, J. H. "An Address to the Graduating Class of the Medical Department of the University of Michigan." *Peninsular and Independent Medical Journal* 1 (May 1858): 65–81.

Christian, Henry A. "The Significance and Relationships of the Thomas Henry Simpson Memorial Institute for Medical Research." *Science* 65 (April 1927): 359–361.

Coggeshall, Lowell T. *Planning for Medical Progress through Education.* Evanston, IL: Association of American Medical Colleges, 1975.

Cooper, John A. "Educational Patterns in Medicine." *University of Michigan Medical Bulletin* 24 (August 1958): 316–324.

Copeland, Royal Samuel. "The New Homoeopathic Hospital and Nurses' Home." *Michigan Alumnus* 7 (November 1900): 54–56.

Dock, George. "Mosquitoes and Malaria: The Present Knowledge of Their Relations, with Some Observations in Ann Arbor and Vicinity." *Journal of the Michigan State Medical Society* 2 (February 1903): 37–45.

Dock, George. "Some Reasons Why There Should Be a Hospital for Consumptives in Connection with the University Hospital." *Physician and Surgeon* 24 (1902): 60–65.

Dock, George. "The University Hospital: Its Past, Present, and Future." *Michigan Alumnus* 9 (1903): 183–192.

Dock, George, and T. L. Chadbourne. "An Etiologic Study of Tuberculosis in Country-People." *Philadelphia Medical Journal* 2 (1898): 966–970.

"Eclecticism." *Michigan Homoeopathic Journal* 2, no. 9 (1854): 163–166.

Eldridge, I. N. "Some Fragmentary Reminiscences of the Early History of Homeopathy in Michigan." *Journal of the American Institute of Homeopathy* 39, no. 3 (1946): 71–75, 86; *Journal of the American Institute of Homeopathy* 39, no. 4 (1946): 112–116, 118.

"The Etiology of Cholera." *Nature* 33 (December 1885): 97–98.

Flexner, Abraham. *Medical Education in the United States and Canada: A Report to the Carnegie Foundation for the Advancement of Teaching.* New York: Carnegie Foundation for the Advancement of Teaching, 1910. http://www.carnegiefoundation.org/sites/default/files/elibrary/Carnegie_Flexner_Report.pdf.

Furstenberg, A. C. "Conclusion." *University of Michigan Medical Bulletin* 24 (August 1958): 337–338.

Furstenberg, A. C. "History and Purpose of the Teaching Institute." *University of Michigan Medical Bulletin* 24 (August 1958): 295–296.

[Gunn, Moses]. "Removal of the Medical Department." *Peninsular and Independent Medical Journal* 1 (May 1858): 106–111.

Harnack, Robert S. "How Do We Go about Doing It?" *University of Michigan Medical Bulletin* 24 (August 1958): 306–311.

Hatcher, Harlan. "Address of Welcome." *University of Michigan Medical Bulletin* 24 (August 1958): 293–294.

Hatcher, Harlan. "Guest Editorial: The University and the Medical School." *University of Michigan Medical Center Journal* 33 (July–August 1967): 151–152.

Haynes, Harley A. "The University Hospital: University of Michigan." *Methods and Problems of Medical Education* 18 (1930): 59–74.

Hewlett, Albion Walter. "Eight Years in the Department of Internal Medicine." *Transactions of the Clinical Society of the University of Michigan* 7 (June 1916): 146–149.

Hinerman, D. L. "Introduction: Our Challenge for the Future of Medical Education." *University of Michigan Medical Bulletin* 24 (August 1958): 291–292.

Hodges, Fred Jenner. "Origin and Growth of Michigan's Medical Center." *University of Michigan Medical Bulletin* 16 (September 1950): 233–242.

Kedzie, Robert C. "The Early Days of the Medical Department." *Michigan Alumnus* 8 (1902): 205–208.

Lewis, Sinclair. *Arrowsmith.* New York: Signet, 1998.

McCotter, Rollo. "A History of the Anatomy Department of the University of Michigan." Address given at honorary dinner, February 7, 1947. Bentley Historical Library.

McGraw, Theodore A. "The Medical Schools of the Last Half-Century." *Journal of the Michigan State Medical Society* 14 (1915): 514–517.

"Milk and Its Relation to the Public Health." Special issue, *Hygienic Laboratory Bulletin*, no. 56 (1909).

Miller, George E. "What Are We Trying to Do?" *University of Michigan Medical Bulletin* 24 (August 1958): 297–303.

Morantz, Regina Markell, Cynthia Stodola Pomerleau, and Carol Hansen Fenichel, eds. *In Her Own Words: Oral Histories of Women Physicians.* New Haven, CT: Yale University Press, 1982.

Mulheron, John J. "Addresses: I." In *Memorial Addresses and Resolutions on George E. Frothingham, M.D.*, 1–7. Detroit: Wayne County Medical Society, [1900?]. http://catalog.hathitrust.org/Record/003200539.

Nightingale, Florence. *Notes on Hospitals.* 3rd ed. London: Longman, Green, Longman, Roberts, and Green, 1863.

Palmer, A. B. "Report to the State Society on the Diseases of Children." *Peninsular and Independent Medical Journal* 1 (May 1858): 89–99.

Peterson, Reuben. "The New Contagious Hospital at the University of Michigan and Its Proposed Plan of Operation." *Journal of the Michigan State Medical Society*, May 1914. https://catalog.hathitrust.org/Record/003304297.

Pitcher, Zina. *An Address to the First Graduates of the Medical Department of the University of Michigan.* Detroit: William Harsha, 1851.

Sewall, Henry. "Experiments on the Preventive Inoculation of Rattlesnake Venom." *Journal of Physiology* 8 (August 1887): 203–210.

Smith, Edgar B. "Addresses: II." In *Memorial Addresses and Resolutions on George E. Frothingham, M.D.*, 7–8. Detroit: Wayne County Medical Society, [1900?]. http://catalog.hathitrust.org/Record/003200539.

The Social Secretary of Detroit. Detroit: Social Secretary, 1922.

"Some Observations on Activities of the Institute Panels." *University of Michigan Medical Bulletin* 24 (August 1958): 312–315.

Sturgis, Cyrus C. *Hematology.* Springfield, IL: Charles C. Thomas, 1947.

Sturgis, Cyrus C. "The Thomas Henry Simpson Memorial Institute for Medical Research." *Phi Chi Quarterly* 25 (May 1928): 602–609.

"Summary of Activities of the Discussion Panels." *University of Michigan Medical Bulletin* 24 (August 1958): 325–337.

Towsley, Harry A. "Introduction: The Goals of Medical Television." *University of Michigan Medical Bulletin* 28 (November 1962): 303–304.

Vaughan, Victor. "Appendix 3: The Michigan State Board of Health." In *A Doctor's Memories.* Indianapolis, IN: Bobbs-Merrill, 1926. http://vaughan.org/bios/vcv/aDoctorsMemories/Text/vcvmemAp3.html.

Vaughan, Victor. "Poisonous Cheese." In *Thirteenth Annual Report of the Secretary of the State Board of Health of the State of Michigan for the Fiscal Year Ending September 30, 1885*, 221–226. Lansing, MI: W. S. George, 1886.

Vaughan, Victor C., and Frederick G. Novy. *Ptomaines and Leucomaines, or the Putrefactive and Physiological Alkaloids.* Philadelphia: Lea Brothers, 1888.

Warthin, Aldred Scott. "The University Medical School and the State." In *Indiana University, 1820–1920: Centennial Memorial Volume*, 157–162. Bloomington: Indiana University, 1921.

Watson, E. H. "By Precept: A Critical Appraisal of Medical Teaching." *Medical Education* 28 (May 1953): 11–16.

Wilkinson, Charles F. "Intern Training in the Hospital System." *Rhode Island Medical Journal* 31 (March 1947): 201–206.

SECONDARY SOURCES

Abowd, Thomas V., Tom R. De Meester, and Donald Lucas. "Our Heritage: A History of the Medical School." *University of Michigan Medical Center Journal* 33 (1967): 172–201.

Ackerknecht, Erwin H. *A Short History of Medicine.* Baltimore: Johns Hopkins University Press, 1982.

Ahuja, Nitin K. "Fordism in the Hospital: Albert Kahn and the Design of Old Main, 1917–25." *Journal of the History of Medicine and Allied Sciences* 67 (2011): 398–427.

Anderson, Fanny J. "The Role of the Physician in the History of the State of Michigan before the Civil War, 1837–1861." Typescript, 1972. Bentley Historical Library.

Ann Arbor District Library. "AACHM Oral History: Rosemarion Blake." February 14, 2013. http://www.aadl.org/aachmvideos/rosemarion_blake.

Ann Arbor District Library. "Ann Arbor: Population and Size." http://www.aadl.org/research/a2populationandsize (accessed February 27, 2017).

Attaway, Doris E., and Marjorie Rabe Barritt, eds. *Women's Voices: Early Years at the University of Michigan.* Ann Arbor, MI: Bentley Historical Library, 2000.

Bass, Christine Kae. "'It Did Not Seem like a Hospital, It Seemed like Home': Women's Experiences as Patients at Peterson's Hospital, Ann Arbor, Michigan, 1902–1933." Ph.D. diss., Program in American Culture, University of Michigan, 1999.

Beecher, Harry K., and Mark D. Altschule. *Medicine at Harvard: The First Three Hundred Years.* Hanover, NH: University Press of New England, 1977.

Beeson, Paul B. "The Changing Role Model, and the Shift in Power." *Daedalus* 115, no. 2 (1986): 83–97.

Bentley Historical Library. "Galens Medical Society Records: 1914–2001." http://quod.lib.umich.edu/b/bhlead/umich-bhl-9859?rgn=Entire+Finding+Aid;view=text;q1=galens (accessed February 27, 2017).

Bloom, Samuel W. "Structure and Ideology in Medical Education: An Analysis of Resistance to Change." *Journal of Health and Social Behavior* 29 (1988): 294–306.

Bonner, Thomas Neville. *Becoming a Physician: Medical Education in Britain, France, Germany, and the United States, 1750–1945.* Baltimore: Johns Hopkins University Press, 1995.

Bonner, Thomas Neville. "Searching for Abraham Flexner." *Academic Medicine* 73 (February 1998): 160–166.

Bonner, Thomas Neville. *To the Ends of the Earth: Women's Search for Education in Medicine.* Cambridge, MA: Harvard University Press, 1992.

Boster, Dea. "Finding the 'Sick' in Cheese: Victor Vaughan and Michigan Public Health in the Late 19th Century." *Medicine at Michigan* 17 (Winter 2015): 14–15.

Boster, Dea. "Founding the Simpson Memorial." *Medicine at Michigan* 17 (Fall–Winter 2015): 12–13.

Boster, Dea. "War of the Pathies: The Conflict around Homeopathic Medicine at Michigan in the Mid-19th Century." *Medicine at Michigan* 17 (Summer 2015): 12–13.

Brandt, Allan M., and Martha Gardner. "Antagonism and Accommodation: Interpreting the Relationship between Public Health and Medicine in the United States during the 20th Century." *American Journal of Public Health* 90 (May 2000): 707–715.

Brinkman, Ferol B., ed. *The University of Michigan: An Encyclopedic Survey*. Vol. 5, *The University of Michigan, 1940–75*. Ann Arbor: University of Michigan Bentley Historical Library, 1977. http://quod.lib.umich.edu/u/umsurvey/AAS3302.0005.001/1:1?rgn=div1;view=fulltext.

Brown, Elizabeth Gaspar. "Notes on the University Hospital: The Early Decades." *Michigan Quarterly Review* 3 (1964): 8–17.

Brown, Ida C. "Introduction." In *Michigan Men in the Civil War: A Guide to the Resources in the Bentley Historical Library (1959–1977)*. Ann Arbor: University of Michigan. http://bentley.umich.edu/legacy-support/civilwar/introduction.php (accessed February 24, 2017).

Burnham, John C. "American Medicine's Golden Age: What Happened to It?" *Science* 225 (March 1982): 1474–1479.

Burnham, John C. *What Is Medical History?* Cambridge, UK: Polity, 2005.

Cornell, Virginia. *Doc Susie: The True Story of a Country Physician in the Colorado Rockies.* New York: Ballantine, 1991.

Crenner, Christopher. *Private Practice: In the Early Twentieth-Century Medical Office of Dr. Richard Cabot.* Baltimore: Johns Hopkins University Press, 2005.

Cummings, Howard H. "The Early History of Psi Chapter of Phi Chi." *Phi Chi Quarterly* 25, no. 4 (1928): 612–621.

Davenport, Horace W. *Doctor Dock: Teaching and Learning Medicine at the Turn of the Century.* New Brunswick, NJ: Rutgers University Press, 1987.

Davenport, Horace W. "George Dock at Michigan, 1891–1908." In *Medical Lives and Scientific Medicine at Michigan, 1891–1969*, edited by Joel D. Howell, 29–44. Ann Arbor: University of Michigan Press, 1993.

Davenport, Horace W. *Not Just Any Medical School: The Science, Practice, and Teaching of Medicine at the University of Michigan, 1850–1941.* Ann Arbor: University of Michigan Press, 1999.

Davenport, Horace W. *University of Michigan Surgeons, 1850–1970.* Ann Arbor: University of Michigan Historical Center for the Health Sciences, 1993.

"Detroit Population History, 1900–2000." *Somacon*, September 7, 2015. http://www.somacon.com/p469.php.

Donnelly, Walter A., Wilfred B. Shaw, and Ruth W. Gjelsness, eds. *The University of Michigan: An Encyclopedic Survey*. Vol. 4. Ann Arbor: University of Michigan Press, 1958. http://quod.lib.umich.edu/u/umsurvey/AAS3302.0004.001/1:1?rgn=div1;view=fulltext.

Doolen, Richard M. "The Founding of the University of Michigan Hospital: An Innovation in Medical Education." *Journal of Medical Education* 39 (January 1964): 50–57.

Duffin, Jacalyn. *History of Medicine: A Scandalously Short Introduction*. Toronto: University of Toronto Press, 2001.

Ebert, Robert H. "Medical Education at the Peak of the Era of Experimental Medicine." *Daedalus* 115, no. 2 (1986): 55–81.

Farley, Reynolds, Sheldon Danziger, and Harry J. Holzer. *Detroit Divided.* New York: Russell Sage Foundation, 2000.

Farmer, Silas. *History of Detroit and Wayne County and Early Michigan: A Chronological Cyclopedia of the Past and Present.* Vol. 1. 3rd ed. Detroit: Silas Farmer, 1890. https://babel.hathitrust.org/cgi/pt?id=mdp.39015071373867;view=1up;seq=15.

Fye, W. Bruce. "Albion Walter Hewlett: Teacher, Clinician, Scientist, and Missionary for 'Pathologic Physiology.'" In *Medical Lives and Scientific Medicine at Michigan, 1891–1969*, edited by Joel D. Howell, 45–72. Ann Arbor: University of Michigan Press, 1993.

Fye, W. Bruce. *The Development of American Physiology: Scientific Medicine in the Nineteenth Century.* Baltimore: Johns Hopkins University Press, 1987.

Geist, Edward. "When Ice Cream Was Poisonous: Adulteration, Ptomaines, and Bacteriology in the United States, 1850–1910." *Bulletin of the History of Medicine* 86 (Fall 2012): 333–360.

Harvey, A. McGhee. *Science at the Bedside: Clinical Research in American Medicine, 1905–1945.* Baltimore: Johns Hopkins University Press, 1981.

Henderson, John W. *The University of Michigan Department of Ophthalmology: A Proud Heritage.* Ann Arbor: Department of Ophthalmology, University of Michigan, 1986.

Howell, Joel D. "Introduction." In *Medical Lives and Scientific Medicine at Michigan, 1891–1969*, edited by Joel D. Howard, 1–11. Ann Arbor: University of Michigan Press, 1993.

Howell, Joel D. "Lowell T. Coggeshall and American Medical Education: 1901–1987." *Academic Medicine* 67 (1992): 711–718.

Howell, Joel D. *Technology in the Hospital: Transforming Patient Care in the Early Twentieth Century.* Baltimore: Johns Hopkins University Press, 1995.

Howell, Joel D. "Telling Michigan's Story." *Medicine at Michigan* 18, no. 1 (2016). http://www.medicineatmichigan.org/history/2016/spring/telling-michigans-story.

Hubbard, William N., Jr., and Nicholas H. Steneck. *The Origins of Michigan's Leadership in the Health Sciences.* Ann Arbor: University of Michigan Historical Center for the Health Sciences, 1995.

Huelke, Donald F. "The History of the Department of Anatomy, the University of Michigan: Part I, 1850 to 1894." *University of Michigan Medical Bulletin* 27 (1961): 1–27.

Humphreys, Margaret. *Marrow of Tragedy: The Health Crisis of the American Civil War.* Baltimore: Johns Hopkins University Press, 2013.

Johnson, Georgia A. Lewis. *Black Graduates of the University of Michigan (1872–1960 Inclusive) and Selected Black Michigan Physicians.* Lansing, MI: Georgia A. Johnson, 1994.

Kaufman, Martin. "American Medical Education." In *The Education of American Physicians: Historical Essays*, edited by Ronald L. Numbers, 7–28. Berkeley: University of California Press, 1980.

Kazanjian, Powel H. "The Beginnings of Bacteriology in American Medicine: Works of Frederick Novy, 1888–1933." Ph.D. diss., University of Michigan, 2012.

Kazanjian, Powel H. *Frederick Novy and the Development of Bacteriology in Medicine.* New Brunswick, NJ: Rutgers University Press, 2017.

Kobayashi, Victor N. "From 'Germ Theory' to Bacteriology: A Case in Academic Freedom at the University of Michigan." Unpublished paper, 1962.

Konnak, John W., and Dev S. Pardanani. *A History of Urology at the University of Michigan 1920–2001.* Ann Arbor: University of Michigan Historical Center for the Health Sciences, 2002.

Lawrence, Susan C. "Iowa Physicians: Legitimacy, Institutions, and the Practice of Medicine; Part One: Establishing a Professional Identity, 1833–1886." *Annals of Iowa* 62 (Spring 2003): 151–200.

Leavitt, Judith Walzer. *Brought to Bed: Childbearing in America, 1750–1950*. New York: Oxford University Press, 1986.

Longo, Lawrence D. "Obstetrics and Gynecology." In *The Education of American Physicians: Historical Essays*, edited by Ronald L. Numbers, 205–225. Berkeley: University of California Press, 1980.

Lubeck, Marvin J. "History of the Galens Honorary Medical Society." *Medical Bulletin* 21 (February 1955): 41–50.

Ludmerer, Kenneth M. *Learning to Heal: The Development of American Medical Education*. New York: Basic Books, 1985.

Ludmerer, Kenneth M. "The Rise of the Teaching Hospital in America." *Journal of the History of Medicine and Allied Sciences* 38 (1983): 389–414.

Ludmerer, Kenneth M. *Time to Heal: American Medical Education from the Turn of the Century to the Era of Managed Care*. Oxford: Oxford University Press, 1999.

Ludmerer, Kenneth M. "The University of Michigan Medical School: A Tradition of Leadership." In *Medical Lives and Scientific Medicine at Michigan, 1891–1969*, edited by Joel D. Howell, 13–27. Ann Arbor: University of Michigan Press, 1993.

Lurie, Stephen. "Innovation and Service Traditional at University of Michigan Medical School." *Journal of the American Medical Association* 283, no. 7 (2000): 865–866.

Marinch, Carol. "A Fair Chance for the Girls: Medical Education for Women at the University of Michigan, 1870–1890." Senior Resident Research Project, Department of Internal Medicine, University of Michigan, 1986.

Markel, Howard. "Foreword." In *Not Just Any Medical School: The Science, Practice, and Teaching of Medicine at the University of Michigan, 1850–1941*, by Horace W. Davenport, v–vii. Ann Arbor: University of Michigan Press, 1999.

Markel, Howard. "The University of Michigan Medical School, 1850–2000: 'An Example Worthy of Imitation.'" *Journal of the American Medical Association* 283, no. 7 (2000): 915–920.

Markel, Howard. "When It Rains It Pours: Endemic Goiter, Iodized Salt, and David Murray Cowie." *American Journal of Public Health* 77 (1987): 219–229.

Martin, Steven C. "Cyrus Cressey Sturgis and American Internal Medicine, 1913–1957." In *Medical Lives and Scientific Medicine at Michigan, 1891–1969*, edited by Joel D. Howell, 73–100. Ann Arbor: University of Michigan Press, 1993.

Marwil, Jonathan. *A History of Ann Arbor*. Ann Arbor: University of Michigan Press, 1990.

Mayer, Frederick W. *A Setting for Excellence: The Story of the Planning and Development of the Ann Arbor Campus of the University of Michigan*. Ann Arbor: University of Michigan Press, 2015.

McGuigan, Dorothy Gies. *A Dangerous Experiment: 100 Years of Women at the University of Michigan*. Benton Harbor: University of Michigan Center for Continuing Education of Women, 1970.

McIntyre, Charles H. "Victor C. Vaughan." In *Builders of American Medicine: Being a Collection of Original Papers Read before the Victor C. Vaughan Society of the*

University of Michigan Medical School, 217–243. Ann Arbor, MI: George Wahr, 1932.

Melosh, Barbara. *"The Physician's Hand": Work Culture and Conflict in American Nursing.* Philadelphia: Temple University Press, 1982.

M.F. "Building the Next Generation of African-American Physicians." *Medicine at Michigan* 4, no. 3 (2002): 34–35.

Morantz-Sanchez, Regina. *Sympathy and Science: Women Physicians in American Medicine*. Chapel Hill: University of North Carolina Press, 1985.

Numbers, Ronald L. "The Fall and Rise of the American Medical Profession." In *The Professions in American History*, edited by Nathan O. Hatch, 51–72. Notre Dame, IN: University of Notre Dame Press, 1988.

Oliver, Robert. *Making the Modern Medical School: The Wisconsin Stories.* Nantucket, MA: Science History, 2002.

Parascandola, John. *The Development of American Pharmacology: John J. Abel and the Shaping of a Discipline.* Baltimore: Johns Hopkins University Press, 1992.

Peckham, Howard H. *The Making of the University of Michigan, 1817–1992.* Edited by Margaret L. Steneck and Nicholas H. Steneck. Ann Arbor: University of Michigan Bentley Historical Library, 1994.

Peitzman, Steven J. "Louis Harry Newburgh and Metabolism at Michigan." In *Medical Lives and Scientific Medicine at Michigan, 1891–1969*, edited by Joel D. Howell, 129–151. Ann Arbor: University of Michigan Press, 1993.

Peterson, Reuben. "Landmarks in the Medical School: A Survey of the History of the University of Michigan Medical School and Its Hospital." *Michigan Alumnus Quarterly Review* 45 (April 1939): 196–202.

Prescott, Albert B. "Silas Hamilton Douglas: Founder of the Chemical Laboratory." Faculty History Project. http://www.lib.umich.edu/faculty-history/faculty/silas-hamilton-douglas/founder-chemical-laboratory (accessed February 24, 2017).

Putnam, Constance E. *The Science We Have Loved and Taught: Dartmouth Medical School's First Two Centuries.* Hanover, NH: University Press of New England, 2004.

Reverby, Susan M. *Ordered to Care: The Dilemma of American Nursing, 1850–1945.* Cambridge: Cambridge University Press, 1987.

Rogers, Naomi. "Thomas Francis, Jr.: From the Bench to the Field." In *Medical Lives and Scientific Medicine at Michigan, 1891–1969*, edited by Joel D. Howell, 161–187. Ann Arbor: University of Michigan Press, 1993.

Rosenberg, Charles E. *The Care of Strangers: The Rise of America's Hospital System.* New York: Basic Books, 1987.

Rosenberg, Charles E. "Martin Arrowsmith: The Scientist as Hero." In *No Other Gods: On Science and American Social Thought*, rev. ed., edited by Charles E. Rosenberg, 123–131. Baltimore: Johns Hopkins University Press, 1997.

Rosner, David. *A Once Charitable Enterprise: Hospitals and Health Care in Brooklyn and New York, 1885–1915*. Cambridge: Cambridge University Press, 1982.

Sappol, Michael. *A Traffic of Dead Bodies: Anatomy and Embodied Social Identity in Nineteenth-Century America.* Princeton, NJ: Princeton University Press, 2002.

Schopieray, Cheney J. "'Col[ore]d Men Are Not Admitted Here.'" *The Quarto* 46 (Fall–Winter 2016): 6–10.

"Section II: Development of the Institute's Research Activities." *Research News* 16, no. 4 (1965): 12–14.

Shaw, Wilfred B., ed. *The University of Michigan: An Encyclopedic Survey*. Vol. 1. Ann Arbor: University of Michigan Press, 1942. http://quod.lib.umich.edu/u/umsurvey/AAS3302.0001.001/1:1?rgn=div1;view=fulltext.

Shaw, Wilfred B., ed. *The University of Michigan: An Encyclopedic Survey*. Vol. 2. Ann Arbor: University of Michigan Press, 1951. http://quod.lib.umich.edu/u/umsurvey/AAS3302.0002.001/1:1?rgn=div1;view=fulltext.

Sicherman, Barbara. *Alice Hamilton: A Life in Letters*. Urbana: University of Illinois Press, 2003.

Stander, Richard W., and Warren H. Pearse. *Obstetrics, Gynecology and the University of Michigan*. Ann Arbor, MI: n.p., 1968.

Starr, Paul. *The Social Transformation of American Medicine*. New York: Basic Books, 1982.

Stephenson, Orlando W. *Ann Arbor: The First Hundred Years*. Ann Arbor, MI: Ann Arbor Chamber of Commerce, 1927.

Stevens, Rosemary. *American Medicine and the Public Interest*. Berkeley: University of California Press, 1998.

Tarolli, Janet. "Epilogue: Building the Modern Medical Center, 1941 to Present." In *Not Just Any Medical School: The Science, Practice, and Teaching of Medicine at the University of Michigan 1850–1941*, by Horace W. Davenport, 297–306. Ann Arbor: University of Michigan Press, 1999.

Tarolli, Janet. "Five Women Determined to Be Doctors and the Role Michigan Played in Helping Them Achieve Their Dream." *Medicine at Michigan* 2, no. 3 (2000): 27–33.

Tobin, James. "Doc Susie." *Medicine at Michigan* 16 (Spring–Summer 2014): 14–15.

Tobin, James. "JFK at the Union: The Unknown Story of the Peace Corps Speech." http://peacecorps.umich.edu/Tobin.html (accessed May 1, 2017).

Tobin, James. "1964: Michigan, LBJ, and the Great Society." *Michigan Today*, May 23, 2012. http://michigantoday.umich.edu/a8273/.

Tomes, Nancy. *The Gospel of Germs: Men, Women, and the Microbe in American Life*. Cambridge, MA: Harvard University Press, 1998.

To Spread the Light of Knowledge: 250 Years of the Nation's First Medical School. Philadelphia: Perelman School of Medicine of the University of Pennsylvania, 2015.

University of Michigan School of Public Health. "1955 Polio Vaccine Trial Announcement." https://sph.umich.edu/polio/ (accessed February 27, 2017).

Voss, Edward G. "Founding of the First University Hospital." *Journal of Medical Education* 39 (August 1964): 797–798.

Warner, John Harley. "Ideals of Science and Their Discontents in Late Nineteenth-Century American Medicine." *Isis* 82 (September 1991): 454–478.

Weisz, George. *Divide and Conquer: A Comparative History of Medical Specialization*. Oxford: Oxford University Press, 2006.

Wells, Susan. *Out of the Dead House: Nineteenth-Century Women Physicians and the Writing of Medicine*. Madison: University of Wisconsin Press, 2001.

White, Casey B. "The Role of Homeopathic Medicine in U.S. Medical Practice and Its Influence on Medical Education at the University of Michigan." Unpublished student paper, n.d.

Wilson, Leonard G. *Medical Revolution in Minnesota: A History of the University of Minnesota Medical School.* St. Paul, MN: Midewiwin, 1989.

Yates, JoAnne. *Control through Communication: The Rise of System in American Management.* Baltimore: Johns Hopkins University Press, 1993.

Index